Bioactive Marine Heterocyclic Compounds

Bioactive Marine Heterocyclic Compounds

Editor

Yoshihide Usami

MDPI • Basel • Beijing • Wuhan • Barcelona • Belgrade • Manchester • Tokyo • Cluj • Tianjin

Editor
Yoshihide Usami
Osaka University of
Pharmaceutical Sciences
Japan

Editorial Office
MDPI
St. Alban-Anlage 66
4052 Basel, Switzerland

This is a reprint of articles from the Special Issue published online in the open access journal *Marine Drugs* (ISSN 1660-3397) (available at: https://www.mdpi.com/journal/marinedrugs/special_issues/Bioactive_Marine_Heterocyclic_Compounds).

For citation purposes, cite each article independently as indicated on the article page online and as indicated below:

LastName, A.A.; LastName, B.B.; LastName, C.C. Article Title. *Journal Name* **Year**, *Volume Number*, Page Range.

ISBN 978-3-0365-2752-9 (Hbk)
ISBN 978-3-0365-2753-6 (PDF)

Contents

About the Editor . . . vii

Preface to "Bioactive Marine Heterocyclic Compounds" . . . ix

Sanghoon Lee, Naonobu Tanaka, Sakura Takahashi, Daisuke Tsuji, Sang-Yong Kim, Mareshige Kojoma, Kohji Itoh, Jun'ichi Kobayashi and Yoshiki Kashiwada
Agesasines A and B, Bromopyrrole Alkaloids from Marine Sponges *Agelas* spp.
Reprinted from: *Mar. Drugs* **2020**, *18*, 455, doi:10.3390/md18090455 . . . 1

Atsushi Nakayama, Hideo Sato, Tenta Nakamura, Mai Hamada, Shuji Nagano, Shuhei Kameyama, Yui Furue, Naoki Hayashi, Go Kamoshida, Sangita Karanjit, Masataka Oda and Kosuke Namba
Synthesis and Antimicrobial Evaluation of Side-Chain Derivatives based on Eurotiumide A
Reprinted from: *Mar. Drugs* **2020**, *18*, 92, doi:10.3390/md18020092 . . . 9

Géraldine Le Goff, Philippe Lopes, Guillaume Arcile, Pinelopi Vlachou, Elsa Van Elslande, Pascal Retailleau, Jean-François Gallard, Michal Weis, Yehuda Benayahu, Nikolas Fokialakis and Jamal Ouazzani
Impact of the Cultivation Technique on the Production of Secondary Metabolites by *Chrysosporium lobatum* TM-237-S5, Isolated from the Sponge *Acanthella cavernosa*
Reprinted from: *Mar. Drugs* **2019**, *17*, 678, doi:10.3390/md17120678 . . . 27

Chunyan Zhang, Wenjuan Ding, Xiangjing Qin and Jianhua Ju
Genome Sequencing of *Streptomyces olivaceus* SCSIO T05 and Activated Production of Lobophorin CR4 via Metabolic Engineering and Genome Mining
Reprinted from: *Mar. Drugs* **2019**, *17*, 593, doi:10.3390/md17100593 . . . 41

Fan-Zhong Zhang, Xiao-Ming Li, Xin Li, Sui-Qun Yang, Ling-Hong Meng and Bin-Gui Wang
Polyketides from the Mangrove-Derived Endophytic Fungus *Cladosporium cladosporioides*
Reprinted from: *Mar. Drugs* **2019**, *17*, 296, doi:10.3390/md17050296 . . . 53

Takeshi Yamada, Asumi Tanaka, Tatsuo Nehira, Takumi Nishii and Takashi Kikuchi
Altercrasins A–E, Decalin Derivatives, from a Sea-Urchin-Derived *Alternaria* sp.: Isolation and Structural Analysis Including Stereochemistry
Reprinted from: *Mar. Drugs* **2019**, *17*, 218, doi:10.3390/md17040218 . . . 67

Rajiv Dahiya, Sunita Dahiya, Neeraj Kumar Fuloria, Suresh Kumar, Rita Mourya, Suresh V. Chennupati, Satish Jankie, Hemendra Gautam, Sunil Singh, Sanjay Kumar Karan, Sandeep Maharaj, Shivkanya Fuloria, Jyoti Shrivastava, Alka Agarwal, Shamjeet Singh, Awadh Kishor, Gunjan Jadon and Ajay Sharma
Natural Bioactive Thiazole-Based Peptides from Marine Resources: Structural and Pharmacological Aspects
Reprinted from: *Mar. Drugs* **2020**, *18*, 329, doi:10.3390/md18060329 . . . 77

About the Editor

Yoshihide Usami (PhD) is a Professor of the Department of Pharmaceutical Organic Chemistry at Osaka University of Pharmaceutical Sciences (OUPS, renamed as Osaka Medical and Pharmaceutical University in April 2021). His research team focuses on natural product chemistry, synthetic organic chemistry, and medicinal chemistry. He received his PhD from Kyoto University under the supervision of Professor Kaoru Fuji in 1989 and worked on the isolation of bioactive marine natural products in OUPS under Professor Atsushi Numata from 1989 to 2004. During the period 2005–2006, he was invited as a Visiting Assistant Professor at the University of North Carolina at Chapel Hill under Professor K. H. Lee. After returning to OUPS, he became an Associate Professor to Professor Shinya Harusawa (Pharmaceutical Organic Chemistry) and was promoted to Full Professor in 2019. He received the Kansai-Branch Award of Society of Synthetic Organic Chemistry, Japan, in 2015 and served as an Editorial Board member of *Chem. Pharm. Bull.*, *Biol. Pharm. Bull.*, and *Yakugaku Zasshi* during 2016–2019. He has been an Editorial Board member of *Marine Drugs* from 2008 to date. Prior to this Special Issue, he has edited two other Special Issues of *Marine Drugs* in 2014 and 2016.

Preface to "Bioactive Marine Heterocyclic Compounds"

Nowadays, the importance of marine-derived heterocyclic natural products is progressively increasing for new drug discovery. This Special Issue of Marine Drugs, entitled "Bioactive Marine Heterocyclic Compounds", aimed to collect excellent original research articles and reviews focused on the isolation of new heterocyclic marine natural products, total synthesis, synthetic modification, or on finding important bioactivities of known heterocyclic marine natural products. As a result, five original papers on isolation and one synthetic study of metabolites from marine-derived bioorganisms or a marine sponge, along with one review paper on thiazole-based peptides, were published. I am proud to show these most recent works of outstanding scientists in this field and hope this Special issue will affect new drug developments or innovation in the future.

Yoshihide Usami
Editor

marine drugs

MDPI

Article

Agesasines A and B, Bromopyrrole Alkaloids from Marine Sponges *Agelas* spp.

Sanghoon Lee [1,2], Naonobu Tanaka [1,*], Sakura Takahashi [1], Daisuke Tsuji [1], Sang-Yong Kim [3], Mareshige Kojoma [3], Kohji Itoh [1], Jun'ichi Kobayashi [4] and Yoshiki Kashiwada [1,*]

1 Graduate School of Pharmaceutical Sciences, Tokushima University, Tokushima 770-8505, Japan; sanghoon_lee@sfu.ca (S.L.); c402031011@tokushima-u.ac.jp (S.T.); dtsuji@tokushima-u.ac.jp (D.T.); kitoh@tokushima-u.ac.jp (K.I.)

2 Department of Chemistry, Simon Fraser University, Burnaby, BC V5A 1S6, Canada

3 Faculty of Pharmaceutical Sciences, Health Sciences University of Hokkaido, Tobetsu 061-0293, Japan; kim@hoku-iryo-u.ac.jp (S.-Y.K.); kojoma@hoku-iryo-u.ac.jp (M.K.)

4 Graduate School of Pharmaceutical Sciences, Hokkaido University, Sapporo 060-0812, Japan; jkobay@pharm.hokudai.ac.jp

* Correspondence: ntanak@tokushima-u.ac.jp (N.T.); kasiwada@tokushima-u.ac.jp (Y.K.)

Received: 29 June 2020; Accepted: 27 August 2020; Published: 30 August 2020

Abstract: Exploration for specialized metabolites of Okinawan marine sponges *Agelas* spp. resulted in the isolation of five new bromopyrrole alkaloids, agesasines A (**1**) and B (**2**), 9-hydroxydihydrodispacamide (**3**), 9-hydroxydihydrooroidin (**4**), and 9*E*-keramadine (**5**). Their structures were elucidated on the basis of spectroscopic analyses. Agesasines A (**1**) and B (**2**) were assigned as rare bromopyrrole alkaloids lacking an aminoimidazole moiety, while **3**–**5** were elucidated to be linear bromopyrrole alkaloids with either aminoimidazolone, aminoimidazole, or *N*-methylated aminoimidazole moieties.

Keywords: agesasines; bromopyrrole alkaloid; marine sponge; *Agelas*

1. Introduction

A number of structurally unique bioactive specialized metabolites have been isolated from marine sources including sponges, algae, cnidarians, and marine microorganisms, etc. [1]. To date, more than 8000 species of marine sponges (phylum Porifera) have been found under the sea throughout tropical, temperate, and polar area [2]. Marine sponges utilize some of their specialized metabolites as chemical defenses against predator attacks, microbial infections, biofouling, and overgrowth of other sessile organisms [3,4]. On the other hand, natural products isolated from marine sponges are recognized as an attractive source of leads for therapeutic agents due to a diversity of their chemical structures and biological activities.

Marine sponges belonging to the genus *Agelas* are known to be a rich source of bromopyrrole alkaloids and diterpene alkaloids that have been used as a taxonomically characteristic maker [5]. In our search for structurally unique marine natural products [6–8], we have recently reported the isolation of diterpene alkaloids from the extracts of a marine sponge *Agelas* spp. [9]. As part of this research project, we have investigated another specimen of Agelas marine sponges, which resulted in the isolation of five new bromopyrrole alkaloids (**1**–**5**). Among others, agesasines A (**1**) and B (**2**) are rare bromopyrrole alkaloids lacking an aminoimidazole moiety, from the point of view that typical bromopyrrole alkaloids consist of a brominated pyrrolecarboxamide moiety and an aminoimidazole moiety linked through a C_3 unit. Herein, we describe the isolation and structure elucidation of **1**–**5**.

2. Results and Discussion

2.1. Isolation of **1–5** from Marine Sponges *Agelas spp.*

Two specimens of the marine sponge *Agelas* spp. (SS-516 and SS-1302) were separately extracted with MeOH to give extracts, each of which was partitioned between *n*-hexane and 90% MeOH aq. Repeated chromatographic separations of the 90% MeOH aq.-soluble materials from SS-516 gave two new bromopyrrole alkaloids, agesasines A (**1**, 2.5 mg) and B (**2**, 2.2 mg) (Figure 1) together with two known bromopyrrole alkaloids, tauroacidin A [10] and taurodispacamide A [11]. In contrast, the 90% MeOH aq.-soluble materials of SS-1302 were further partitioned with *n*-BuOH and water. The *n*-BuOH-soluble materials were separated by column chromatographies to give three new bromopyrrole alkaloids, 9-hydroxydihydrodispacamide (**3**, 5.0 mg), 9-hydroxydihydrooroidin (**4**, 2.1 mg), and 9*E*-keramadine (**5**, 3.1 mg) (Figure 1), together with four known alkaloids, oroidin [12,13], keramadine [14], 2-bromo-9,10-dihydrokeramadine [15], and nagelamide L [16].

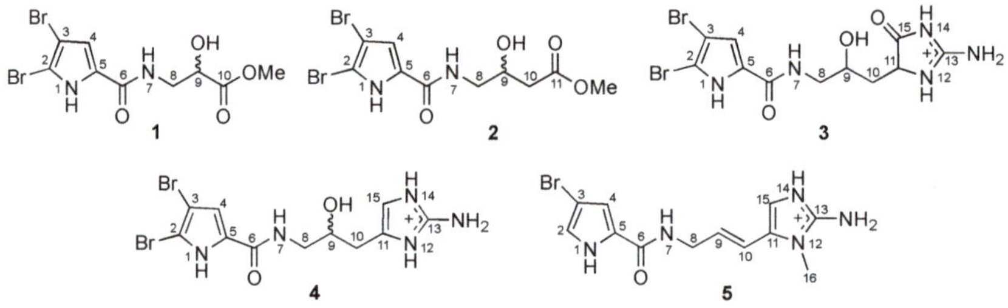

Figure 1. Structures of agesasines A (**1**) and B (**2**), 9-hydroxydihydrodispacamide (**3**), 9-hydroxydihydrooroidin (**4**), and 9*E*-keramadine (**5**).

2.2. Structure Elucidation of **1–5**

Agesasine A (**1**) displayed ion peaks at *m/z* 391, 393, and 395 (1:2:1), suggesting the presence of two bromine atoms in **1**. The molecular formula of **1**, $C_9H_{10}N_2O_4Br_2$, was determined by the high-resolution electrospray ionization mass spectrometry (HRESIMS) (*m/z* 390.89045 $[M + Na]^+$, $\Delta - 0.05$ mmu). The ^1H and ^{13}C NMR spectra (Table 1) displayed the signals of one sp^3 methine, one sp^3 methylene, one methoxy group, and one carboxy carbon as well as resonances assignable to a 2,3-dibromopyrrole carboxamide moiety (N-1~N-7). Analysis of the ^1H-^1H correlation spectroscopy (COSY) spectrum revealed the connectivities from 7-NH to 9-OH (Figure 2), while heteronuclear multiple bond coherence (HMBC) correlations for methoxy protons and H_2-8 with C-10 suggested the presence of a methoxy carbonyl group at C-9. Thus, the planar structure of agesasine A (**1**) was elucidated as shown in Figure 2. Agesasine B (**2**) showed an ion peak at *m/z* 380.9088 ($[M - H]^-$, $\Delta + 0.2$ mmu), corresponding to the molecular formula of $C_{10}H_{12}N_2O_4Br_2$. The 1D NMR spectra of **2** (Table 1) were closely correlated to those of **1**, except for the presence of an additional sp^3 methylene signal (CH_2-10) in **2**. The methylene protons (H_2-10) showed a ^1H-^1H COSY cross-peak with H-9 and an HMBC correlation with a methoxy carbonyl carbon (C-11), suggesting the planar structure of **2** as shown in Figure 2.

Table 1. One-dimensional (1D) NMR data for agesasines A (**1**) and B (**2**) in DMSO-d_6.

Position	**1**		**2**	
	^{13}C	^{1}H (*J* in Hz)	^{13}C	^{1}H (*J* in Hz)
1	–	12.67 (brs)	–	12.65 (brs)
2	104.8	–	104.7	–
3	98.0	–	98.0	–
4	113.1	6.93 (brs)	113.0	6.93 (d, 2,7)
5	128.1	–	128.3	–
6	159.3	–	159.3	–
7	–	8.20 (t, 5.8)	–	8.12 (t, 5.5)
8	42.7	3.46, 3.36 (each 1 H, m)	44.9	3.20 (2 H, m)
9	69.3	4.17 (q, 6.1)	66.6	3.99 (m)
10	173.1	–	40.6	2.49 (m), 2.27 (dd, 15.2, 8.8)
11	–	–	171.8	–
9-OH	–	5.71 (d, 5.9)	–	nd
OMe	51.8	3.61 (3 H, brs)	51.4	3.56 (3 H, brs)

nd: Not detected.

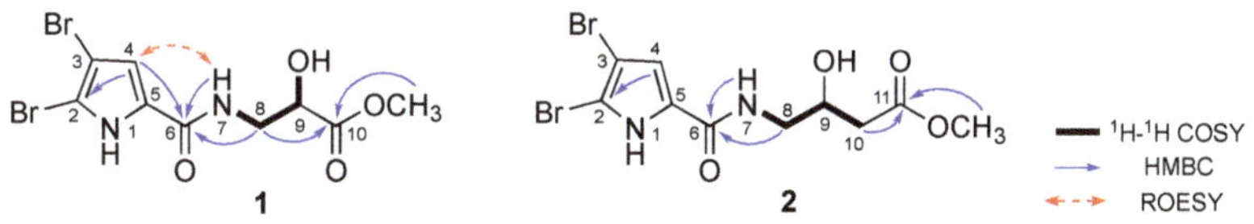

Figure 2. Key two-dimensional (2D) NMR correlations for agesasines A (**1**) and B (**2**).

The racemic nature of agesasines A (**1**) and B (**2**) indicated by their specific rotation values being nearly zero prompted us to perform the optical resolutions of **1** and **2**. The analysis of **1** using the reversed phase chiral high performance liquid chromatography (HPLC) gave a pair of peaks in the integral ratio of ca. 1:1, indicating agesasine A (**1**) to be a racemate. Agesasine B (**2**) was also deduced to be a racemate, although the optical resolution could not be achieved in spite of attempts being made at various separation conditions.

9-Hydroxydihydrodispacamide (**3**) was obtained as a pale yellow amorphous solid. The HRESIMS showed an ion peak at *m/z* 443.92824 ($[M - H + Na]^+$, $\Delta - 0.04$ mmu), suggesting the molecular formula of $C_{11}H_{14}N_5O_3Br_2$. The ^{1}H and ^{13}C NMR spectra of **3** (Table 2) were similar to those of a known linear bromopyrrole alkaloid, dihydrodispacamide [17], except for the presence of an oxygenated methine signal (CH-9) in **3**. Therefore, **3** was deduced to be a hydroxylated derivative of dihydrodispacamide. The presence of the hydroxy group at C-9 was confirmed by ^{1}H-^{1}H COSY cross-peaks of H$_2$-8/H-9 and H-9/H$_2$-10 (Figure 3). The relative configuration of **3** was not assigned in this study, while the racemic nature of **3** was confirmed by HPLC analysis with chiral column with a similar manner as for **1**.

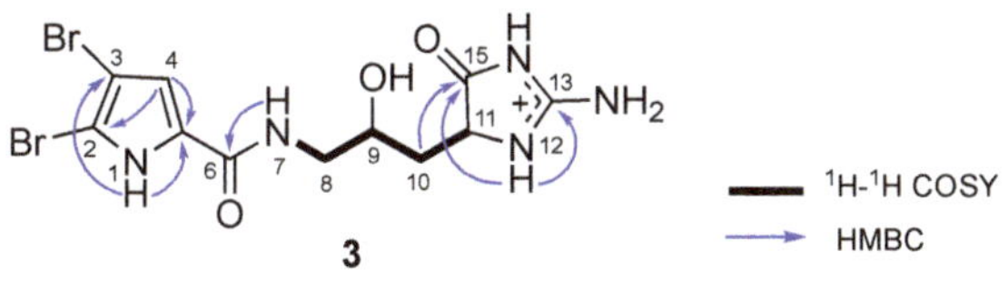

Figure 3. Selected 2D NMR correlations for 9-hydroxydihydrodispacamide (**3**).

Table 2. 1D NMR data for 9-hydroxydihydrodispacamide (**3**), 9-hydroxydihydrooroidin (**4**), and 9*E*-keramadine (**5**) in DMSO-d_6.

Position	3		4		5	
	^{13}C	^{1}H (*J* in Hz)	^{13}C	^{1}H (*J* in Hz)	^{13}C	^{1}H (*J* in Hz)
1	–	12.66 (brs)	–	12.66 (brs)	–	11.83 (brs)
2	104.7	–	104.8	–	121.6	6.98 (dd, 2.9, 1.6)
3	98.0	–	98.2	–	95.2	–
4	113.1	6.94 (d, 2.8)	113.2	6.86 (s)	111.8	6.92 (s)
5	128.3	–	128.4	–	126.9	–
6	159.3	–	159.4	–	159.7	–
7	–	8.15 (t, 5.9)	–	8.19 (t, 5.6)	–	8.40 (t, 5.5)
8	45.3	3.18 (2 H, m)	44.8	3.23 (m), 3.16 (m)	40.4	3.99 (2 H, t, 5.5)
9	66.3	3.79 (m)	68.4	3.76 (m)	130.8	6.19 (dt, 16.1, 5.5)
10	34.8	1.96 (ddd, 14.4, 5.5, 2.6) 1.71 (ddd, 14.4, 10.9, 5.5)	30.1	2.57 (dd, 15.2, 4.2) 2.40 (dd, 15.2, 7.8)	115.3	6.30 (d, 16.1)
11	56.8	4.34 (t, 5.5)	124.3	–	126.6	–
12	–	9.47 (brs)	–	11.95 (brs)		
13	158.2	–	147.1	–	146.9	–
14	–	nd	–	11.87 (brs)	–	12.35 (brs)
15	175.6	–	110.1	6.58 (brs)	109.4	7.14 (brs)
N-Me					29.8	3.38 (3 H, s)
13-NH$_2$	–	nd	–	7.35 (2 H, brs)	–	7.71 (2 H, brs)

nd: Not detected.

9-Hydroxydihydrooroidin (**4**) was obtained as a pale yellow amorphous solid. Although the ^{1}H and ^{13}C NMR spectra (Table 2) implied that **4** was a bromopyrrole alkaloid related to dihydrooroidin [17], the signals of an oxygenated methine (CH-9, δ_H 3.76, and δ_C 68.4) were observed in **4**. In the ^{1}H-^{1}H COSY spectrum, the oxygenated methine proton (H-9) showed cross-peaks with H_2-8 and H_2-10 (Figure 4). Based on the above findings and the molecular formula of **4**, $C_{11}H_{14}N_5O_2Br_2$, obtained by the HRESIMS (*m/z* 405.9510 [M]$^+$, Δ – 0.4 mmu), **4** was assigned as 9-hydroxydihydrooroidin (Figure 1). A nearly zero value of the specific rotation indicated **4** to be a racemate, which was supported by the fact that **4** showed no cotton effect in the electronic circular dichroism (ECD) spectrum.

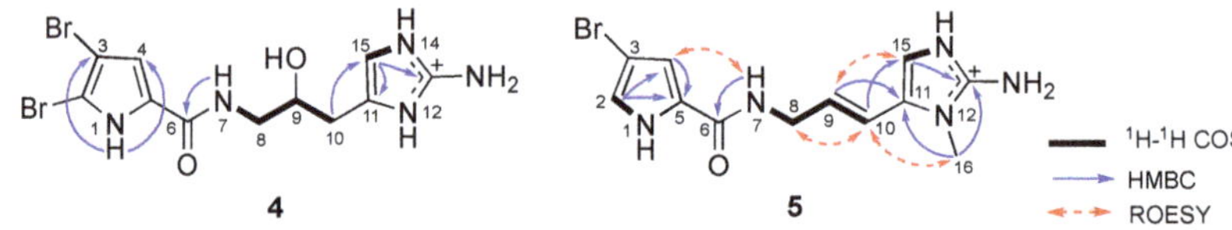

Figure 4. Selected 2D NMR correlations for 9-hydroxydihydrooroidin (**4**) and 9*E*-keramadine (**5**).

9*E*-Keramadine (**5**) displayed the ^{1}H and ^{13}C NMR spectra (Table 2) similar to those of a known bromopyrrole alkaloid possessing a 3-bromopyrrolecarboxamide moiety, keramadine [14]. The HRESIMS revealed the molecular formula of **5** to be $C_{12}H_{15}N_5OBr$, which was identical to that of keramadine. However, the ^{3}J (H-9/H-10) value (J = 16.1 Hz) in **5** indicated the geometry of the double bond to be *E*, whereas keramadine has the *Z*-olefin. The *E*-geometry was further underpinned by rotating frame nuclear Overhauser effect spectroscopy (ROESY) correlations for H-9/H-15 and H_2-8/H-10 (Figure 4). This is the first report of 9*E*-keramadine from a natural source, although the synthesis of 9*E*-keramadine has been reported to date [18].

Bromopyrrole alkaloids isolated from marine sponges have attracted the interest of researchers due to their diverse chemical structures. Various intriguing biological activities of bromopyrrole alkaloids leading drug discovery such as cytotoxic, antibacterial (antibiofilm), and protein kinase C modulating activities have been reported [19,20]. We have also reported the isolation of antimicrobial bromopyrrole alkaloids to date [6]. In this study, the antiproliferative activity of **1**–**5** against human cancer cell lines (HeLa, A549, and MCF7) were evaluated, showing no cytotoxicity against all cell lines (IC_{50} > 100 μM) (Figures S43–S45).

In conclusion, five new bromopyrrole alkaloids, agesasines A (**1**) and B (**2**), 9-hydroxydihydrodispacamide (**3**), 9-hydroxydihydrooroidin (**4**), and 9*E*-keramadine (**5**) were isolated from Okinawan marine sponges *Agelas* spp. Typical bromopyrrole alkaloids such as oroidin [12,13] and keramadine [14] consist of a mono or dibrominated pyrrolecarboxamide moiety and an aminoimidazole moiety linked through a C_3 unit. In contrast, agesasines A (**1**) and B (**2**) are rare bromopyrrole alkaloids lacking an aminoimidazole moiety, whereas **1** and **2** might be artifacts during the extraction and isolation process with acidic condition. Few alkaloids with such structural feature have been isolated from marine sponges *Agelas* spp. collected off the South China Sea [21,22].

3. Materials and Methods

3.1. General Procedures

Optical rotations were obtained on a JASCO P-2200 digital polarimeter (JASCO Co., Tokyo, Japan). UV spectra were recorded on a Hitachi U-3900H spectrophotometer (Hitachi, Ltd., Tokyo, Japan). NMR spectra were measured by a Bruker AVANCE-500 instrument (Bruker, Billerica, MA, USA) using tetramethylsilane as an internal standard. HRESIMS were recorded on a Waters LCT PREMIER 2695 (Waters Co., Milford, MA, USA) and a JEOL JMS-T100LP (JEOL, Ltd., Tokyo, Japan). Column chromatography was performed with silica gel 60 N (Kanto Kagaku, Tokyo, Japan) and Diaion HP-20 (Mitsubishi Chemical, Tokyo, Japan). Medium pressure liquid chromatography (MPLC) was carried out on Toyopearl HW-40F (TOSOH Co., Tokyo, Japan), MCI gel CHP20P (Mitsubishi Chemical, Tokyo, Japan), and Biotage SNAP Cartridge KP-C18-HS (Biotage, Uppsala, Sweden).

3.2. Materials

The marine sponges *Agelas* spp. were collected off Kerama Islands, Okinawa, and identified by one of the authors (N.T.). The voucher specimens (SS-516 and SS-1302) were deposited in the Graduate School of Pharmaceutical Sciences, Tokushima University.

3.3. Extraction and Isolation

The marine sponges *Agelas* spp. SS-516 (5.22 kg, wet weight) and SS-1302 (3.42 kg, wet weight) were separately extracted with MeOH to give the extracts (197.1 and 376.3 g, respectively), each of which was partitioned with *n*-hexane and 90% MeOH aq. The 90% MeOH aq.-soluble materials of SS-516 were separated by column chromatography on Diaion HP-20 (MeOH/H_2O, 0:100–100:0) to give six fractions (frs. 1–6). Fr. 3 was subjected to silica gel column chromatography ($CHCl_3$/MeOH/TFA, 95:5:0.1–80:20:0.1) to yield 12 fractions (frs. 3.1–3.12). Fr. 3.7 was applied to ODS MPLC (MeCN/H_2O/TFA, 5:95:0.1–80:20:0.1), and then purified by ODS HPLC (YMC Hydrosphere C18, ϕ20 × 250 mm, MeCN/H_2O/TFA, 35:65:0.1) to furnish agesasines A (**1**, 2.5 mg) and B (**2**, 2.2 mg). Separation of fr. 3.11 by ODS MPLC (MeCN/H_2O/TFA, 5:95:0.1–80:20:0.1) gave five fractions (frs. 3.11.1–3.11.5). Tauroacidin A (124.1 mg) and taurodispacamide A (34.5 mg) were purified from fr. 3.11.3 by ODS MPLC (MeCN/H_2O/TFA, 20:80:0.1).

The 90% MeOH aq.-soluble materials of SS-1302 were further partitioned between *n*-BuOH and water. The *n*-BuOH-soluble materials (58.0 g) were applied to silica gel column chromatography ($CHCl_3$/MeOH/TFA, 9:1:0.1–5:5:0.1) to give six fractions (frs. 1′–6′) including oroidin (17.1 g, fr. 3′). Fr. 4′ was subjected to MPLC on a Toyopearl HW-40F column (MeOH/H_2O/TFA, 10:90:0.1–90:10:0.1), an MCI gel CHP 20P column (MeOH/H_2O/TFA, 10:90:0.1–90:10:0.1) to yield seven fractions (frs. 4′.4.1–4′.4.7). Fr. 4′.4.3 was loaded to MPLC on an ODS column (MeCN/H_2O/TFA, 10:90:0.1–60:40:0.1) to give six fractions (frs. 4′.4.3.1–4′.4.3.6), and then fr. 4′.4.3.3 was purified by ODS HPLC (COSMOSIL 5C_{18}-MS-II, ϕ 20 × 250 mm, MeCN/H_2O/TFA, 17:83:0.1). Further purification of fr. 4′.4.3.3.2 on ODS HPLC (YMC Hydrosphere C18, ϕ 10 × 250 mm, MeCN/H_2O/TFA, 13:87:0.1) afforded 9-hydroxydihydrodispacamide (**3**, 5.0 mg), 9*E*-keramadine (**5**, 3.1 mg), and keramadine (6.7 mg). 9-Hydroxydihydrooroidin (**4**, 2.1 mg) was isolated from fr. 4′4.3.3.3 by ODS HPLC (YMC Hydrosphere

C18, ϕ 10 × 250 mm, $MeCN/H_2O/TFA$, 13:87:0.1). Fr. 4′.4.4 was subjected to ODS MPLC ($MeCN/H_2O/TFA$, 10:90:0.1–50:50:0.1) and then ODS HPLC (YMC Hydrosphere C18, ϕ 10 × 250 mm, $MeCN/H_2O/TFA$, 15:85:0.1) to furnish 2-bromo-9,10-dihydrokeramadine (2.1 mg). Fr. 5′ was applied to MPLC on a Toyopearl HW-40F column ($MeOH/H_2O/TFA$, 10:90:0.1–90:10:0.1) to give eight fractions (frs. 5′.1–5′.8). Fr. 5′ was passed through an MCI gel CHP 20P column ($MeOH/H_2O/TFA$, 10:90:0.1–100:0:0.1) and an ODS column ($MeOH/H_2O/TFA$, 10:90:0.1–0:10:0.1) to afford nagelamide L (187.5 mg). Tauroacidin A and nagelamide L did not show optical rotations.

Agesasine A (**1**): Pale yellow amorphous solid; $[\alpha]_D^{28}$ 0 (*c* 0.10, MeOH); UV (MeOH) λ_{max} 275 (ε 4900) nm; ^{1}H and ^{13}C NMR data (Table 1); ESIMS: *m/z* 391, 393, and 395 (1:2:1), $[M + Na]^+$; HRESIMS: *m/z* 390.89045 $[M + Na]^+$ (calcd for $C_9H_{10}N_2O_4Na^{79}Br_2$, 390.89050).

Agesasine B (**2**): Pale yellow amorphous solid; $[\alpha]_D^{28}$ 0 (*c* 0.10, MeOH); UV (MeOH) λ_{max} 274 (ε 3100) nm; ^{1}H and ^{13}C NMR data (Table 1); ESIMS: *m/z* 381, 383, and 385 (1:2:1), $[M - H]^-$; HRESIMS: *m/z* 380.9088 $[M - H]^-$ (calcd for $C_{10}H_{11}N_2O_4{}^{79}Br_2$, 380.9086).

9-Hydroxydihydrodispacamide (**3**): Pale yellow amorphous solid; $[\alpha]_D^{27}$ 0 (*c* 0.10, MeOH); UV (MeOH) λ_{max} 223 (ε 3900) and 275 (3400) nm; ^{1}H and ^{13}C NMR data (Table 2); ESIMS: *m/z* 444, 446, and 448 (1:2:1), $[M - H + Na]^+$; HRESIMS: *m/z* 443.92824 $[M - H + Na]^+$ (calcd for $C_{11}H_{13}N_5O_3Na^{79}Br_2$, 443.92828).

9-Hydroxydihydrooroidin (**4**): Pale yellow amorphous solid; $[\alpha]_D^{27}$ 0 (*c* 0.10, MeOH); UV (MeOH) λ_{max} 276 (ε 3900) nm; ^{1}H and ^{13}C NMR data (Table 2); ESIMS: *m/z* 406, 408, and 410 (1:2:1), $[M]^+$; HRESIMS: *m/z* 405.9510 $[M]^+$ (calcd for $C_{11}H_{14}N_5O_2{}^{79}Br_2$, 405.9514).

9E-Keramadine (**5**): Pale yellow amorphous solid; UV (MeOH) λ_{max} 271 (ε 3300) nm; ^{1}H and ^{13}C NMR data (Table 2); ESIMS: *m/z* 324 and 326 (1:1), $[M]^+$; HRESIMS: *m/z* 324.04592 $[M]^+$ (calcd for $C_{12}H_{15}N_5O^{79}Br$, 324.04600).

3.4. Optical Resolutions of 1–3

Optical resolutions of agesasine A (**1**) and 9-hydroxydihydrodispacamide (**3**), were performed on chiral HPLC (Chiral ART Cellulose-SB, YMC, ϕ 4.6 × 250 mm, flow rate 0.5 mL/min, UV detection 254 nm) at 35 °C with elution of $MeOH/MeCN/H_2O/H_3PO_4$ (30:10:60:0.1 for **1**; 8:2:90:0.1 for **3**) to give enantiomers in the integral ratio of ca. 1:1 (t_R 27.5 and 29.0 min for **1**; t_R 12.5 and 14.3 min for **3**) in each case. The separations of enantiomers were confirmed by MS analyses. Separated peaks for enantiomers of agesasine B (**2**) could not be obtained in any condition in this study.

3.5. Evaluation for Antiproliferative Activity of 1–5

New bromopyrrole alkaloids **1–5** were evaluated for their antiproliferative activity against human cancer cell lines (HeLa, A549, and MCF7) according to the following procedure. The human cancer cell lines were cultured in Dulbecco's modified eagle medium (DMEM) supplemented with 5% fetal bovine serum (FBS). All cells were incubated at 37 °C in a humidified atmosphere with 5% CO_2–95% air. Cells were seeded at 1×10^4 cells/well in a 96-well plate and preincubated for 24 h. Test samples were dissolved in small amounts of DMSO and diluted in the appropriate culture medium (final concentration of DMSO < 1%). After removal of the preincubated culture medium, 100 μL of medium containing various concentrations of test compound was added and further incubated for 48 h. A cell proliferation assay was performed with the Cell Counting Kit-8 (WST-8; Dojindo, Japan) according to the manufacturer's instruction. Briefly, the WST-8 reagent solution (10 μL) was added to each well of a 96-well microplate containing 100 μL of cells in the culture medium at various densities, and the plate was incubated for 2 h at 37 °C. Absorbance was measured at 450 nm using a microplate reader. Cisplatin was used as a positive control, whose IC_{50} values against HeLa, A549, and MCF7 cells were 11.7, 7.2, and 52.4 mM, respectively.

Supplementary Materials: The following are available online at http://www.mdpi.com/1660-3397/18/9/455/s1. Figure S1: ^{1}H NMR spectrum of agesasine A (**1**) in DMSO-d_6 (500 MHz), Figure S2: ^{13}C NMR spectrum of agesasine A (**1**) in DMSO-d_6 (125 MHz), Figure S3: ^{1}H-^{1}H COSY spectrum of agesasine A (**1**) in DMSO-d_6 (500 MHz), Figure S4: HSQC spectrum of agesasine A (**1**) in DMSO-d_6 (500 MHz), Figure S5: HMBC spectrum of agesasine A (**1**) in DMSO-d_6 (500 MHz), Figure S6: ROESY spectrum of agesasine A (**1**) in DMSO-d_6 (500 MHz), Figure S7: HRESIMS spectrum (pos.) of agesasine A (**1**), Figure S8: Chiral HPLC chart of agesasine A (**1**), Figure S9: ^{1}H NMR spectrum of agesasine B (**2**) in DMSO-d_6 (500 MHz), Figure S10: ^{13}C NMR spectrum of agesasine B (**2**) in DMSO-d_6 (125 MHz), Figure S11: ^{1}H-^{1}H COSY spectrum of agesasine B (**2**) in DMSO-d_6 (500 MHz), Figure S12: HSQC spectrum of agesasine B (**2**) in DMSO-d_6 (500 MHz), Figure S13: HMBC spectrum of agesasine B (**2**) in DMSO-d_6 (500 MHz), Figure S14: HRESIMS spectrum (neg.) of agesasine B (**2**), Figure S15: ^{1}H NMR spectrum of 9-hydroxydihydrodispacamide (**3**) in DMSO-d_6 (500 MHz), Figure S16: ^{13}C NMR spectrum of 9-hydroxydihydrodispacamide (**3**) in DMSO-d_6 (125 MHz), Figure S17: ^{1}H-^{1}H COSY spectrum of 9-hydroxydihydrodispacamide (**3**) in DMSO-d_6 (500 MHz), Figure S18: HSQC spectrum of 9-hydroxydihydrodispacamide (**3**) in DMSO-d_6 (500 MHz), Figure S19: HMBC spectrum of 9-hydroxydihydrodispacamide (**3**) in DMSO-d_6 (500 MHz), Figure S20: HRESIMS spectrum (pos.) of 9-hydroxydihydrodispacamide (**3**), Figure S21: Chiral HPLC chart of 9-hydroxydihydrodispacamide (**3**), Figure S22: ^{1}H NMR spectrum of 9-hydroxydihydrooroidin (**4**) in DMSO-d_6 (500 MHz), Figure S23: ^{13}C NMR spectrum of 9-hydroxydihydrooroidin (**4**) in DMSO-d_6 (125 MHz), Figure S24: ^{1}H-^{1}H COSY spectrum of 9-hydroxydihydrooroidin (**4**) in DMSO-d_6 (500 MHz), Figure S25: HSQC spectrum of 9-hydroxydihydrooroidin (**4**) in DMSO-d_6 (500 MHz), Figure S26: HMBC spectrum of 9-hydroxydihydrooroidin (**4**) in DMSO-d_6 (500 MHz), Figure S27: HRESIMS spectrum (pos.) of 9-hydroxydihydrooroidin (**4**), Figure S28: ECD spectrum of 9-hydroxydihydrooroidin (**4**) in MeOH, Figure S29: ^{1}H NMR spectrum of 9*E*-keramadine (**5**) in DMSO-d_6 (500 MHz), Figure S30: ^{13}C NMR spectrum of 9*E*-keramadine (**5**) in DMSO-d_6 (125 MHz), Figure S31: ^{1}H-^{1}H COSY spectrum of 9*E*-keramadine (**5**) in DMSO-d_6 (500 MHz), Figure S32: HSQC spectrum of 9*E*-keramadine (**5**) in DMSO-d_6 (500 MHz), Figure S33: HMBC spectrum of 9*E*-keramadine (**5**) in DMSO-d_6 (500 MHz), Figure S34: ROESY spectrum of 9*E*-keramadine (**5**) in DMSO-d_6 (500 MHz), Figure S35: HRESIMS spectrum (pos.) of 9*E*-keramadine (**5**), Figure S36: ^{1}H NMR spectrum of tauroacidin A in DMSO-d_6 (500 MHz), Figure S37: ^{1}H NMR spectrum of taurodispacamide A in DMSO-d_6 (500 MHz), Figure S38: ^{1}H NMR spectrum of oroidin in DMSO-d_6 (500 MHz), Figure S39: ^{1}H NMR spectrum of keramadine in DMSO-d_6 (500 MHz), Figure S40: ^{1}H NMR spectrum of 2-bromo-9,10-dihydrokeramadine in DMSO-d_6 (500 MHz), Figure S41: ^{1}H NMR spectrum of nagelamide L in DMSO-d_6 (500 MHz), Figure S42: Structures of known bromopyrrole alkaloids, tauroacidin A, taurodispacamide A, oroidin, keramadine, 2-bromokeramadine, and nagelamide L, Figure S43: Antiproliferative activity of **1–5** against HeLa cells, Figure S44: Antiproliferative activity of **1–5** against A549 cells, Figure S45: Antiproliferative activity of **1–5** against MCF7 cells, Table S1: 1D and 2D NMR data for agesasine A (**1**) in DMSO-d_6, Table S2: 1D and 2D NMR data for agesasine B (**2**) in DMSO-d_6, Table S3: 1D and 2D NMR data for 9-hydroxydihydrodispacamide (**3**) in DMSO-d_6, Table S4: 1D and 2D NMR data for 9-hydroxydihydrooroidin (**4**) in DMSO-d_6, Table S5: 1D and 2D NMR data for 9*E*-keramadine (**5**) in DMSO-d_6, Table S6: ^{1}H NMR data for tauroacidin A and taurodispacamide A in DMSO-d_6, Table S7: ^{1}H NMR data for oroidin, keramadine, and 2-bromo-9,10-dihydrokeramadine in DMSO-d_6, Table S8: ^{1}H NMR data for nagelamide L in DMSO-d_6.

Author Contributions: Conceptualization, S.L., N.T., D.T., S.-Y.K., M.K., K.I., J.K., and Y.K.; methodology, S.L. and N.T.; validation, S.L. and N.T.; formal analysis, S.L., N.T., and Y.K.; investigation, S.L., S.T., D.T., and S.-Y.K.; resources, J.K.; writing—original draft preparation, S.L.; writing—review and editing, N.T., M.K., K.I., and Y.K. All authors have read and agreed to the published version of the manuscript.

Funding: This work was partly supported by JSPS KAKENHI, grant number JP17K08337.

Acknowledgments: We thank Z. Nagahama for his help with the sponge collection.

Conflicts of Interest: The authors declare no conflict of interest.

References

1. Carroll, A.R.; Copp, B.R.; Davis, R.A.; Keyzers, R.A.; Prinsep, M.R. Marine natural products. *Nat. Prod. Rep.* **2020**, *37*, 175–223. [CrossRef] [PubMed]
2. Laport, M.S.; Santos, O.C.S.; Muricy, G. Marine sponges: Potential sources of new antimicrobial drugs. *Curr. Pharm. Biotechnol.* **2009**, *10*, 86–105. [CrossRef] [PubMed]
3. Paul, V.J.; Puglisi, M.P. Chemical mediation of interactions among marine organisms. *Nat. Prod. Rep.* **2004**, *21*, 189–209. [CrossRef] [PubMed]
4. Paul, V.J.; Puglisi, M.P.; Ritson-Williams, R. Marine chemical ecology. *Nat. Prod. Rep.* **2006**, *23*, 153–180. [CrossRef]
5. Braekman, J.-C.; Daloze, D.; Stoller, C.; Van Soest, R.W.M. Chemotaxonomy of *Agelas* (Polifera: Demospongiae). *Biochem. Syst. Ecol.* **1992**, *20*, 417–431. [CrossRef]

6. Tanaka, N.; Kusama, T.; Kashiwada, Y.; Kobayashi, J. Bromopyrrole alkaloids from Okinawan marine sponges *Agelas* spp. *Chem. Pharm. Bull.* **2016**, *64*, 691–694. [CrossRef]
7. Kusama, T.; Tanaka, T.; Sakai, K.T.; Gonoi, T.; Fromont, J.; Kashiwada, Y.; Kobayashi, J. Agelamadins A and B, dimeric bromopyrrole alkaloids from a marine sponge *Agelas* sp. *Org. Lett.* **2014**, *16*, 3916–3918. [CrossRef]
8. Kusama, T.; Tanaka, N.; Sakai, K.; Gonoi, T.; Fromont, J.; Kashiwada, Y.; Kobayashi, J. Agelamadins C-E, bromopyrrole alkaloids comprising oroidin and 3-hydroxykynurenine from a marine sponge *Agelas* sp. *Org. Lett.* **2014**, *16*, 5176–5179. [CrossRef]
9. Lee, S.; Tanaka, N.; Kobayashi, J.; Kashiwada, Y. Agelamasines A and B, diterpene alkaloids from an Okinawan marine sponge *Agelas* sp. *J. Nat. Med.* **2018**, *72*, 364–368. [CrossRef]
10. Kobayashi, J.; Inaba, K.; Tsuda, M. Tauroacidins A and B, new bromopyrrole alkaloids possessing a taurine residue from *Hymeniacidon* sponge. *Tetrahedron* **1997**, *53*, 16679–16682. [CrossRef]
11. Fattorusso, E.; Taglialatela-Scafati, O. Two novel pyrrole-imidazle alkaloids from the Mediterranean sponge *Agelas oroides*. *Tetrahedron Lett.* **2000**, *41*, 9917–9922. [CrossRef]
12. Forenza, S.; Minale, L.; Riccio, R.; Fattorusso, E. New bromo-pyrrole derivatives from the sponge *Agelas oroides*. *J. Chem. Soc. D Chem. Commun.* **1971**, 1129–1130. [CrossRef]
13. Ando, N.; Terashima, S. A novel synthesis of the 2-amino-1*H*-imidazol-4-carbaldehyde derivatives and its application to the efficient synthesis of 2-aminoimidazole alkaloids, oroidin, hymenidin, dispacamide, monobromodispacamide, ageladine A. *Tetrahedron* **2010**, *66*, 6224–6237. [CrossRef]
14. Nakamura, H.; Ohizumi, Y.; Kobayashi, J.; Hirata, Y. Keramadine, a novel antagonist of serotonergic receptors isolated from the Okinawan sea sponge *Agelas* sp. *Tetrahedron Lett.* **1984**, *25*, 2475–2478. [CrossRef]
15. Kusama, T.; Tanaka, N.; Takahashi-Nakaguchi, A.; Gonoi, T.; Fromont, J.; Kobayashi, J. Bromopyrrole alkaloids from a marine sponge *Agelas* sp. *Chem. Pharm. Bull.* **2014**, *62*, 499–503. [CrossRef]
16. Araki, A.; Kubota, T.; Tsuda, M.; Mikami, Y.; Fromont, J.; Kobayashi, J. Nagelamides K and L, Dimeric Bromopyrrole Alkaloids from Sponge *Agelas* Species. *Org. Lett.* **2008**, *10*, 2099–2102. [CrossRef]
17. Olofson, A.; Yakushijin, K.; Horne, D.A. Synthesis of marine sponge alkaloids oroidin, clathrodin, and dispacamides. Preparation and transformation of 2-amino-4,5-dialkoxy-4,5-dihydroimidazolines from 2-aminoimidazoles. *J. Org. Chem.* **1998**, *63*, 1248–1253. [CrossRef]
18. Daninos-Zeghal, S.; Al Mourabit, A.; Ahond, A.; Poupat, C.; Potier, P. Synthèse de metabolites marins 2-aminoimidazoliques: Hyménidine, oroïdine et kéramadine. *Tetrahedron* **1997**, *53*, 7605–7614. [CrossRef]
19. Zhang, H.; Dong, M.; Chen, J.; Wang, H.; Tenney, K.; Crews, P. Bioactive secondary metabolites from the marine sponge genus Agelas. *Mar. Drugs* **2017**, *15*, 351. [CrossRef]
20. Al-Mourabit, A.; Zancanella, M.A.; Tilvi, S.; Romo, D. Biosynthesis, asymmetric synthesis, and pharmacology, including cellular targets, of the pyrrole-2-aminoimidazole marine alkaloids. *Nat. Prod. Rep.* **2011**, *28*, 1229–1260. [CrossRef]
21. Zhu, Y.; Wang, Y.; Gu, B.-B.; Yang, F.; Jiao, W.-H.; Hu, G.-H.; Yu, H.-B.; Han, B.-N.; Zhang, W.; Shen, Y.; et al. Antifungal bromopyrrole alkaloids from the South China sea sponge *Agelas* sp. *Tetrahedron* **2016**, *72*, 2964–2971. [CrossRef]
22. Chu, M.-J.; Tang, X.-L.; Qin, G.-F.; de Voogd, N.J.; Li, P.-L. Three new non-brominated pyrrole alkaloids from the South China sea sponge *Agelas nakamurai*. *Chin. Chem. Lett.* **2017**, *28*, 1210–1213. [CrossRef]

marine drugs

MDPI

Article

Synthesis and Antimicrobial Evaluation of Side-Chain Derivatives based on Eurotiumide A

Atsushi Nakayama [1,*], Hideo Sato [1], Tenta Nakamura [1], Mai Hamada [1], Shuji Nagano [1], Shuhei Kameyama [1], Yui Furue [2], Naoki Hayashi [2], Go Kamoshida [2], Sangita Karanjit [1], Masataka Oda [2] and Kosuke Namba [1,*]

1 Graduate School of Pharmaceutical Sciences and Research Cluster on "Innovative Chemical Sensing", Tokushima University, 1-78-1 Shomachi, Tokushima 770-8505, Japan; hideo1995214@gmail.com (H.S.); c401603069@tokushima-u.ac.jp (T.N.); c401403070@tokushima-u.ac.jp (M.H.); c401941004@tokushima-u.ac.jp (S.N.); c401931030@tokushima-u.ac.jp (S.K.); karanjit@tokushima-u.ac.jp (S.K.)

2 Department of Microbiology and Infection Control Sciences, Kyoto Pharmaceutical University, Misasaginakauchi-cho, Yamashita-Ku, Kyoto 607-8414, Japan; mametty1214@gmail.com (Y.F.); nhayashi@mb.kyoto-phu.ac.jp (N.H.); kamoshida@mb.kyoto-phu.ac.jp (G.K.); moda@mb.kyoto-phu.ac.jp (M.O.)

* Correspondence: anakaya@tokushima-u.ac.jp (A.N.); namba@tokushima-u.ac.jp (K.N.)

Received: 30 November 2019; Accepted: 29 January 2020; Published: 30 January 2020

Abstract: Side-chain derivatives of eurotiumide A, a dihydroisochroman-type natural product, have been synthesized and their antimicrobial activities described. Sixteen derivatives were synthesized from a key intermediate of the total synthesis of eurotiumide A, and their antimicrobial activities against two Gram-positive bacteria, methicillin-susceptible and methicillin-resistant *Staphylococcus aureus* (MSSA and MRSA), and a Gram-negative bacterium, *Porphyromonas gingivalis*, were evaluated. The results showed that derivatives having an iodine atom on their aromatic ring instead of the prenyl moiety displayed better antimicrobial activity than eurotiumide A against MSSA and *P. gingivalis*. Moreover, we discovered that a derivative with an isopentyl side chain, which is a hydrogenated product of eurotiumide A, is the strongest antimicrobial agent against all three strains, including MRSA.

Keywords: antibiotics; natural product; *P. gingivalis*; methicillin-resistant *S. aureus*

---

1. Introduction

Humans have always struggled against infectious diseases [1–5] and in relatively recent times have developed various antimicrobial therapies [6–8]. Since the discovery of penicillin [9], various natural products having antimicrobial activity have been discovered [10–16], and the majority of clinically used antibiotics are either natural products, semisynthetic derivatives, or compounds derived from them [17–19]. Despite the presence of many excellent antibiotics, multidrug-resistant bacterial pathogens have emerged all over the world [20–22], and the development of novel and effective antimicrobial agents against many kinds of pathogenic bacteria, including methicillin-resistant *Staphylococcus aureus* (MRSA), should remain a continuous mission for medicinal chemists. In 2014, Wang and co-workers discovered eurotiumides, which are novel dihydroisocoumarin-type natural products, from a gorgonian-derived fungus, *Eurotium* sp. XS-200900E6 [23]. Among the series of eurotiumides, eurotiumide A (**1**), having *cis* configurations at H3/H4, exhibited potent antimicrobial activities against *Staphylococcus epidermidis*, *Bacillus cereus*, *Vibrio anguillarum*, and *Escherichia coli*. Based on that report, although **1** seems to be an attractive seed compound for antibiotics, further antimicrobial investigation and a structure–activity relationship study of **1** are needed. In particular, because there is a chance that modification of the side chain of the aromatic ring could improve antimicrobial activity and the spectrum, a structure–activity relationship study of the substituent effect of the aromatic ring is essential for discovering promising candidates for antimicrobial agents. Recently, we reported the first asymmetric total syntheses of (−)-eurotiumide A (**1**) and (+)-eurotiumide B and revised their reported structures [24]. In our synthetic route, the prenyl side chain of the aromatic ring was introduced in the late stage by the Stille coupling reaction with the key intermediate **2**. Based on our previous results, we considered that a number of derivatives of **1**, which have a variety of kinds of side-chain moiety, could be obtained from the common intermediate **2** and non-substituted compound **3** in the late stage of synthesis (Figure 1).

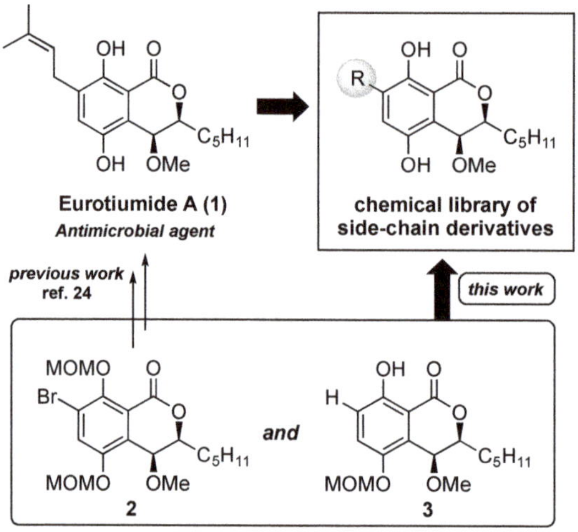

Figure 1. Concept of construction of the chemical library of the side chain-derivatives of eurotiumide A (**1**).

In this work, as part of our continuing research [24,25], we constructed a chemical library of the side-chain derivatives of eurotiumide A (**1**) to elucidate the effects of the side chains of the aromatic rings and to develop antimicrobial agents against methicillin-susceptible *S. aureus* (MSSA) and methicillin-resistant *S. aureus* (both Gram-positive bacteria), as well as *Porphyromonas gingivalis* (a Gram-negative bacterium).

2. Results and Discussion

2.1. Synthesis of the Side-Chain Derivatives of Eurotiumide A

Our synthetic plan is shown in Figure 2. We planned to introduce three types of functional groups: a hydrocarbon group, including hydrogen, alkyl, and aromatic rings (Type A); a heteroatom and heteroatom-containing alkyl group (Type B); and halogen atoms group (Type C). The derivatives of groups A and B could be derived from **2** by the cross-coupling reaction and functional group transformation. The halogenated derivatives (Type C) would be obtained from **3** by direct introduction of the halogen atoms. Although Wang et al. isolated the natural eurotiumide A (**1**) as a racemic form, they evaluated the antimicrobial activities of its enantiomers after separation by chiral HPLC and revealed that there was no significant difference between the enantiomers [23]. From the viewpoint of the efficiency of compound supply, we decided to make racemic compounds.

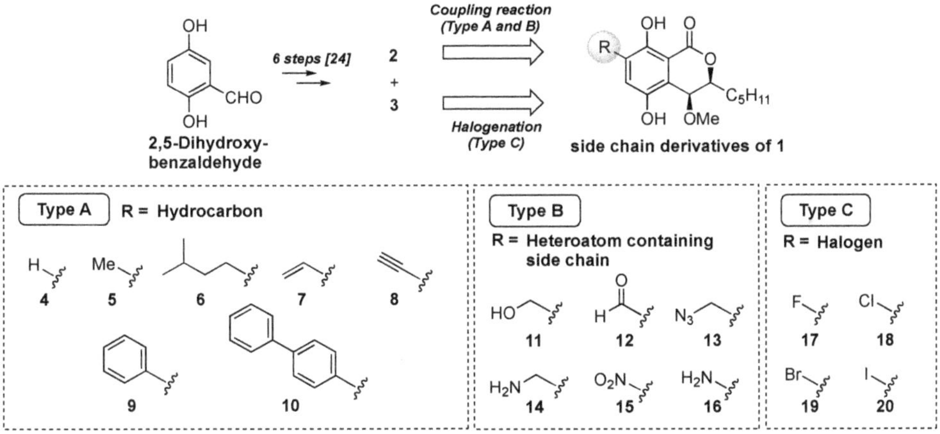

Figure 2. Synthetic plan of the side-chain derivatives of eurotiumide A (**1**).

First, we initiated the syntheses of the derivatives of group A (Scheme 1). The non-substituted derivative **4** was obtained from **3** by deprotection of the diMOM group with aqueous 6 M HCl in methanol at 40 °C in 79% yield. Catalytic hydrogenation of eurotiumide A (**1**) gave the isopentyl derivative **6** in quantitative yield. Methyl and vinyl groups were introduced by the Stille coupling reaction with **2** to afford methyl derivative **5a** and styrene derivative **7a** in 83% and quantitative yields, respectively. Phenyl derivative **9a** and biphenyl derivative **10a** were obtained from **2** by the Suzuki–Miyaura cross coupling reaction with the corresponding boronic acids in 75% and 77% yields, respectively. Deprotection of the diMOM group of derivatives **5a**, **7a**, **9a**, and **10a** then gave the corresponding desired products (**5**, **7**, **9**, and **10**). We tried to introduce the alkyne group by the Sonogashira coupling reaction; however, the desired alkyne product was obtained in only 12% yield. To improve the reaction yield, the Seyferth–Gilbert homologation using the Ohira–Bestmann reagent **21** was applied to the aldehyde derivative **12a** (vide infra) and afforded the desired alkyne **8a** in quantitative yield. After acidic treatment of **8a**, the alkyne derivative **8** was obtained in 68% yield.

With type A derivatives in hand, we turned our attention to preparing type B derivatives having heteroatom-containing side chains (Scheme 2). For the introduction of an alkyl group containing heteroatoms, we chose the styrene derivative **7a** as a starting point. Ozonolysis of the alkene moiety of **7a** afforded the diMOM-protected benzaldehyde **12a** in excellent yield. Acidic treatment of **12a** gave the desired deprotected benzaldehyde derivative **12** in 77%. On the other hand, reduction of the aldehyde moiety of **12a** with sodium borohydride to give the benzyl alcohol **11a** and the deprotection furnished the hydroxymethyl derivative **11** in moderate yield. To introduce a nitrogen group at the benzyl position of **11a**, the primary alcohol moiety was converted to a mesyl group (**22**) and a nucleophilic substitution reaction with sodium azide afforded diMOM-protected azide **13a** in good yield. Derivative **13a** was treated with aqueous 6 M HCl in MeOH to furnish the desired dihydroxy azide derivative **13**. We then tried to convert the azide into an amine functionality. After several attempts, we found that addition of triethylamine was crucial to keep the reaction clean and we succeeded to get **14a**. Then, deprotection of the diMOM group gave the desired aminomethyl derivative **14**.

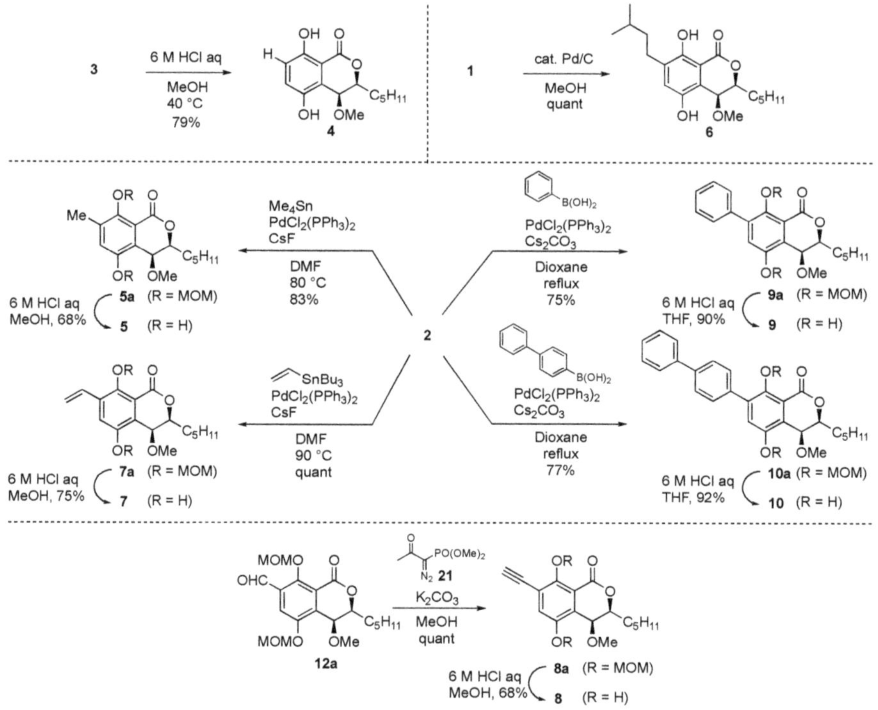

Scheme 1. Synthesis of the hydrocarbon derivatives (type A).

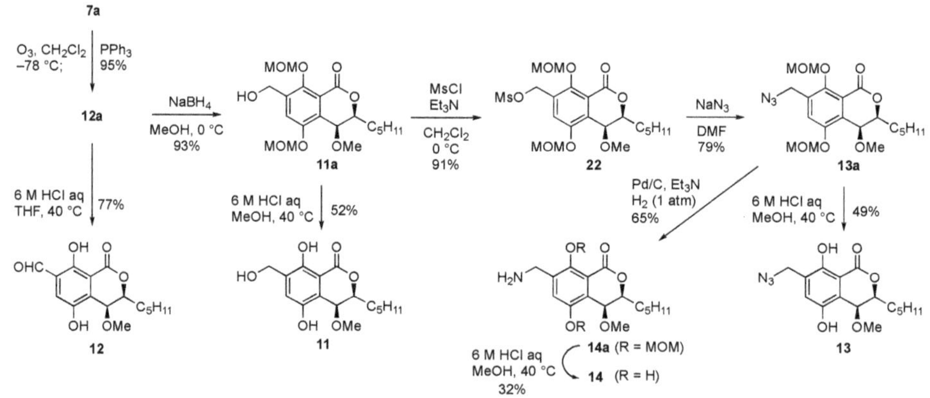

Scheme 2. Synthesis of the derivatives having heteroatom-containing side chains (type B).

Next, a nitration reaction was conducted with non-substituted derivative **3** by adding HNO_3 in AcOH to afford monoMOM-protected nitro derivative **15a** as a crude product; then it was deprotected under acidic condition to give the nitro derivative **15** (Scheme 3). After that, hydrogenation with Adam's catalyst produced the aniline derivative **16** from **15**.

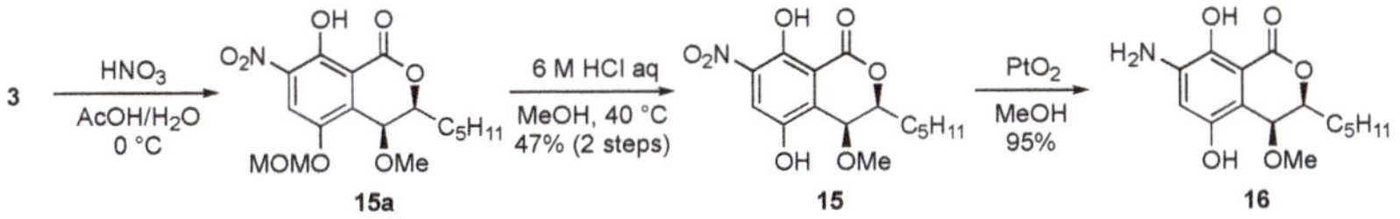

Scheme 3. Synthesis of nitro and aniline derivatives.

Finally, we tried to synthesize the halogenated derivatives (Scheme 4). Chloro and iodo groups were introduced to treat **3** with *N*-chlorosuccinimide and *N*-iodosuccinimide in DMF to afford the chloro derivative **18a** and the iodo derivative **20a**, respectively. The diMOM groups of **18a** and **20a** were then deprotected under acidic conditions to afford the desired **18** and **20**. Bromo derivative **19** was obtained from **2** in 97% yield by acid treatment to cleave the diMOM group. However, despite several efforts to introduce fluorine to the aromatic ring from **3**, we could not get the desired fluoro derivative **17**. We also tried the Sandmeyer reaction with **16** but did not obtain the desired **17**.

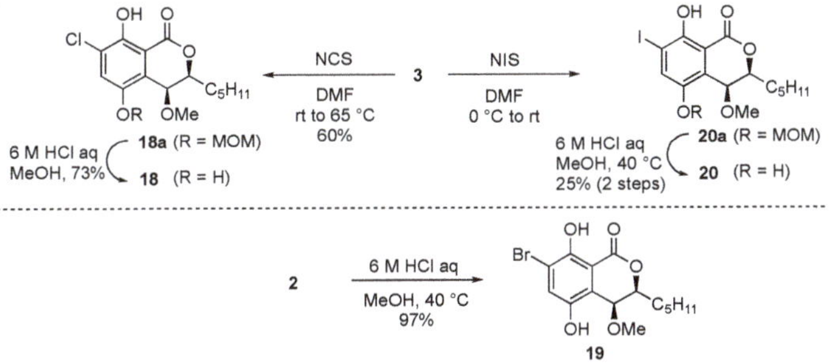

Scheme 4. Synthesis of halogenated derivatives (type C).

2.2. Antimicrobial Evaluation of Synthesized Derivatives

After the initially set derivatives of eurotiumide A were synthesized, the first antimicrobial activity screening was conducted against the Gram-positive MSSA and MRSA as well as the Gram-negative *P. gingivalis* in 10 μM solutions of the synthesized derivatives to narrow down the promising antimicrobial candidates. The results are depicted in Figure 3. (+/−)-Eurotiumide A (**1**) exhibited mild antimicrobial activity against MSSA at this concentration (Figure 3a). While most of the derivatives did not show antimicrobial activity against this strain, the isopentyl derivative **6** and the iodo derivative **20** exhibited more potent antimicrobial activity than **1**. Next, we tested the same screening against MRSA (Figure 3b). Most of the derivatives that displayed good activity against MSSA showed no antimicrobial activity against MRSA. Even natural product **1** and the iodo derivative **20** also did not show good antimicrobial activity against MRSA. Surprisingly, only the isopentyl derivative **6**, which was a reduced derivative of **1**, was found to have good antimicrobial activity against MRSA. We also conducted antimicrobial screening against *P. gingivalis* (Figure 3c). Unlike the case with *S. aureus*, many derivatives, specifically eurotiumide A (**1**), isopentyl derivative **6**, vinyl derivative **7**, aniline derivative **16**, and three halogenated derivatives (**18**, **19**, **20**), were effective against *P. gingivalis*.

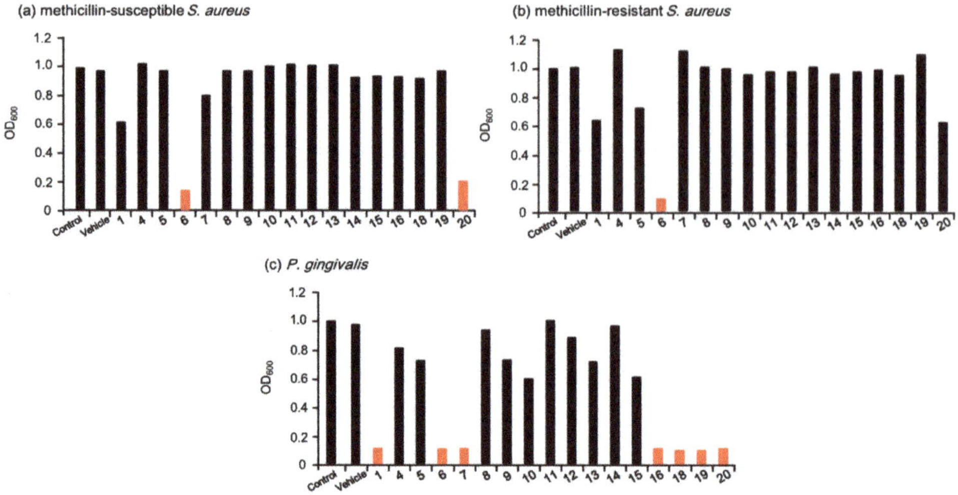

Figure 3. Initial screening of antimicrobial activity against (**a**) methicillin-susceptible *S. aureus*, (**b**) methicillin-resistant *S. aureus*, and (**c**) *P. gingivalis*. The terminal concentration was 10 μM.

Since we acquired promising agents against all three strains, we determined the IC_{50} values of these candidates (Table 1). The IC_{50} values of the isopentyl derivative **6** and the iodo derivative **20** against MSSA were 5.6 μM (2.0 μg/mL) and 9.0 μM (3.7 μg/mL), respectively. Moreover, the IC_{50} value of **6** against MRSA was 4.3 μM (1.5 μg/mL), which is the same level of activity against MSSA. The IC_{50} values of these seven candidates (**1**, **6**, **7**, **16**, **18**, **19**, and **20**) against *P. gingivalis* ranged from 2.0 to 7.0 μM. We also checked the cytotoxicity of three compounds (**1**, **6**, and **20**) against the A549 cell line, and these three compounds were non-toxic in 10 μM.

Table 1. The IC_{50} values (μM) of the selected side chain derivatives against methicillin-susceptible *S. aureus* (MSSA), methicillin-resistant *S. aureus* (MRSA), and *P. gingivalis*. Vancomycin (VCM) was used as a positive control against MSSA and MRSA. Cefcapene pivoxyl (CFPN-PI) was used as a positive control against *P. gingivalis*.

Strains	1	6	7	16	18	19	20	VCM	CFPN-PI
Methicillin-susceptible *S. aureus* (MSSA)	–	5.6	–	–	–	–	9.0	1.3	–
Methicillin-resistant *S. aureus* (MRSA)	–	4.3	–	–	–	–	–	1.5	–
P. gingivalis	3.6	2.0	3.5	6.7	6.4	7.0	3.5	–	0.03

In this study, we discovered that the isopentyl derivative **6**, which is a one-point modified compound of natural product **1**, and the iodo derivative **20** have superior antimicrobial activity to **1** against MSSA and *P. gingivalis*. Although **20** did not exhibit good efficacy against MRSA, **6** was found to maintain antimicrobial activity against these three strains, including MRSA. These results indicate that *S. aureus* is sensitive to changes in the side chain of the aromatic ring and that MRSA can distinguish the subtle difference between prenyl and isopentyl moieties. Moreover, the weak antimicrobial activity of **1** against MRSA suggests a binding affinity between **1** and the penicillin binding protein 2′ [26], which is the main resistance mechanism of MRSA against antibiotics. The inhibition of cell wall synthesis seems to be the mode of action of **1**, although a more detailed study is needed to clarify the mode of action of **6** and **20**. On the other hand, we found that several compounds having alkyl and halogenated side chains well suppressed the increase in *P. gingivalis*.

3. Materials and Methods

3.1. Preparation of Eurotiumide A Derivatives.

3.1.1. General Procedure

All the reactions were carried out in a round-bottomed flask with an appropriate number of necks and side arms connected to a three-way stopcock and/or a rubber septum cap under an argon atmosphere. All vessels were first evacuated by rotary pump and then flushed with argon prior to use. Solutions and solvents were introduced by hypodermic syringe through a rubber septum. During the reaction, the vessel was kept under a positive pressure of argon. Dry THF was freshly prepared by distillation from benzophenone ketyl before use. Anhydrous CH_2Cl_2, DMF, ethanol, MeCN, methanol, pyridine, and toluene were purchased from Kanto Chemical Co. Inc. Infrared (IR) spectra were recorded on a JASCO FT/IR-4100 spectrophotometer using a 5 mm KBr plate. Wavelengths of maximum absorbance are quoted in cm^{-1}. 1H-NMR spectra were recorded on a JEOL ECA–400 (400 MHz), Bruker AV-400N (400 MHz), and Bruker AV–500 (500 MHz) in $CDCl_3$. Chemical shifts are reported in parts per million (ppm), and signals are expressed as singlet (s), doublet (d), triplet (t), multiplet (m), broad (br), and overlapped. 13C-NMR spectra were recorded on a JEOL ECA–400 (100 MHz), Bruker AV–400N (100 MHz), and Bruker AV–500 (125 MHz) in $CDCl_3$. Chemical shifts are reported in parts per million (ppm) (see Supplementary Materials). High resolution mass (HRMS) spectra were recorded on a Thermo Scientific Exactive. All melting points were measured with a Yanaco MP-500D. Analytical thin layer chromatography (TLC) was performed using 0.25 mm E. Merck Silica gel (60F-254) plates. Reaction components were visualized phosphomolybdic acid or ninhydrin or *p*-anisaldehyde in 10% sulfuric acid in ethanol. Kanto Chem. Co. Silica Gel 60N (particle size 0.040–0.050 mm) was used for column chromatography.

3.1.2. Synthesis of (3*S*,4*S*)-5,8-dihydroxy-4-methoxy-3-pentylisochroman-1-one (**4**)

To a solution of bromo compound **3** (10.0 mg, 30.8 μmol) in MeOH (2.3 mL) was added 6 M aqueous HCl (0.77 mL) at 0 °C. After stirring for 30 min at 40 °C, the reaction was quenched by adding saturated aqueous $NaHCO_3$ at 0 °C. The mixture was extracted with EtOAc (×3) and the combined organic layers were washed with brine, dried over Na_2SO_4, filtered, and concentrated under reduced pressure. The residue was purified by preparative thin layer chromatography (PTLC) (EtOAc:*n*-hexane = 3:7) to give non-substituted derivative **4** (6.8 mg, 79%) as a white solid. m.p. 120–121 °C; 1H-NMR (400 MHz, $CDCl_3$) δ 10.62 (1H, s), 7.06 (1H, d, *J* = 9.0 Hz), 6.91 (1H, d, *J* = 9.0 Hz), 5.89 (1H, br-s), 4.77 (1H, d, *J* = 2.7 Hz), 4.50 (1H, ddd, *J* = 2.7, 5.4, 8.3 Hz), 3.40 (3H, s), 1.95 (1H, m), 1.85 (1H, m), 1.70–1.50 (1H, overlapped), 1.46 (1H, m), 1.40–1.25 (4H, overlapped), 0.91 (3H, t, *J* = 6.8 Hz); 13C-NMR (100 MHz, $CDCl_3$) δ 169.0, 156.2, 145.7, 125.1, 121.7, 118.8, 107.6, 81.4, 69.8, 56.8, 31.6, 29.8, 24.9, 22.5, 14.0.; IR (KBr) 3219, 2955, 2924, 2860, 1661, 1586, 1471, 1293, 1204, 905 cm^{-1}; HRMS (ESI) *m*/*z* $(M + Na)^+$ calculated for $(C_{15}H_{20}O_5Na)^+$ 303.1208, found 303.1200.

3.1.3. Synthesis of (3*S*,4*S*)-5,8-dihydroxy-7-isopentyl-4-methoxy-3-pentylisochroman-1-one (**6**)

To a solution of eurotiumide A (**1**) (1.6 mg, 4.6 μmol) in MeOH (0.23 mL) was added Pd/C (1.6 mg, 100 w/w%) at room temperature. After stirring for 1.5 h under hydrogen atmosphere (balloon), the reaction mixture was passed through Celite and the organic solvent was removed under reduced pressure. The residue was purified with flash column chromatography (EtOAc:*n*-hexane = 2:3) to give isopentyl derivative **6** (1.4 mg, 88%) as a white wax. 1H-NMR (500 MHz, $CDCl_3$) δ 10.91 (1H, s), 6.93 (1H, s), 5.62 (1H, br-s), 4.74 (1H, d, *J* = 2.5 Hz), 4.48 (1H, ddd, *J* = 2.6, 5.4, 8.6 Hz), 3.38 (3H, s), 2.62 (2H, m), 1.95 (1H, m), 1.85 (1H, m), 1.65–1.50 (2H, overlapped), 1.50–1.40 (3H, overlapped), 1.40–1.30 (4H, overlapped), 0.95 (6H, d, *J* = 6.3 Hz), 0.90 (3H, *J* = 6.9 Hz); 13C-NMR (125 MHz, $CDCl_3$) δ 169.4, 154.7, 145.0, 133.6, 124.8, 118.6, 106.8, 81.4, 69.9, 56.6, 38.4, 31.6, 29.8, 29.7, 27.9, 27.5, 14.9, 22.5, 14.0.;

IR (KBr) 3290, 2956, 2927, 2870, 1761, 1445, 1171, 807 cm^{-1}; HRMS (ESI) *m/z* $(M + H)^+$ calculated for $(C_{20}H_{31}O_5)^+$ 351.2171, found 351.2177.

3.1.4. (3*S*,4*S*)-4-methoxy-5,8-bis(methoxymethoxy)-7-methyl-3-pentylisochroman-1-one (**5a**)

To a solution of bromo compound **3** (40.0 mg, 89.4 μmol) and CsF (16.3 mg, 107 μmol) in degassed DMF (0.45 mL) were added Me_4Sn (15 μL, 107 μmol) and $PdCl_2(PPh_3)_2$ (6.3 mg, 8.94 μmol) at room temperature. After stirring for 50 min at 80 °C, the reaction was quenched by adding water. The mixture was extracted with EtOAc (×3) and the combined organic layers were washed with brine, dried over Na_2SO_4, filtered, and concentrated under reduced pressure. The residue was purified with flash column chromatography (EtOAc:*n*-hexane = 3:7) to give diMOM-protected methyl derivative **5a** (28.5 mg, 83%) as a yellow amorphous. 1H-NMR (400 MHz, $CDCl_3$) δ 7.255 (1H, s), 5.21 (2H, s), 5.10 (1H, d, *J* = 6.8 Hz), 5.07 (1H, d, *J* = 6.8 Hz), 4.59 (1H, d, *J* = 1.5 Hz), 4.26 (1H, ddd, *J* = 1.5, 5.9, 7.5 Hz), 3.60 (3H, s), 3.50 (3H, s), 3.30 (3H, s), 2.39 (3H, s), 2.02 (1H, m), 1.81 (1H, m), 1.70–1.50 (1H, overlapped), 1.43 (1H, m), 1.40–1.25 (4H, overlapped), 0.91 (3H, t, *J* = 6.8 Hz); 13C-NMR (125 MHz, $CDCl_3$) δ 162.4, 152.3, 149.8, 135.7, 126.3, 121.3, 118.7, 101.5, 95.0, 80.9, 68.2, 57.5, 56.7, 56.4, 31.6, 30.6, 24.9, 22.6, 17.6, 14.0.; IR (KBr) 2958, 2927, 2858, 2828, 1728, 1478, 1153 cm^{-1}; HRMS (ESI) *m/z* $(M + H)^+$ calculated for $(C_{20}H_{31}O_7)^+$ 383.2070, found 383.2069.

3.1.5. (3*S*,4*S*)-5,8-dihydroxy-4-methoxy-7-methyl-3-pentylisochroman-1-one (**5**)

To a solution of diMOM-protected methyl derivative **5a** (10.0 mg, 26.0 μmol) in MeOH (2.0 mL) was added 6 M aqueous HCl (0.65 mL) at 0 °C. After stirring for 1 h at 40 °C, the reaction was quenched by adding saturated aqueous $NaHCO_3$. The mixture was extracted with EtOAc (×3) and the combined organic layers were washed with brine, dried over Na_2SO_4, filtered, and concentrated under reduced pressure. The residue was purified with PTLC (EtOAc:*n*-hexane = 3:7) to give methyl derivative **5** (5.2 mg, 68%) as a yellow solid. m.p. 113 °C; 1H-NMR (400 MHz, $CDCl_3$) δ 10.89 (1H, s), 6.93 (1H, s), 5.59 (1H, br-s), 4.75 (1H, d, *J* = 2.7 Hz), 4.48 (1H, ddd, *J* = 2.7, 5.4, 8,3 Hz), 3.37 (3H, s), 2.25 (3H, s), 1.93 (1H, m), 1.84 (1H, m), 1.70-1.50 (1H, overlapped), 1.45 (1H, m), 1.40–1.25 (4H, overlapped), 0.91 (3H, t, *J* = 6.6 Hz); 13C-NMR (125 MHz, $CDCl_3$) δ 169.4, 154.9, 144.9, 128.7, 125.8, 118.6, 106.6, 81.4, 69.8, 56.5, 31.6, 29.8, 24.9, 22.5, 15.8, 14.0.; IR (KBr) 3340, 2957, 2928, 2859, 1682, 1654, 1604, 1296, 1172 cm^{-1}; HRMS (ESI) *m/z* $(M + Na)^+$ calculated for $(C_{16}H_{22}O_5Na)^+$ 317.1365, found 317.1350.

3.1.6. (3*S*,4*S*)-4-methoxy-5,8-bis(methoxymethoxy)-3-pentyl-7-vinylisochroman-1-one (**7a**)

To a solution of bromo compound **3** (200 mg, 0.447 mmol) and CsF (135.8 mg, 0.894 mmol) in degassed DMF (2.2 mL) were added tributylvinyltin (0.26 mL, 0.894 mmol) and $PdCl_2(PPh_3)_2$ (62.8 mg, 89.0 μmol) at room temperature. After stirring for 1 h at 80 °C, the reaction was quenched by adding water. The mixture was extracted with EtOAc (×3) and the combined organic layers were washed with brine, dried over Na_2SO_4, filtered, and concentrated under reduced pressure. The residue was purified with flash column chromatography (EtOAc:*n*-hexane = 3:7) to give diMOM-protected vinyl derivative **7a** (185.1 mg, quant) as a yellow solid. m.p. 63–64 °C; 1H-NMR (500 MHz, $CDCl_3$) δ 7.56 (1H, s), 7.14 (1H, dd, *J* = 11.1, 17.7 Hz), 5.76 (1H, d, *J* = 17.7 Hz), 5.40 (1H, d, *J* = 11.1 Hz), 5.24 (2H, s), 5.08 (1H, d, *J* = 6.3 Hz), 5.05 (1H, d, *J* = 6.3 Hz), 4.60 (1H, d, *J* = 1.3 Hz), 4.26 (1H, ddd, *J* = 1.3, 5.8, 7.4 Hz), 3.58 (3H, s), 3.50 (3H, s), 3.31 (3H, s), 2.03 (1H, m), 1.81 (1H, m), 1.56 (1H, m), 1.43 (1H, m), 1.40–1.25 (4H, overlapped), 0.90 (3H, t, *J* = 6.9 Hz); 13C-NMR (125 MHz, $CDCl_3$) δ 162.0, 150.7, 150.2, 134.9, 131.3, 128.5, 119.7, 116.7, 116.0, 101.5, 95.2, 80.8, 68.3, 57.9, 56.8, 56.4, 31.6, 30.6, 24.9, 22.5, 14.0.; IR (KBr) 2953, 2931, 2861, 2829, 1730, 1471, 1426, 1155, 929 cm^{-1}; HRMS (ESI) *m/z* $(M + H)^+$ calculated for $(C_{21}H_{31}O_7)^+$ 395.2070, found 395.2078.

3.1.7. (3*S*,4*S*)-5,8-dihydroxy-4-methoxy-3-pentyl-7-vinylisochroman-1-one (**7**)

To a solution of diMOM-protected methyl derivative **7a** (13.7 mg, 34.7 μmol) in MeOH (2.6 mL) was added 6 M aqueous HCl (0.87 mL) at 0 °C. After stirring for 3 h at 40 °C, the reaction was quenched by adding saturated aqueous $NaHCO_3$. The mixture was extracted with EtOAc (×3) and the combined organic layers were washed with brine, dried over Na_2SO_4, filtered, and concentrated under reduced pressure. The residue was purified with PTLC (EtOAc:*n*-hexane = 3:7) to give vinyl derivative **7** (8.5 mg, 75%) as a yellow wax. 1H-NMR (500 MHz, $CDCl_3$) δ 11.10 (1H, s), 7.23 (1H, s), 7.01 (1H, dd, *J* = 11.4, 17.7 Hz), 5.82 (1H, br-s), 5.80 (1H, d, *J* = 18.0 Hz), 5.37 (1H, d, *J* = 11.0 Hz), 4.77 (1H, br-s), 4.50 (1H, br-s), 3.40 (3H, s), 1.95 (1H, m), 1.85 (1H, m), 1.58 (1H, m), 1.45 (1H,m), 1.40–1.25 (4H, overlapped), 0.90 (3H, br-s); 13C-NMR (125 MHz, $CDCl_3$) δ 169.3, 153.9, 145.4, 129.8, 128.0, 121.4, 120.9, 116.5, 107.7, 81.5, 69.7, 56.8, 31.6, 29.8, 24.9, 22.5, 14.0.; IR (KBr) 3311, 2956, 2930, 2859, 1659, 1438, 1171 cm^{-1}; HRMS (ESI) *m/z* $(M + Na)^+$ calculated for $(C_{17}H_{22}O_5Na)^+$ 329.1365, found 329.1368.

3.1.8. (3*S*,4*S*)-4-methoxy-5,8-bis(methoxymethoxy)-3-pentyl-7-phenylisochroman-1-one (**9a**)

Bromo compound **3** (10.0 mg, 22.4 μmol), Cs_2CO_3 (21.9 mg, 67.1 μmol), phenylboronic acid (5.5 mg, 44.7 μM), and $PdCl_2(PPh_3)_2$ (3.1 mg, 44.7 μmol) were dissolved in degassed dioxane (0.22 mL) at room temperature. After stirring for 1 h under reflux condition, the reaction was quenched by adding saturated aqueous NH_4Cl. The mixture was extracted with EtOAc (×3) and the combined organic layers were washed with brine, dried over Na_2SO_4, filtered, and concentrated under reduced pressure. The residue was purified with flash column chromatography (EtOAc:*n*-hexane = 3:7) to give diMOM-protected phenyl derivative **9a** (7.4 mg, 75%) as a white wax. 1H-NMR (500 MHz, $CDCl_3$) δ 7.55 (1H, d, *J* = 7.6 Hz), 7.50-7.38 (3H, overlapped), 7.36 (1H, dd, *J* = 7.3 Hz), 5.25 (2H, s), 4.80 (2H, s), 4.66 (1H, s), 4.33 (1H, t, *J* = 7.0 Hz), 3.50 (3H, s), 3.37 (3H, s), 2.92 (3H, s), 2.06 (1H, m), 1.85 (1H, m), 1.70–1.50 (1H, overlapped), 1.50–1.25 (5H, overlapped), 0.92 (3H, br-s); 13C-NMR (125 MHz, $CDCl_3$) δ 162.1, 150.5, 150.0, 139.5, 137.9, 129.8, 128.3, 128.1, 127.7, 121.0, 119.9, 101.0, 95.1, 80.8, 68.3, 57.1, 56.4, 31.6, 30.6, 24.9, 22.5, 14.0.; IR (KBr) 2956, 2927, 2859, 2828, 1728, 1467, 1152, 1008, 932 cm^{-1}; HRMS (ESI) *m/z* $(M + Na)^+$ calculated for $(C_{25}H_{32}O_7Na)^+$ 467.2046, found 467.2043.

3.1.9. (3*S*,4*S*)-5,8-dihydroxy-4-methoxy-3-pentyl-7-phenylisochroman-1-one (**9**)

To a solution of diMOM-protected methyl derivative **9a** (7.4 mg, 16.8 μmol) in THF (1.0 mL) was added 6 M aqueous HCl (0.50 mL) at 0 °C. After stirring for 6 h at room temperature, the reaction was quenched by adding saturated aqueous $NaHCO_3$. The mixture was extracted with EtOAc (×3) and the combined organic layers were washed with brine, dried over Na_2SO_4, filtered, and concentrated under reduced pressure. The residue was purified with PTLC (EtOAc:*n*-hexane = 3:7) to give phenyl derivative **9** (6.0 mg, 90%) as a yellow solid. m.p. 173–174 °C; 1H-NMR (400 MHz, $CDCl_3$) δ 11.21 (1H, s), 7.58 (2H, d, *J* = 7.3 Hz), 7.44 (2H, t, *J* = 7.3 Hz), 7.38 (1H, d, *J* = 7.6 Hz), 7.13 (1H, s), 5.76 (1H, br-s), 4.82 (1H, d, *J* = 2.7 Hz), 4.55 (1H, ddd, *J* = 2.7, 5.1, 8.3 Hz), 3.44 (3H, s), 1.98 (1H, m), 1.89 (1H, m), 1.70–1.40 (2H, overlapped), 1.40–1.25 (4H, overlapped), 0.92 (3H, t, *J* = 6.8 Hz); 13C-NMR (125 MHz, $CDCl_3$) δ 169.5, 153.7, 145.4, 136.2, 131.8, 129.2, 128.3, 127.9, 125.5, 121.1, 107.8, 81.6, 69.6, 56.9, 31.6, 29.8, 24.9, 22.5, 14.0.; IR (KBr) 3307, 2955, 2928, 2859, 1650, 1425, 1295, 1194 cm^{-1}; HRMS (ESI) *m/z* $(M + H)^+$ calculated for $(C_{21}H_{25}O_5)^+$ 357.1702, found 357.1707.

3.1.10. (3*S*,4*S*)-7-([1,1′-biphenyl]-4-yl)-4-methoxy-5,8-bis(methoxymethoxy)-3-pentylisochroman-1-one (**10a**)

Bromo compound **3** (20.0 mg, 44.7 μmol), Cs_2CO_3 (21.9 mg, 67.1 μmol), 4-biphenylboronic acid (5.5 mg, 44.7 μmol), and $PdCl_2(PPh_3)_2$ (3.2 mg, 4.47 μmol) were dissolved in degassed dioxane (0.23 mL) at room temperature. After stirring for 1 h under reflux condition, the reaction was quenched by adding saturated aqueous NH_4Cl. The mixture was extracted with EtOAc (×3) and the combined organic layers were washed with brine, dried over Na_2SO_4, filtered, and concentrated under reduced pressure. The residue was purified with PTLC (EtOAc:*n*-hexane = 3:7) to give diMOM-protected biphenyl derivative **10a** (18.0 mg, 88%) as a white solid. 1H-NMR (500 MHz, $CDCl_3$) δ 7.74–7.60 (6H, overlapped), 7.53–7.40 (3H, overlapped), 7.38 (1H, t, *J* = 7.3 Hz), 5.28 (2H, s), 4.85 (1H, d, *J* = 7.0 Hz), 4.84 (1H, d, *J* = 7.0 Hz), 4.68 (1H, d, *J* = 1.3 Hz), 4.35 (1H, ddd, *J* = 1.3, 6.0, 7.6 Hz), 3.51 (3H, s), 3.38

(3H, s), 2.99 (3H, s), 2.08 (1H, m), 1.86 (1H, m), 1.70-1.50 (1H, overlapped), 1.46 (1H, m), 1.40–1.25 (4H, overlapped), 0.92 (3H, t, J = 6.9 Hz); 13C-NMR (125 MHz, $CDCl_3$) δ 162.1, 150.6, 150.0, 140.5, 140.4, 139.1, 136.8, 130.2, 128.9, 128.1, 127.5, 127.0, 126.9, 120.9, 120.0, 101.1, 95.1, 80.8, 68.3, 57.2, 56.9, 56.4, 31.6, 30.6, 24.9, 22.5, 14.0.; IR (KBr) 2956, 2927, 2858, 2827, 1728, 1467, 1152, 1007, 931 cm^{-1}; HRMS (ESI) m/z $(M + H)^+$ calculated for $(C_{31}H_{37}O_7)^+$ 521.2539, found 521.2539.

3.1.11. (3*S*,4*S*)-7-([1,1′-biphenyl]-4-yl)-5,8-dihydroxy-4-methoxy-3-pentylisochroman-1-one (**10**)

To a solution of diMOM-protected biphenyl derivative **10a** (12.9 mg, 24.8 µmol) in THF (1.7 mL) was added 6 M aqueous HCl (0.83 mL) at 0 °C. After stirring for 17 h at room temperature, the reaction was quenched by adding saturated aqueous $NaHCO_3$ at 0 °C. The mixture was extracted with EtOAc (×3) and the combined organic layers were washed with brine, dried over Na_2SO_4, filtered, and concentrated under reduced pressure. The residue was purified with PTLC (EtOAc:*n*-hexane = 3:7) to give biphenyl derivative **10** (9.9 mg, 92%) as a yellow solid. m.p. 181–182 °C; 1H-NMR (400 MHz, $CDCl_3$) δ 11.28 (1H, s), 7.67 (4H, s), 7.64 (2H, d, J = 7.3 Hz), 7.46 (2H, t, J = 7.3 Hz), 7.37 (1H, t, J = 7.3 Hz), 7.19 (1H, s), 5.75 (1H, br-s), 4.84 (1H, d, J = 2.7 Hz), 4.56 (1H, ddd, J = 2.7, 5.4, 8.3 Hz), 3.46 (3H, s), 1.98 (1H, m), 1.89 (1H, m), 1.70–1.50 (2H, overlapped), 1.45–1.25 (4H, overlapped), 0.92 (3H, t, J = 6.8 Hz); 13C-NMR (125 MHz, $CDCl_3$) δ 169.4, 153.8, 145.5, 140.7, 135.2, 131.4, 129.6, 128.8, 127.5,127.15, 127.07, 125.3, 121.0, 107.9, 81.5, 69.8, 56.9, 31.6, 29.8, 24.9, 22.5, 14.0.; IR (KBr) 3283, 2954, 2929, 2863, 1668, 1595, 1295, 1220, 772 cm^{-1}; HRMS (ESI) m/z $(M + Na)^+$ calculated for $(C_{27}H_{28}O_5Na)^+$ 455.1834, found 455.1831.

3.1.12. (3*S*,4*S*)-7-ethynyl-4-methoxy-5,8-bis(methoxymethoxy)-3-pentylisochroman-1-one (**8a**)

To a solution of aldehyde **12a** (5.4 mg, 13.6 µmol) in MeOH (0.14 mL) were added K_2CO_3 (5.7 mg, 40.9 µmol) and Ohira–Bestmann reagent (3.9 mg, 20.4 µmol) at room temperature. After stirring for 40 min at the same temperature, the mixture was concentrated under reduced pressure. The residue was purified with column chromatography (EtOAc:*n*-hexane = 1:4 to 1:1) to give diMOM alkyne derivative **8a** (6.3 mg, quant) as a yellow oil. 1H-NMR (500 MHz, $CDCl_3$) δ 7.52 (1H, s), 5.27 (1H, d, J = 6.0 Hz), 5.22 (2H, s), 5.17 (1H, d, J = 6.0 Hz), 4.59 (1H, d, J = 1.3 Hz), 4.27 (1H, ddd, J = 1.3, 5.8, 7.4 Hz), 3.65 (3H, s), 3.49 (3H, s), 3.32 (3H, s), 2.05 (1H, m), 1.82 (1H, m), 1.65–1.50 (1H, overlapped), 1.42 (1H, m), 1.40–1.25 (4H, overlapped), 0.91 (3H, t, J = 7.1 Hz); 13C-NMR (125 MHz, $CDCl_3$) δ 161.2, 154.6, 149.5, 130.0, 123.5, 120.4, 120.1, 101.0, 95.2, 82.7, 80.7, 79.3, 68.3, 58.1, 57.0, 56.5, 31.6, 30.5, 24.8, 22.5, 14.0.; IR (KBr) 3260, 2954, 2932, 2861, 2830, 1730, 1155, 1012, 931 cm^{-1}; HRMS (ESI) m/z $(M + H)^+$ calculated for $(C_{21}H_{29}O_7)^+$ 393.1913, found 393.1903.

3.1.13. (3*S*,4*S*)-7-ethynyl-5,8-dihydroxy-4-methoxy-3-pentylisochroman-1-one (**8**)

To a solution of diMOM alkyne derivative **8a** (6.3 mg, 13.6 µmol) in MeOH (1.2 mL) was added 6 M aqueous HCl (0.40 mL) at room temperature. After stirring for 24 h at the same temperature, the reaction was quenched by adding saturated aqueous $NaHCO_3$ at 0 °C. The mixture was extracted with EtOAc (×3) and the combined organic layers were washed with brine, dried over Na_2SO_4, filtered, and concentrated under reduced pressure. The residue was purified with column chromatography (EtOAc:*n*-hexane = 1:4 to 1:1) to give alkyne derivative **8** (3.3 mg, 67%) as a yellow solid. m.p. 132–133 °C; 1H-NMR (500 MHz, $CDCl_3$) δ 11.20 (1H, s), 7.22 (1H, s), 6.03 (1H, br-s), 4.76 (1H, d, J = 2.5 Hz), 4.51 (1H, ddd, J = 2.5, 5.1, 8.2 Hz), 3.40 (3H, s), 3.39 (1H, s), 1.94 (1H, m), 1.84 (1H, m), 1.70–1.50 (1H, overlapped), 1.45 (1H, m), 1.40–1.25 (4H, overlapped), 0.91 (3H, t, J = 7.0 Hz); 13C-NMR (125 MHz, $CDCl_3$) δ 168.6, 157.3, 145.1, 127.8, 123.4, 112.6, 108.0, 83.2, 81.4, 77.7, 69.7, 57.0, 31.5, 29.7, 24.8, 22.5, 14.0.; IR (KBr) 3294, 2956, 2930, 2859, 1679, 1434, 1172 cm^{-1}; HRMS (ESI) m/z $(M + H)^+$ calculated for $(C_{17}H_{21}O_5)^+$ 305.1389, found 305.1391.

3.1.14. (3*S*,4*S*)-4-methoxy-5,8-bis(methoxymethoxy)-1-oxo-3-pentylisochromane-7-carbaldehyde (**12a**)

A stirred solution of **7a** (185.1 mg, 0.469 mmol) in CH_2Cl_2 (10.0 mL) was cooled to −78 °C and a stream of ozone was passed through it for 30 min. At this time, ozone gas was bubbled into the reaction mixture until the color of the reaction mixture turned to blue. After completion of the reaction, the mixture was purged with oxygen gas for 30 min before being treated with PPh_3 (246.2 mg, 0.939 mmol) and allowed to warm to room temperature. After stirring at the same temperature for 12 h, the mixture was concentrated under reduced pressure and the resultant mixture was purified with column chromatography (EtOAc:*n*-hexane = 1:4 to 2:3) to give diMOM benzaldehyde derivative **12a** (177.4 mg, 95%) as a white solid. m.p. 38–39 °C; 1H-NMR (400 MHz, $CDCl_3$) δ 10.42 (1H, s), 7.83 (1H, s), 5.29 (2H, s), 5.2 (2H, s), 4.65 (1H, d, *J* = 1.0 Hz), 4.29 (1H, *J* = 1.0, 5.6, 8.3 Hz), 3.59 (3H, s), 3.50 (3H, s), 3.35 (3H, s), 2.06 (1H, m), 1.83 (1H, m), 1.70-1.50 (1H, overlapped), 1.44 (1H, m), 1.40-1.30 (4H, overlapped), 0.91 (3H, t, *J* = 7.1 Hz); 13C-NMR (125 MHz, $CDCl_3$) δ 189.9, 161.4, 156.6, 150.6, 135.8, 132.5, 120.8, 116.9, 103.0, 95.4, 81.0, 68.7, 58.4, 57.8, 57.0, 31.9, 30.8, 25.2, 22.8, 14.3.; IR (KBr) 2957, 2929, 2859, 2829, 1730, 1691, 1379, 1155, 930 cm^{-1}; HRMS (ESI) *m*/*z* $(M + H)^+$ calculated for $(C_{20}H_{29}O_8)^+$ 397.1862, found 397.1866.

3.1.15. (3*S*,4*S*)-5,8-dihydroxy-4-methoxy-1-oxo-3-pentylisochromane-7-carbaldehyde (**12**)

To a solution of diMOM aldehyde derivative **12a** (10.0 mg, 25.2 μmol) in THF (1.9 mL) was added 6 M aqueous HCl (0.63 mL) at 0 °C. After stirring for 4 h at room temperature, the reaction was quenched by adding saturated aqueous $NaHCO_3$ at 0 °C. The mixture was extracted with EtOAc (×3) and the combined organic layers were washed with brine, dried over Na_2SO_4, filtered, and concentrated under reduced pressure. The residue was purified with PTLC (EtOAc:*n*-hexane = 2:3) to give benzaldehyde derivative **12** (6.0 mg, 77%) as a pale yellow solid. m.p. 170 °C (dec); 1H-NMR (400 MHz, $CDCl_3$) δ 11.33 (1H, s), 10.47 (1H, s), 7.70 (1H, d, *J* = 1.5 Hz), 6.62 (1H, br-s), 4.75 (1H, d, *J* = 2.2 Hz), 4.49 (1H, ddd, *J* = 2.2, 5.6, 8.0 Hz), 3.43 (3H, s), 2.03 (1H, s), 1.88 (1H, m), 1.61 (1H, m), 1.48 (1H, m), 1.42–1.30 (4H, overlapped), 0.92 (3H, t, *J* = 6.8 Hz); 13C-NMR (125 MHz, $CDCl_3$) δ 189.0, 168.8, 158.9, 146.0, 131.3, 124.9, 121.5, 110.2, 82.2, 69.2, 57.9, 31.9, 30.3, 25.1, 22.8, 14.3.; IR (KBr) 3444, 3169, 2953, 2940, 2920, 1676, 1455, 1395, 1299 cm^{-1}; HRMS (ESI) *m*/*z* $(M + H)^+$ calculated for $(C_{16}H_{21}O_6)^+$ 309.1338, found 309.1342.

3.1.16. (3*S*,4*S*)-7-(hydroxymethyl)-4-methoxy-5,8-bis(methoxymethoxy)-3-pentylisochroman-1-one (**11a**)

To a solution of diMOM aldehyde derivative **12a** (20.0 mg, 50.5 μmol) in MeOH (0.25 mL) was added $NaBH_4$ (2.1 mg, 55.5 μmol) at 0 °C. After stirring for 15 min at the same temperature, the reaction was quenched by adding water at 0 °C. The mixture was extracted with EtOAc (×3) and the combined organic layers were washed with brine, dried over Na_2SO_4, filtered, and concentrated under reduced pressure. The residue was purified with PTLC (EtOAc:*n*-hexane = 1:1) to give diMOM hydroxymethyl derivative **11a** (18.6 mg, 93%) as a white wax. 1H-NMR (400 MHz, $CDCl_3$) δ 7.46 (1H, s), 5.25 (1H, d, *J* = 6.8 Hz), 5.24 (1H, d, *J* = 6.8 Hz), 5.15 (2H, s), 4.72 (1H, dd, *J* = 6.4, 12.5 Hz), 4.62 (1H, d, *J* = 1.2 Hz), 4.58 (1H, dd, *J* = 7.8, 12.5 Hz), 4.25 (1H, ddd, *J* = 1.2, 5.8, 8.0 Hz), 3.64 (3H, s), 3.55 (1H, t, *J* = 6.8 Hz), 3.50 (3H, s), 3.31 (3H, s), 2.05 (1H, m), 1.83 (1H, m), 1.65-1.50 (1H, overlapped), 1.43 (1H, m), 1.42–1.30 (4H, overlapped), 0.91 (3H, t, *J* = 6.8 Hz); 13C-NMR (125 MHz, $CDCl_3$) δ 162.4, 152.7, 150.7, 138.7, 128.9, 120.8, 119.3, 102.2, 95.4, 81.2, 68.4, 61.4, 57.8, 57.2, 56.8, 31.9, 30.9, 25.2, 22.9, 14.4.; IR (KBr) 3443, 2957, 2928, 2859, 2828, 1724, 1153, 1012 cm^{-1}; HRMS (ESI) *m*/*z* $(M + H)^+$ calculated for $(C_{20}H_{31}O_8)$+ 399.2019, found 399.2017.

3.1.17. (3*S*,4*S*)-5,8-dihydroxy-7-(hydroxymethyl)-4-methoxy-3-pentylisochroman-1-one (**11**)

To a solution of diMOM hydroxymethyl derivative **11a** (7.2 mg, 24.1 μmol) in MeOH (1.8 mL) was added 6 M aqueous HCl (0.45 mL) at 0 °C. After stirring for 4 h at 40 °C, the reaction was quenched by adding saturated aqueous $NaHCO_3$ at 0 °C. The mixture was extracted with EtOAc (×3) and the combined organic layers were washed with brine, dried over Na_2SO_4, filtered, and concentrated under reduced pressure. The residue was purified with PTLC (EtOAc:*n*-hexane = 1:1) to give hydroxymethyl derivative **11** (3.9 mg, 52%) as a white solid. m.p. 143–145 °C; 1H-NMR (400 MHz, $CDCl_3$) δ 10.99 (1H, s), 7.12 (1H, s), 6.03 (1H, br-s), 4.74 (1H, d, *J* = 2.4 Hz), 4.72 (2H, br-s), 4.48 (1H, ddd, *J* = 2.4, 5.2, 8.0 Hz), 3.38 (3H, s), 2.53 (1H, br-s), 1.96 (1H, m), 1.86 (1H, m), 1.70–1.50 (1H, overlapped), 1.46 (1H, m), 1.40–1.25 (4H, overlapped), 0.91 (3H, t, *J* = 6.8 Hz); 13C-NMR (125 MHz, $CDCl_3$) δ 169.5, 154.2, 145.8, 130.8, 123.8, 121.4, 107.8, 82.1, 69.8, 61.2, 57.2, 31.9, 30.2, 25.2, 22.8, 14.3.; IR (KBr) 2951, 2921, 2854, 1682, 1440, 1302 cm^{-1}; HRMS (ESI) *m/z* $(M + H)^+$ calculated for $(C_{16}H_{23}O_6)^+$ 311.1495, found 311.1498.

3.1.18. ((3*S*,4*S*)-4-methoxy-5,8-bis(methoxymethoxy)-1-oxo-3-pentylisochroman-7-yl) methylmethanesulfonate (**22**)

To a solution of diMOM hydroxymethyl derivative **11a** (7.2 mg, 24.1 μmol) in CH_2Cl_2 (0.47 mL) were added Et_3N (10.8 μL, 77.5 μmol) and MsCl (6.0 μL, 77.5 μmol) at 0 °C. After stirring for 40 min at the same temperature, the reaction was quenched by adding water at 0 °C. The mixture was extracted with EtOAc (×3) and the combined organic layers were washed with brine, dried over Na_2SO_4, filtered, and concentrated under reduced pressure. The residue was purified with PTLC (EtOAc:*n*-hexane = 2:3) to give diMOM mesylated derivative **22** (30.4 mg, 91%) as a white wax. 1H-NMR (400 MHz, $CDCl_3$) δ 7.51 (1H, s), 5.45 (1H, d, *J* = 12.0 Hz), 5.37 (1H, d, *J* = 12.2 Hz), 5.25 (2H, s), 5.14 (1H, d, *J* = 6.6 Hz), 5.12 (1H, d, *J* = 6.6 Hz), 4.62 (1H, d, *J* = 1.4 Hz), 4.27 (1H, ddd, *J* = 1.2, 5.6, 7.8 Hz), 3.59 (3H, s), 3.50 (3H, s), 3.33 (3H, s), 3.07 (3H, s), 2.03 (1H, m), 1.82 (1H, m), 1.58 (1H, m), 1.44 (1H, m), 1.40–1.25 (4H, overlapped), 0.91 (3H, t, *J* = 6.8 Hz); 13C-NMR (100 MHz, $CDCl_3$) δ 161.9, 152.2, 150.5, 131.3, 130.5, 120.3, 119.7, 102.8, 95.5, 81.2, 68.6, 66.9, 58.1, 57.4, 56.9, 38.2, 31.9, 30.9, 25.2, 22.8, 14.3.; IR (KBr) 2958, 2930, 2860, 1829, 1681, 1440, 1358, 1175, 933 cm^{-1}; HRMS (ESI) *m/z* $(M + Na)^+$ calculated for $(C_{21}H_{32}O_{10}SNa)^+$ 499.1614, found 499.1616.

3.1.19. (3*S*,4*S*)-7-(azidomethyl)-4-methoxy-5,8-bis(methoxymethoxy)-3-pentylisochroman-1-one (**13a**)

To a solution of diMOM mesylated derivative **22** (5.3 mg, 11.1 μmol) in DMF (55 μL) was added NaN_3 (0.79 mg, 12.1 μmol) at room temperature. After stirring for 6 h at the same temperature, the reaction was quenched by adding water at 0 °C. The mixture was extracted with EtOAc (×3) and the combined organic layers were washed with brine, dried over Na_2SO_4, filtered, and concentrated under reduced pressure. The residue was purified with PTLC (EtOAc:*n*-hexane = 3:7) to give diMOM azide derivative **13a** (3.7 mg, 79%) as a pale-yellow oil. 1H-NMR (500 MHz, $CDCl_3$) δ 7.44 (1H, s), 5.26 (1H, d, *J* = 6.9 Hz), 5.25 (1H, d, *J* = 6.9 Hz), 5.13 (1H, d, *J* = 6.9 Hz), 5.11 (1H, d, *J* = 6.9 Hz), 4.65 (1H, d, *J* = 14.5 Hz), 4.62 (1H, d, *J* = 1.3 Hz), 4.53 (1H, d, *J* = 14.5 Hz), 4.27 (1H, ddd, *J* = 1.3, 5.7, 7.3 Hz), 3.60 (3H, s), 3.51 (3H, s), 3.32 (3H, s), 2.04 (1H, m), 1.82 (1H, m), 1.65–1.50 (1H, overlapped), 1.43 (1H, m), 1.40–1.30 (4H, overlapped), 0.91 (3H, t, *J* = 7.0 Hz); 13C-NMR (125 MHz, $CDCl_3$) δ 162.2, 152.1, 150.5, 133.5, 129.1, 119.7, 119.5, 102.6, 95.5, 81.2, 68.6, 57.9, 57.3, 56.8, 50.2, 31.9, 30.9, 25.2, 22.9, 14.4.; IR (KBr) 2957, 2928, 2858, 2829, 2105, 1729, 1153, 1009 cm^{-1}; HRMS (ESI) *m/z* $(M + H)^+$ calculated for $(C_{20}H_{30}N_3O_7)^+$ 424.2084, found 424.2085.

3.1.20. (3*S*,4*S*)-7-(azidomethyl)-5,8-dihydroxy-4-methoxy-3-pentylisochroman-1-one (**13**)

To a solution of diMOM azide derivative **13a** (8.3 mg, 19.6 μmol) in MeOH (1.5 mL) was added 6 M aqueous HCl (0.49 mL) at room temperature. After stirring for 4 h at 40 °C, the reaction was quenched by adding saturated aqueous $NaHCO_3$ at 0 °C. The mixture was extracted with EtOAc (×3) and the combined organic layers were washed with brine, dried over Na_2SO_4, filtered, and concentrated under reduced pressure. The residue was purified with PTLC (EtOAc:*n*-hexane = 3:7) to give nitro derivative **13** (3.1 mg, 49%) as a white solid. m.p. 98–99 °C; 1H-NMR (400 MHz, $CDCl_3$) δ 10.98 (1H, s), 7.10 (1H, s), 5.81 (1H, br-s), 4.78 (1H, d, *J* = 2.9 Hz), 4.52 (1H, ddd, *J* = 2.9, 5.4, 8.5 Hz), 4.45 (1H, d, *J* = 14.4 Hz), 4.42 (1H, d, *J* = 14.4 Hz), 3.41 (3H, s), 1.93 (1H, m), 1.86 (1H, m), 1.70-1.50 (1H, overlapped), 1.47 (1H, m), 1.40–1.25 (4H, overlapped), 0.91 (3H, t, *J* = 7.1 Hz); 13C-NMR (125 MHz, $CDCl_3$) δ 169.1, 154.4, 145.7, 126.2, 124.6, 121.8, 108.0, 81.7, 70.4, 57.2, 49.3, 31.9, 30.0, 25.2, 22.8, 14.3.; IR (KBr) 2959, 2924, 2857,

2108, 1654, 1441, 1293, 1170 cm^{-1}; HRMS (ESI) *m/z* $(M + H)^+$ calculated for $(C_{16}H_{22}N_3O_5)^+$ 336.1559, found 336.1563.

3.1.21. (3*S*,4*S*)-7-(aminomethyl)-4-methoxy-5,8-bis(methoxymethoxy)-3-pentylisochroman-1-one (**14a**)

To a solution of diMOM azide derivative **13a** (3.3 mg, 7.8 µmol) in MeOH (0.78 mL) was added Et_3N (0.10 mL, 7.35 mmol) and Pd/C (1.6 mg, 1.5 µmol) at room temperature. After stirring for 1 h at the same temperature, the mixture was filtered, and the filtrate was concentrated under reduced pressure. The residue was purified with PTLC ($MeOH:CH_2Cl_2$ = 1:9) to give diMOM amine derivative **14a** (2.0 mg, 65%) as brown oil. 1H-NMR (400 MHz, $CDCl_3$) δ 7.49 (1H, s), 5.26 (2H, s), 5.16 (1H, d, *J* = 7.2 Hz), 5.07 (1H, d, *J* = 6.8 Hz), 4.61 (1H, d, *J* = 1.2 Hz), 4.27 (1H, ddd, *J* = 1.2, 6.0, 7.6 Hz), 4.00 (2H, s), 3.61 (3H, s), 3.50 (3H, s), 3.32 (3H, s), 2.59 (1H, br-s), 2.03 (1H, m), 1.82 (1H, m), 1.57 (1H, m), 1.43 (1H, m), 1.40-1.25 (1H, overlapped), 0.91 (3H, t, *J* = 6.8 Hz); 13C-NMR (125 MHz, $CDCl_3$) δ 162.6, 152.6, 150.5, 128.1, 120.0, 119.0, 102.4, 95.4, 81.2, 68.5, 57.9, 57.2, 56.8, 42.5, 32.0, 30.9, 30.0, 25.2, 22.9, 14.4.; IR (KBr) 2957, 2925, 2857, 2827, 1726, 1470, 1153, 1005 cm^{-1}; HRMS (ESI) *m/z* $(M + H)^+$ calculated for $(C_{20}H_{32}NO_7)^+$ 398.2179, found 398.2178.

3.1.22. (3*S*,4*S*)-7-(aminomethyl)-5,8-dihydroxy-4-methoxy-3-pentylisochroman-1-one (**14**)

To a solution of diMOM amine derivative **14a** (4.4 mg, 11.1 µmol) in MeOH (0.83 mL) was added 6 M aqueous HCl (0.28 mL) at 0 °C. After stirring for 5 h at room temperature, the reaction was quenched by adding saturated aqueous $NaHCO_3$ at 0 °C. The mixture was extracted with the mixture of MeOH and CH_2Cl_2 ($MeOH:CH_2Cl_2$ = 1:4) (×4) and the combined organic layers were dried over Na_2SO_4, filtered and concentrated under reduced pressure. The residue was purified with PTLC ($MeOH:CHCl_3$ saturated with NH_3 = 1:9) to give amiomethyl derivative **14** (1.1 mg, 32%) as brown solid. m.p. 78–80 °C; 1H-NMR (400 MHz, $CDCl_3$) δ 6.98 (1H, s), 4.59 (1H, d, *J* = 1.8 Hz), 4.35 (1H, ddd, *J* = 1.8, 6.0, 8.0 Hz), 3.97 (1H, d, *J* = 13.3 Hz), 3.88 (1H, d, *J* = 13.3 Hz), 3.19 (3H, s), 1.98 (1H, m), 1.83 (1H, m), 1.56 (1H, m), 1.43 (1H, m), 1.40–1.25 (4H, overlapped), 0.90 (3H, t, *J* = 7.0 Hz) ; 13C-NMR (125 MHz, $CDCl_3$) δ 169.9, 154.2, 146.2, 130.0, 125.8, 122.9, 108.1, 82.8, 68.5, 56.9, 42.3, 31.9, 30.6, 25.1, 22.8, 14,3.; IR (KBr) 2956, 2921, 2857, 1676, 1441, 1171 cm^{-1}; HRMS (ESI) *m/z* $(M + Na)^+$ calculated for $(C_{16}H_{23}NO_5Na)^+$ 332.1474, found 332.1474.

3.1.23. ((3*S*,4*S*)-5,8-dihydroxy-4-methoxy-7-nitro-3-pentylisochroman-1-one (**15**)

To a solution of **3** (28.9 mg, 89.1 µmol) in AcOH (0.50 mL) was added the mixture of AcOH and 70% HNO_3 (0.80 mL:0.20 mL) at 0 °C. After stirring for 10 min at the same temperature, the reaction was quenched by adding saturated aqueous $NaHCO_3$ at 0 °C. The mixture was extracted with EtOAc (×3) and the combined organic layers were washed with saturated aqueous $NaHCO_3$ and brine, dried over Na_2SO_4, filtered, and concentrated under reduced pressure. The residue was pathed through SiO_2 plug and the resultant mixture of monoMOM nitro derivative **15a** was used for the next reaction without further purification. To a solution of **15a** mixture in MeOH (7.5 mL) was added 6 M aqueous HCl (2.4 mL) at 0 °C. After stirring for 5 h at 40 °C, the reaction was quenched by adding saturated aqueous $NaHCO_3$ at 0 °C. The mixture was extracted with EtOAc (×3) and the combined organic layers were washed with brine, dried over Na_2SO_4, filtered, and concentrated under reduced pressure. The residue was purified with PTLC (EtOAc:*n*-hexane = 1:1) to give nitro derivative **15** (21.5 mg, 74%) as a yellow solid. m.p. 158-159; 1H-NMR (400 MHz, $CDCl_3$) δ 11.89 (1H, s), 7.78 (1H, s), 6.80 (1H, br-s), 4.82 (1H, d, *J* = 2.6 Hz), 4.55 (1H, ddd, *J* = 2.6, 5.2, 8.3 Hz), 3.46 (3H, s), 1.96 (1H, m), 1.86 (1H, m), 1.59 (1H, m), 1.47 (1H, m), 1.40–1.25 (4H, overlapped), 0.91 (3H, t, *J* = 7.1 Hz); 13C-NMR (125 MHz, $CDCl_3$) δ 167.5, 150.4, 144.9, 137.6, 129.4, 119.7, 110.7, 81.0, 70.3, 57.6 , 31.4, 29.4, 24.7, 22.4, 14.0; IR (KBr) 3416, 2962, 2927, 2857, 1679, 1445, 1261, 1018, 800 cm^{-1}; HRMS (ESI) *m/z* $(M + H)^+$ calculated for $(C_{15}H_{20}NO_7)^+$ 326.1240, found 326.1224.

3.1.24. (3*S*,4*S*)-7-amino-5,8-dihydroxy-4-methoxy-3-pentylisochroman-1-one (**16**)

To a solution of nitro derivative **15** (5.0 mg, 15.4 μmol) in THF (0.62 mL) and MeOH (80 μL) was added PtO_2 (0.3 mg, 1.54 μmol) at room temperature. After stirring for 1.5 h at the same temperature under hydrogen atmosphere (1 atm), the mixture was passed through a membrane filter to remove PtO_2. The mixture was concentrated under reduced pressure and the residue was purified with PTLC (EtOAc:*n*-hexane = 3:7, developed by three times) to give nitro derivative **16** (4.3 mg, 95%) as a yellow solid. m.p. 118–119 °C; 1H-NMR (500 MHz, $CDCl_3$) δ 10.72 (1H, s), 6.45 (1H, s), 5.68 (1H, br-s), 4.67 (1H, d, *J* = 2.5 Hz), 4.46 (1H, ddd, *J* = 2.5, 5.5, 8.3 Hz), 4.05 (1H, br-s), 3.32 (3H, s), 1.94 (1H, m), 1.84 (1H, m), 1.75–1.50 (1H, overlapped), 1.45 (1H, m), 1.40–1.25 (4H, overlapped), 0.90 (3H, t, *J* = 7.0 Hz); 13C-NMR (125 MHz, $CDCl_3$) δ 169.8, 145.9, 144.5, 137.2, 109.8, 108.4, 106.8, 82.4, 69.1, 56.1, 31.6, 30.1, 24.9, 22.5, 14.0; IR (KBr) 3378, 2957, 2926, 2858, 1681, 1464, 1217, 1171 cm^{-1}; HRMS (ESI) *m*/*z* $(M + Na)^+$ calculated for $(C_{15}H_{21}NO_5Na)^+$ 318.1317, found 318.1321.

3.1.25. (3*S*,4*S*)-7-chloro-8-hydroxy-4-methoxy-5-(methoxymethoxy)-3-pentylisochroman-1-one (**18a**)

To a solution of **3** (5.0 mg, 15.4 μmol) in DMF (0.18 mL) was added the solution of *N*-chlorosuccinimide (4.1 mg, 30.8 μmol) in DMF (31 μL) at room temperature. After stirring for 5 h at 65 °C, the reaction was quenched by adding saturated aqueous $NaHCO_3$ at 0 °C. The mixture was extracted with EtOAc (×3) and the combined organic layers were washed with brine, dried over Na_2SO_4, filtered, and concentrated under reduced pressure. The residue was purified with PTLC (EtOAc:*n*-hexane = 1:9) to give monoMOM chloro derivative **18a** (3.3 mg, 60%) as a brown solid. m.p. 79–81 °C; 1H-NMR (400 MHz, $CDCl_3$) δ 11.23 (1H, s), 7.55 (1H, s), 5.18 (1H, d, *J* = 7.0 Hz), 5.16 (1H, d, *J* = 7.0 Hz), 4.59 (1H, d, *J* = 1.7 Hz), 4.39 (1H, ddd, *J* = 1.7, 6.0, 8.0 Hz), 3.50 (3H, s), 3.30 (3H, s), 2.07 (1H, m), 1.86 (1H, m), 1.70-1.50 (1H, overlapped), 1.47 (1H, m), 1.45-1.25 (4H, overlapped), 0.92 (3H, t, *J* = 7.1 Hz); 13C-NMR (125 MHz, $CDCl_3$) δ 168.7, 152.8, 146.3, 125.1, 123.6, 123.0, 109.0, 95.7, 82.7, 67.4, 56.8, 56.4, 31.5, 30.4, 24.7, 22.5, 14.0.; IR (KBr) 2955, 2927, 2853, 2826, 1681, 1453, 1433, 1206 cm^{-1}; HRMS (ESI) *m*/*z* $(M + Na)^+$ calculated for $(C_{17}H_{23}O_6ClNa)^+$ 381.1081, found 381.1088.

3.1.26. (3*S*,4*S*)-7-chloro-5,8-dihydroxy-4-methoxy-3-pentylisochroman-1-one (**18**)

To a solution of monoMOM chloro derivative **18a** (3.3 mg, 9.20 μmol) in MeOH (0.69 mL) was added 6 M aqueous HCl (0.23 mL) at 0 °C. After stirring for 2 h at 40 °C, the reaction was quenched by adding saturated $NaHCO_3$ at 0 °C. The mixture was extracted with EtOAc (×3) and the combined organic layers were washed with brine, dried over Na_2SO_4, filtered, and concentrated under reduced pressure. The residue was purified with PTLC (EtOAc:*n*-hexane = 1:9) to give chloro derivative **18** (2.1 mg, 73%) as a brown solid. m.p. 119-120 °C; 1H-NMR (400 MHz, $CDCl_3$) δ 11.17 (1H, br-s), 7.34 (1H, s), 6.34 (1H, br-s), 4.82 (1H, br-s), 4.59 (1H, ddd, *J* = 2.8, 5.6, 8.4 Hz), 3.48 (3H, s), 2.03 (1H, m), 1.93 (1H, m), 1.64 (1H, m), 1.53 (1H, m), 1.51–1.35 (4H, overlapped), 0.98 (3H, t, *J* = 7.2 Hz); 13C-NMR (100 MHz, $CDCl_3$) δ 168.7, 152.1, 145.6, 124.9, 122.8, 121.1, 108.5, 81.8, 69.6, 57.0, 31.5, 29.8, 24.8, 22.5, 14.0.; IR (KBr) 3282, 2958, 2929, 2860, 1681, 1437, 1198 cm^{-1}; HRMS (ESI) *m*/*z* $(M + H)^+$ calculated for $(C_{15}H_{20}O_5Cl)^+$ 315.0999, found 315.0998.

3.1.27. (3*S*,4*S*)-7-bromo-5,8-dihydroxy-4-methoxy-3-pentylisochroman-1-one (**19**)

To a solution of bromo derivative **2** (11.0 mg, 24.6 μmol) in MeOH (1.8 mL) was added 6 M aqueous HCl (0.62 mL) at 0 °C. After stirring for 3.5 h at 40 °C, the reaction was quenched by adding saturated aqueous $NaHCO_3$ at 0 °C. The mixture was extracted with EtOAc (×3) and the combined organic layers were washed with brine, dried over Na_2SO_4, filtered, and concentrated under reduced pressure. The residue was purified with PTLC (EtOAc:*n*-hexane = 1:9) to give bromo derivative **19** (8.6 mg, 97%) as a white solid. m.p. 132 °C; 1H-NMR (400 MHz, $CDCl_3$) δ 11.26 (1H, s), 7.36 (1H, s), 6.00 (1H, br-s), 4.76 (1H, d, *J* = 2.7 Hz), 4.52 (1H, ddd, *J* = 2.7, 5.1, 8.3 Hz), 3.41 (3H, s), 1.95 (1H, m), 1.86 (1H, m), 1.70-1.50 (2H, overlapped), 1.40–1.25 (4H, overlapped), 0.91 (3H, t, *J* = 7.0 Hz); 13C-NMR

(125 MHz, $CDCl_3$) δ 168.4, 153.0, 145.8, 127.9, 121.5, 111.6, 108.2, 81.4, 70.0, 57.0, 31.5, 29.6, 24.8, 22.5, 14.0.; IR (KBr) 3296, 2955, 2930, 2859, 1679, 1432, 1197 cm^{-1}; HRMS (ESI) m/z $(M + Na)^+$ calculated for $(C_{15}H_{19}O_5BrNa)^+$ 381.0314, found 381.0322.

3.1.28. (3*S*,4*S*)-5,8-dihydroxy-7-iodo-4-methoxy-3-pentylisochroman-1-one (**20**)

To a solution of **3** (12.6 mg, 38.8 μmol) in DMF (0.35 mL) was added the solution of *N*-iodosuccinimide (17.5 mg, 77.6 μmol) in DMF (50 μL) at room temperature. After stirring for 3 h at room temperature, the reaction was quenched by adding saturated aqueous $NaHCO_3$ at 0 °C. The mixture was extracted with CH_2Cl_2 (×3) and the combined organic layers were washed with brine, dried over Na_2SO_4, filtered, and concentrated under reduced pressure. The residue was pathed through SiO_2 plug and the resultant mixture of monoMOM iodo derivative **20a** was used for the next reaction without further purification. To a solution of crude mixture of **20a** in MeOH (0.83 mL) was added 6 M aqueous HCl (0.30 mL) at 0 °C. After stirring for 5 h at 40 °C, the reaction was quenched by adding saturated aqueous $NaHCO_3$ at 0 °C. The mixture was extracted with EtOAc (×3) and the combined organic layers were washed with brine, dried over Na_2SO_4, filtered, and concentrated under reduced pressure. The residue was purified with PTLC (EtOAc:*n*-hexane = 1:9) to give iodo derivative **20** (4.0 mg, 87%) as a pale-yellow oil. m.p. 109–110 °C; 1H-NMR (500 MHz, $CDCl_3$) δ 11.44 (1H, s), 7.57 (1H, s), 6.11 (1H, br-s), 4.51 (1H, ddd, J = 2.8, 5.4, 8.5 Hz), 3.40 (3H, s), 1.94 (1H, m), 1.85 (1H, m), 1.75–1.50 (4H, overlapped), 1.45 (1H, m), 1.40–1.30 (4H, overlapped), 0.91 (3H, t, J = 7.0 Hz); 13C-NMR (125 MHz, $CDCl_3$) δ 168.3, 155.3, 146.3, 133.8, 122.6, 107.1, 85.5, 81.5, 69.8, 56.9, 31.5, 29.7, 24.8, 22.5, 14.0; IR (KBr) 3293, 2977, 298, 2857, 1674, 1427, 1197 cm^{-1}; HRMS (ESI) m/z $(M + Na)^+$ calculated for $(C_{15}H_{19}O_5Ina)^+$ 429.0175, found 429.0174.

3.2. Bactericidal Assay

Methicillin-susceptible *Staphylococcus aureus* (MSSA) ATCC25923 and methicillin-resistant *Staphylococcus aureus* (MRSA) ATCC 33,591 were aerobically incubated at 37 °C in Luria–Bertani medium (LB, Nippon Becton Dickinson Company, Tokyo, Japan). *Porphyromonas gingivalis* W83 was anaerobically incubated at 37 °C in Gifu anaerobic medium (GAM, Nissui, Tokyo, Japan). Each culture (20 μL) prepared to an optical density of 1.5 at 600 nm were appropriately incubated with various concentrations of synthesized compounds in 200 μL of culture medium at 37 °C for 24 h in 96-well plate (Thermo scientific, MA, USA). Compounds were dissolved in DMSO (Wako, Osaka, Japan). The degree of turbidity in the broth culture was measured at absorbance 600 nm using microplate reader (Thermo scientific, MA, USA).

3.3. Cellular Toxicity

Human lung adenocarcinoma epithelial cell line A549 cells were cultured at 37 °C in growth medium (DMEM with 10% fetal bovine serum) in 5% CO_2, and then seeded into 96-well plates at a density of 1×10^5 cells/mL. Once the cells reached 80%–90% confluence, they were treated with or without 10 μM of various compounds at 37 °C for 12 h. Next, 10 μL Cell Counting Kit-8 (Dojindo Molecular Technologies, Kumamoto, Japan) solution was added to each well, and the plate was incubated for 2 h at 37 °C. Cell viability was determined by measuring the absorbance at 450 nm using a fluorimeter (Varioscan, Thermo, USA).

4. Conclusions

We constructed a chemical library of the side-chain derivatives of eurotiumide A, which is a dihydroisocoumarin-type marine natural product. The antimicrobial evaluation of these compounds was conducted against MSSA, MRSA, and *P. gingivalis*. We discovered several compounds to be effective against these strains; among them, the isopentyl derivative **6** is especially more active against all three strains than **1**. Continuous research to clarify the modes of action of these derivatives is under way in our laboratory.

Supplementary Materials: The following are available online at http://www.mdpi.com/1660-3397/18/2/92/s1, 1H- and 13C-NMR charts of all new compounds.

Author Contributions: A.N. conceived and designed this research and analyzed the experimental data; H.S., T.N., M.H., S.N., and S.K. (Shuhei Kameyama) prepared compounds and collected their spectral data; S.K. (Sangita Karanjit) checked the experimental data; Y.F., N.H., G.K. and M.O. evaluated the antimicrobial activity; A.N., M.O. and K.N. wrote the paper; all of the authors reviewed and approved the manuscript. All authors have read and agreed to the published version of the manuscript.

Funding: This work was supported by JSPS KAKENHI Grant Nos. 17K08365 (A.N.), 18H02657 (M.O.), JP19H02851 (K.N.), and JP16H01156 (K.N.), as well as the Kurita Water and Environment Foundation. We also acknowledge Tokushima University for their financial support of the Research Clusters program of Tokushima University (No. 1802001).

Conflicts of Interest: The authors declare no conflict of interest.

References

1. Ma, B.; Forney, L.; Ravel, J. Vaginal microbiology: Rethinking health and disease. *Annu. Rev. Microbiol.* **2012**, *66*, 371–389. [CrossRef] [PubMed]
2. Buffie, C.G.; Parker, E.G. Microbiota-mediated colonization resistance against intestinal pathogens. *Nat. Rev. Immunol.* **2013**, *13*, 790–801. [CrossRef] [PubMed]
3. MCKenney, P.T.; Palmer, E.G. From hype to hope: The gut microbiome in Health and Disease. *Cell* **2015**, *163*, 1326–1332. [CrossRef] [PubMed]
4. Lynch, S.V.; Petersen, O. The Human Intestinal Microbiome in Health and Disease. *N. Eng. J. M.* **2016**, *375*, 371–389. [CrossRef] [PubMed]
5. Ma, W.H.; Piters, W.A.A.S.; Bogaert, D. The microbiota of the respiratory tract: Gatekeeper to respiratory health. *Nat. Rev. Microbiol.* **2017**, *13*, 259–270.
6. Lewis, K. Platforms for Antibiotic Discovery. *Nat. Rev. Drug Discovery* **2013**, *12*, 371–387. [CrossRef] [PubMed]
7. Becattini, S.; Taru, Y.; Palmer, E.G. Antibiotic-induced changes in the intestinal microbiota and disease. *Trends Mol. Med.* **2016**, *22*, 458–478. [CrossRef]
8. Brown, E.D.; Wright, G.D. Antibacterial Drug Discovery in the Resistance Era. *Nature* **2016**, *529*, 336–343. [CrossRef]
9. Fleming, A. On the antibacterial action of cultures of a penicillium with special reference to their use in the isolation of B. influenzae. *Br. J. Exp. Pathol.* **1929**, *10*, 226–236. [CrossRef]
10. Chu, D.T.W.; Plattner, J.J.; Katz, L. New Directions in Antibacterial Research. *J. Med. Chem.* **1996**, *39*, 3853–3874. [CrossRef]
11. Saleem, M.; Nazir, M.; Ali, M.S.; Hussain, H.; Lee, Y.S.; Riaz, N.; Jabbar, A. Antimicrobial natural products: An update on future antibiotic drug candidates. *Nat. Prod. Rep.* **2010**, *27*, 238–254. [CrossRef] [PubMed]
12. Bologa, C.G.; Ursu, O.; Oprea, T.I.; Melancon, C.E., III; Tegos, G.P. Emerging trends in the discovery of natural product antibacterials. *Curr. Opin. Pharmacol.* **2013**, *13*, 678–687. [CrossRef] [PubMed]
13. Butler, M.S.; Robertson, A.A.B.; Cooper, M.A. Natural product and natural product derived drugs in clinical trials. *Nat. Prod. Rep.* **2014**, *31*, 1612–1661. [CrossRef]
14. Szychowski, J.; Truchon, J.-F.; Bennani, Y.L. Natural Products in Medicine: Transformational Outcome of Synthetic Chemistry. *J. Med. Chem.* **2014**, *57*, 9292–9308. [CrossRef] [PubMed]
15. Sclinke, C.; Martins, T.; Queiroz, S.C.; Melo, I.S.; Reyes, F.G.R. Antibacterial Compounds from Marine Bacteria, 2010–2015. *J. Nat. Prod.* **2017**, *80*, 1215–1228. [CrossRef] [PubMed]
16. Masscheletin, J.; Henner, M.; Challis, G.L. Antibiotics from Gram-negative bacteria: A comprehensive overview and selected biosynthetic highlights. *Nat. Prod. Rep.* **2017**, *34*, 712–783. [CrossRef]
17. Von Nussbaum, F.; Brands, M.; Hizen, B.; Weigand, S.; Habich, D. Antibacterial natural products in medicinal chemistry-exodus or revival? *Angew, Chem. Int. Ed.* **2006**, *45*, 5072–5129. [CrossRef]
18. Clardy, J.; Fischbach, M.A.; Walsh, C.T. New antibiotics from bacterial natural product. *Nat. Biotechnol.* **2006**, *24*, 1541–1550. [CrossRef]
19. Abouelhassan, Y.; Garrison, A.T.; Yang, H.; Riveros, A.C.; Burch, G.M.; Huigens, R.W., III. Recent Progress in Natural-Product-Inspired Progra,s Aimed To Address Antibiotic Resistance and Tolerance. *J. Med. Chem.* **2019**, *62*, 7618–7642. [CrossRef]

20. Blair, J.M.; Webber, M.A.; Baylay, A.J.; Ogbolu, D.O.; Piddock, L.J.V. Molecular Mechanisms of Antibiotic Resistance. *Nat. Rev. Microbiol.* **2015**, *13*, 42–51. [CrossRef]
21. Ali, J.; Rafiq, Q.A.; Ratcliffe, E. Antimicrobial Resistance Mechanisms and Potential Synthetic Treatments. *Futur. Sci. OA* **2018**, *4*, FSO290. [CrossRef]
22. Francino, M.P. Antibiotics and the human gut microbiome: Dysbioses and accumulation of resistances. *Front. Microbiol.* **2016**, *6*, 1543. [CrossRef] [PubMed]
23. Chen, M.; Shao, C.-L.; Wang, K.-L.; Xu, Y.; She, Z.-G.; Wang, C.-Y. Dihydroisocoumarin derivatives with antifouling activities from a gorgonian-derived *Eurotium* sp. fungus. *Tetrahedron* **2014**, *70*, 9132–9138. [CrossRef]
24. Nakayama, A.; Sato, H.; Karanjit, S.; Hayashi, N.; Oda, M.; Namba, K. Asymmetric Total Syntheses and Structure Revisions of Eurotiumide A and Eurotiumide B, and Their Evaluation as Natural Fluorescent Probes. *Eur. J. Org. Chem.* **2018**. [CrossRef]
25. Nakayama, A.; Sato, H.; Nagano, S.; Karanjit, S.; Imagawa, H.; Namba, K. Asymmetric Total Syntheses and Structure Elucidations of (+)-Eurtiumide F and (+)-Eurotiumide G. *Chem. Pharm. Bull.* **2019**, *67*, 953–958. [CrossRef] [PubMed]
26. Katayama, Y.; Ito, T.; Hiramatsu, K. A new class of genetic element, *Staphylococcus* cassette chromosome *mec*, encodes methicillin resistance in *Staphylococcus aureus*. *Antimicrob. Agents Chemother.* **2000**, *44*, 1549–1555. [CrossRef]

marine drugs

Article

Impact of the Cultivation Technique on the Production of Secondary Metabolites by *Chrysosporium lobatum* TM-237-S5, Isolated from the Sponge *Acanthella cavernosa*

Géraldine Le Goff [1,*], Philippe Lopes [1], Guillaume Arcile [1], Pinelopi Vlachou [2], Elsa Van Elslande [1], Pascal Retailleau [1], Jean-François Gallard [1], Michal Weis [3], Yehuda Benayahu [3], Nikolas Fokialakis [2] and Jamal Ouazzani [1]

1 Institut de Chimie des Substances Naturelles ICSN, Centre National de la Recherche Scientifique CNRS, Avenue de la Terrasse, 91198 Gif-sur-Yvette, France; Philippe.lopes@cnrs.fr (P.L.); Guillaume.arcile@cnrs.fr (G.A.); elsa.van-elslande@cnrs.fr (E.V.E.); Pascal.retailleau@cnrs.fr (P.R.); jean-francois.gallard@cnrs.fr (J.-F.G.); jamal.ouazzani@cnrs.fr (J.O.)

2 Division of Pharmacognosy and Chemistry of Natural Products, Department of Pharmacy, National and Kapodistrian University of Athens, 15771 Athens, Greece; pvlachou@pharm.uoa.gr (P.V.); fokialakis@pharm.uoa.gr (N.F.)

3 School of Zoology, George S. Wise Faculty of Life Sciences, Tel Aviv University, Ramat Aviv, Tel Aviv 69978, Israel; mich9@tauex.tau.ac.il (M.W.); yehudab@tauex.tau.ac.il (Y.B.)

* Correspondence: geraldine.legoff@cnrs.fr; Tel.: +33-1-69-82-30-05

Received: 8 November 2019; Accepted: 26 November 2019; Published: 30 November 2019

Abstract: The fungi *Chrysosporium lobatum* TM-237-S5 was isolated from the sponge *Acanthella cavernosa*, collected from the mesophotic coral ecosystem of the Red Sea. The strain was cultivated on a potato dextrose agar (PDA) medium, coupling solid-state fermentation and solid-state extraction (SSF/SSE) with a neutral macroreticular polymeric adsorbent XAD Amberlite resin (AMBERLITE XAD1600N). The SSF/SSE lead to high chemodiversity and productivity compared to classical submerged cultivation. Ten phenalenone related compounds were isolated and fully characterized by one-dimensional and two-dimensional NMR and HRMS. Among them, four were found to be new compounds corresponding to isoconiolactone, (-)-peniciphenalenin F, (+)-8-hydroxyscleroderodin, and (+)-8-hydroxysclerodin. It is concluded that SSF/SSE is a powerful strategy, opening a new era for the exploitation of microbial secondary metabolites.

Keywords: solid-state fermentation; solid-state extraction; *Chrysosporium lobatum*; marine fungi; phenalenone derivatives

1. Introduction

The symbiosis between marine sponges and microorganisms is of considerable interest, both biologically and chemically [1,2]. Sponges are benthic organisms that have been colonizing different marine ecosystems, including coral reefs, for 600 million years [3,4]. Their survival under drastically changing conditions requires a variety of adaptations, including the evolving strategy of symbiosis with beneficial microorganisms, which has been taking place since the Precambrian Age [5]. The mutualism between marine sponges and microbial symbionts is mainly related to nutrition and defense [1,6], under the control of dedicated enzymes and active secondary metabolites [2]. Although sponges are the main source of bioactive molecules isolated from marine organisms, a certain amount of evidence indicates that they are biosynthesized by microbial symbionts [7,8]. This has also been corroborated by the massive presence of microorganisms in the mesophyl matrix of the sponges, representing around 50% of their biomass [9–11].

Fungi in the marine environment, and especially those associated with marine invertebrates, have been extensively investigated and reviewed [12,13]. A 2019 collaborative review highlighted the present state of knowledge and raised a multitude of open questions regarding the diversity and function of fungi in marine ecosystems [13].

The symbiont assemblages inside the sponge are well organized in biofilms or dense colonies and are stabilized in the skeleton network over time [14,15]. This certainly impacts their development steps and the expression of biosynthetic clusters of secondary metabolites because it is now well documented that, in fungi, secondary metabolism and life cycle among fungi are co-regulated at the genomic level [16–18].

This idea drives us to compare the metabolic profile of fungi cultivated on a gar slants and in liquid state. The result is that solid-state cultivation often leads to larger molecular diversity than classical liquid state fermentation LSF [19–21]. The major obstacle that stands against agar cultivation is the scale-up. In order to overcome such a challenge, we have developed specific innovative technologies, namely Platotex [22,23] and, more recently, Unifertex [24]. As we systematically coupled the culture of microorganisms with in-situ solid phase extraction (SPE), we also developed a specific SPE procedure for agar cultivation, termed solid-solid extraction (SSE) [25].

In the present study, we report the impact of agar-supported cultivation on the production of secondary metabolites by the marine fungi *Chrysosporium lobatum* TM-237-S5, isolated from the Red Sea sponge *Acanthella cavernosa*. *Chrysosporium lobatum* was previously reported in the literature as a mosquito pathogenic fungus [26]. However, a very limited number of secondary metabolites have been reported in the literature for the genus *Chrysosporium*. Thus, the strain *Chrysosporium queenslandicum* IFM produced naphthaquinone-type altersolanols A, B, and C, the antifungal queenslandon, a representative of the zearalenone family of mycotoxin, and the antibacterial dihydronaphthaquinones chrysoqueen and chrysolandol [27]. The diterpenoid derivative RPR113228, a farnesyl transferase inhibitor, was also attributed to *Chrysosporium lobatum*, yet the identification of the strain was only based on morphological analysis [28]. Furthermore, curvularin and dehydroculvilarin were isolated from *Chrysosporium lobatum* BK-3 [29].

2. Results and Discussion

2.1. The Context of This Work

The TASCMAR project (Tools And Strategies to access to original bioactive compounds from Cultivation of MARine invertebrates and associated symbionts), funded by the European Union in the frame of the Horizon 2020 framework program, offered the opportunity to investigate the molecules produced by marine invertebrates and their symbionts from mesophotic coral ecosystems (MCEs) (30 to 150 m depth). Among the invertebrates investigated, the sponge *Acanthella cavernosa* was collected on the upper mesophotic reef of Eilat at Dekel Beach (51 m depth), in the Gulf of Aqaba (Israel, 2 April 2017, 29°32′12.48″N; 34°56′55.656″E). The area is characterized by a moderate slope covered with dense patches of hard substrate, mostly calcareous, and is also inhabited by other invertebrates such as octocorals, stony corals, black corals, and sea anemones (Figure 1).

The strain *Chrysosporium lobatum* TM-237-S5 (Figure 2) was among the strains isolated and identified based on its ITS rDNA sequence (Nuclear ribosomal internal transcribed spacer).

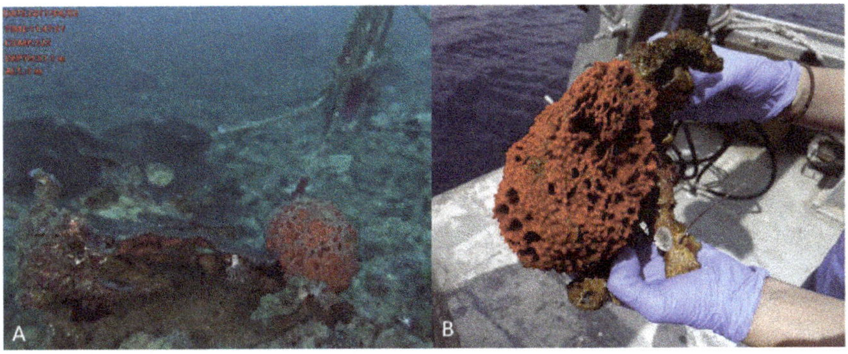

Figure 1. *Acanthella cavernosa* was collected at 51 m depth in Eilat, Gulf of Aqaba (Israel). (**A**) The sponge in its natural environment, (**B**) The sponge was collected by the remote operating vehicle (ROV) arm, introduced in-situ to the collection basket, and brought to the boat for immediate processing. Two representative pieces were recovered, one for taxonomic identification and the other for symbiont isolation. Both samples were immediately frozen on the boat and shipped in dry ice.

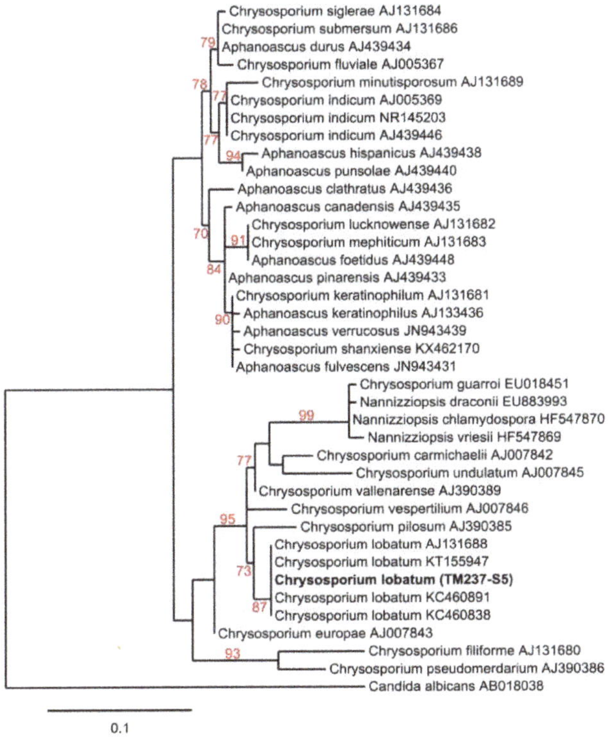

Figure 2. Maximum-likelihood tree obtained from ITS rDNA sequence alignment of the strain TM237-S5 and *Chrysosporium* spp. Reliability of the internal branch is represented in red. *Candida albicans* was used as the outgroup. Numbers are Genbank accessions. Th estrain in bold font is the one described in this study. Scale represents substitutions per site.

The strain was cultivated on potato dextrose broth (PDB), potato dextrose agar (PDA), marine broth (MB), and marine agar (MA). Solid phase extraction (SPE) with XAD resin (AMBERLITE™ *XAD™16HP* N) was applied in-situ to both liquid (LSF/SPE) and agar-supported cultures (solid-state fermentation and solid-state extraction (SSF/SSE)). It has been previously reported that in-situ XAD extraction coupled to agar-supported cultivation prevents the diffusion of target compounds to the agar layer and traps the target compounds on the resin beads [25].

On day four of incubation (Figure 3E), the resin beads became colored, but were not yet covered by the mycelium (white filaments). On day seven (Figure 3F), the resin beads became darker and the mycelium surface increased. On day 10 (Figure 3G), the recovery time, the resin beads were totally covered by the mycelium. We previously reported that such phenomenon is probably due to the lack of oxygen in the viscous resin layer, which pushes the mycelium to reach the surface to access more oxygen. However, the mycelia remained in contact with the agar to access nutriments, as shown on the agar layer, following the recovery of the resin beads (Figure 3H).

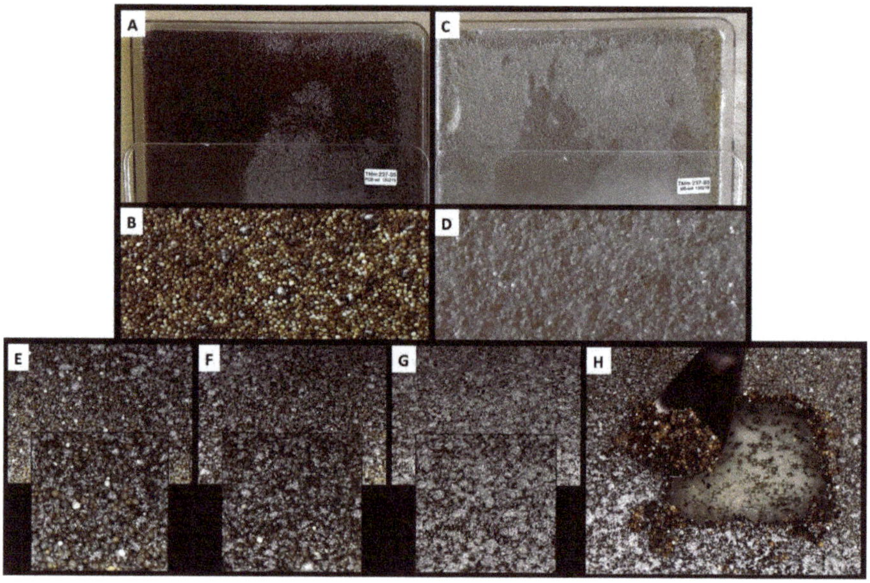

Figure 3. 10 days culture of *Chrysosporium lobatum* TM-237-S5 on potato dextrose agar (PDA) (**A**,**B**) and marine agar (MA) (**C**,**D**) coupled to solid-solid extraction (SSE) with XAD resin (AMBERLITE™ *XAD™16HP* N). The resin beads remained white to light beige on the marine broth (MB) (**D**), while they turned dark brown on the PDA (**B**), showing that the resin beads trapped the colored compounds secreted by the strain. (**E**–**G**) present the coverage of the resin beads by the mycelium at four, seven, and 10 days. (**H**) depicts the easy recovery of the resin biofilm layers; the mycelium is not incrusted and no compounds flow to the agar. The resin beads, as revealed by the dark brown color, trapped all the produced compounds.

After 10 days of incubation, the resin beads were recovered by filtration from the liquid cultures (10 L), and by scraping the surface of the agar cultures (10 × 625 cm^2 petri plates), and washed extensively with water to remove medium residues and any compounds not trapped by the XAD. Resin beads from the PDB, MB, and MA cultures had a light beige color, while the PDA culture was dark brown; most of the color being trapped by the resin beads (Figure 3A–D and Figure 4).

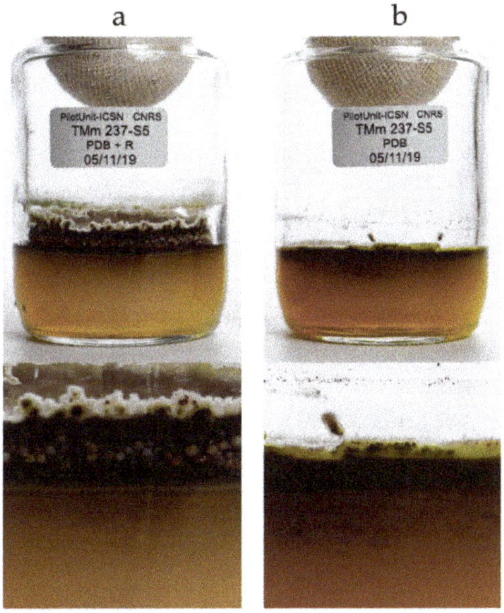

Figure 4. 10 days culture of *Chrysosporium lobatum* TM-237-S5 on PDA coupled to SSE with *XAD™16HP* N (**a**) and the control culture on PDA without resin (**b**). Without the resin (**b**), the colored compounds were spread in the agar, and their extraction was difficult. With the resin (**a**), the agar remained clear as the resin beads trapped all the colored target compounds.

The compounds trapped in the XAD were eluted with ethyl acetate and analyzed by HPLC coupled to photodiode array PDA, light-scattering LSD, and mass spectrometry MS detectors (Figure 5). According to the recovered quantities of extracts and the diversity of metabolites observed in the chromatograms, the current study focused on the extract from agar-supported cultivation coupled to in-situ solid-state extraction (SSF/SSE, Figure 5B). This SSF/SSE on PDA lead to an overall extract yield of 872 mg/m^2 of cultivation surface, corresponding to 2 L of medium (200 mL per plate). HPLC analysis revealed 10 peaks with specific UV absorption spectra (Figure 6), which were totally absent in the liquid culture (LSF/SPE) (Figure 5C).

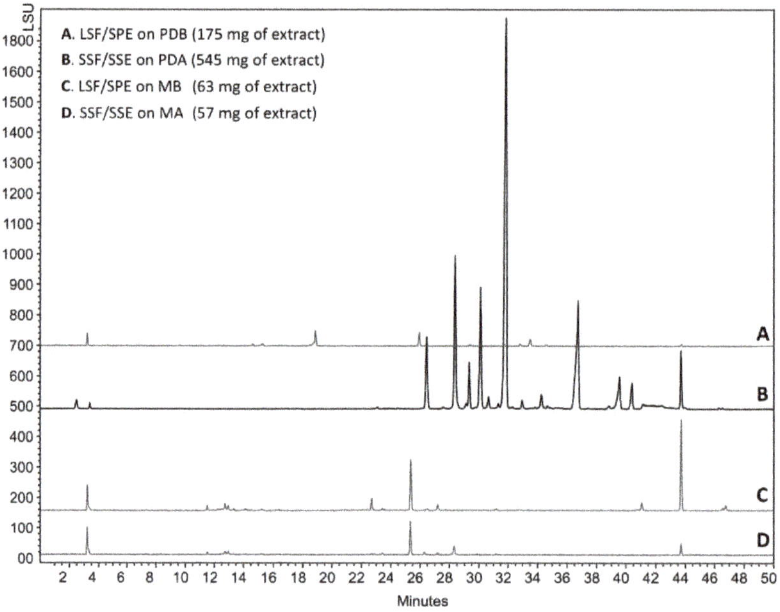

Figure 5. HPLC analysis of the ethyl acetate extract of *C. lobatum* TM-237-S5 cultivated on different media and support.

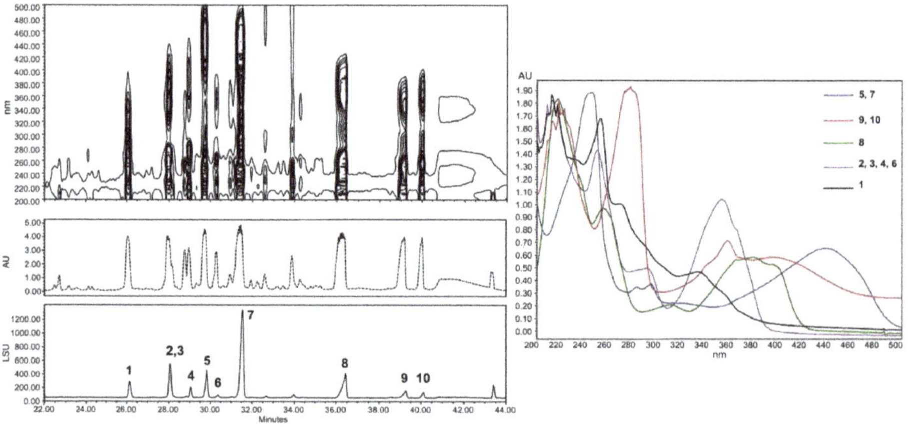

Figure 6. HPLC analysis with LSD and one-dimensional/two-dimensional PDA detections (right). Absorbance spectrum of the compounds investigated.

2.2. *Structural Identification of Compounds **1** to **10***

Compounds **1** to **10** in Figure 7 were purified and submitted to one-dimensional and two-dimensional NMR and HRMS analysis. Six compounds were unambiguously identified as peniciphenalenin D (**1**), isolated from *Pebnicillium* sp. ZZ901 [30], coniolactone (**3**), (-)-7,8-Dihydro-3,6-dihydroxy-1,7,7,8-tetramethyl-5H-furo-[2′,3′:5,6] naphtho[1,8-bc]furan-5-one (**6**), coniosclerodin (**9**), isolated from *Coniothyrium cereale* [30,31], (+)-scleroderolide (**7**), isolated from *Gremmeniella abietina* [32,33], and (+)-sclerodin (**10**), isolated from *Aspergillus silvaticus* [34].

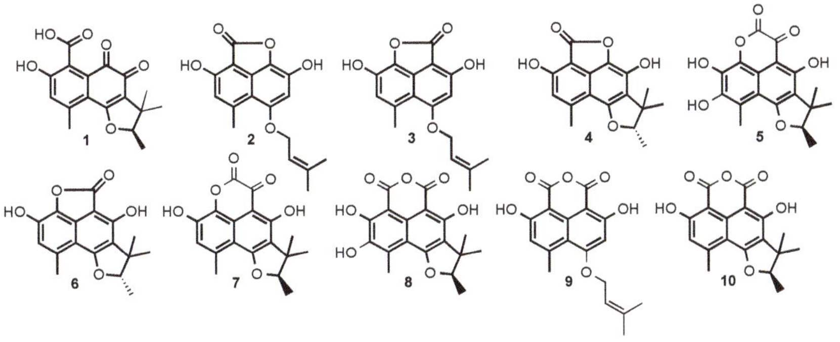

Figure 7. Structures of the compounds produced by *Chrysosporium lobatum* TM-237-S5, cultivated for 10 days on PDA medium coupling solid-state fermentation with solid-state extraction (SSF/SSE).

Compounds **2**, **4**, **5**, and **8** were submitted to dereplication based on the Antibase database of microbial compounds (Wiley–VCH) and the natural compounds Reaxys database (Elsevier). Spectroscopic data of these compounds did not match the previously reported compounds or present significant differences, and were submitted to de-novo structural elucidation. Their ^{1}H and ^{13}C NMR data are shown in Tables 1 and 2.

Table 1. ^{13}C NMR (125 and 150 MHz) of compounds **2**, **4**, **5**, and **8**.

Position	δ_C, Type			
	2 [a]	**4** [a]	**5** [a]	**8** [b]
1	160.2, C	160.2, C	138.9, C	160.0, C
2	118.9, CH	118.5, C	144.9, C	140.4, C
3	149.1, C	147.8, C	120.5, C	130.3, C
4	112.5, C	108.2, C	109.3, C	108.9, C
5	140.2, C	132.9, C	132.9, C	131.9, C
6	100.0, C	100.1, C	117.4, C	92.9, C
7	168.1, C	168.7, C	170.8, C	165.7, C
8	-	-	171.2, C	165.7, C
9	126.5, C	127.4, C	108.1, C	91.8, C
10	139.5, C	139.3, C	166.7, C	162.8, C
11	99.8, CH	122.1, C	120.5, C	119.8, C
12	156.4, C	153.8, C	158.5, C	153.9, C
13	66.8, CH_2	91.4, CH	93.7, CH	91.7, CH
14	120.8, CH	46.0, C	44.3, C	43.4, C
15	139.2, C	14.6, CH_3	14.9, CH_3	14.1, CH_3
16	25.8, CH_3	21.3, CH_3	21.2, CH_3	20.3, CH_3
17	18.3, CH_3	26.3, CH_3	25.9, CH_3	25.2, CH_3
18	23.0, CH_3	21.4, CH_3	13.7, CH_3	13.9, CH_3

[a,b]; the spectra were recorded in MeOD and CD_2Cl_2, respectively.

The peak at 28 min exhibits a molecular formula of $C_{17}H_{16}O_5$, determined by HRESIMS (*m*/*z* 301.1076 $[M + H]^+$). A careful ^{1}H and ^{13}C NMR analysis of the peak at 28 min revealed a mixture of two compounds with indistinguishable HRMS. De-replication and comparison with published results showed that one of the constituents was unambiguously coniolactone (**3**). As well as **3**, HMBC correlations showed that compound **2** differs only at the ring C configuration. A key HMBC correlation from H-2 (δ_H 6.70, s) to the carbonyl C-7 (δ_C 168.1) indicated that, in **2**, the carbonyl at C-7 is connected to C-6 rather than to C-9 in coniolactone (**3**) (Figure 8). So far, all our attempts to separate **2** and **3** by different chromatographic techniques have failed. Compound **2** was named isoconiolactone.

Table 2. ^{1}H NMR (500 and 600 MHz) of compounds **2**, **4**, **5** and **8**.

Position	δ_H, Mult. (*J* in Hz)			
	2 [a]	**4** [a]	**5** [a]	**8** [b]
1	-	-	-	
2	6.70, s	6.70, s	-	
3	-	-	-	
4	-	-	-	
5	-	-	-	
6	-	-	-	
7	-	-	-	
8	-	-	-	
9	-	-	-	
10	-	-	-	
11	6.35,s	-	-	
12	-	-	-	
13	4.60, d (*6.4*)	4.50, q (*6.5*)	4.78, q (*6.6*)	4.71, q (*6.6*)
14	5.57, br m	-	-	-
15	-	1.43, d (*6.5*)	1.52, d (*6.7*)	1.50, d (*6.6*)
16	1.83, s	1.23, s	1.31, s	1.30, s
17	1.80, s	1.50, s	1.56, s	1.54, s
18	2.76, s	2.73, s	2.61, s	2.79, s
OH-10				11.36, s

[a,b]; the spectra were recorded in MeOD and CD_2Cl_2, respectively.

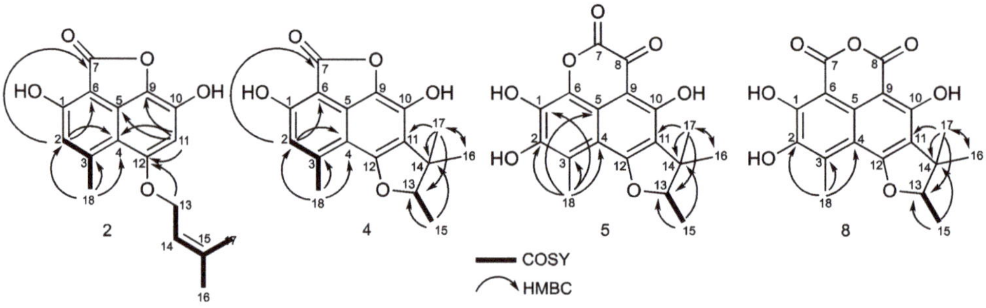

Figure 8. COSY and key HMBC correlations for compounds **2**, **4**, **5**, and **8**.

Compound **4** has a molecular formula $C_{17}H_{16}O_5$, deduced from HRESIMS and NMR data (Tables 1 and 2). According to NMR and MS data, **4** has the same planar structure as the already known fungal metabolite peniciphenalenin F [30]. However, compound **4** and peniciphenalenin F have an opposite optical rotation; negative for **4** (−36.10° (c 0.10, MeOH)) and positive for the reported peniciphenalenin F (+16.50° (c 0.50, MeOH)). Subsequently, **4** was named (-)-peniciphenalenin F.

Compound **5** had a molecular formula of $C_{18}H_{16}O_7$, deduced from HRESIMS and NMR data (Tables 1 and 2). The NRM data of **5** indicates the presence of two carbonyls, eight aromatic carbons, one oxymethine, one quaternary carbon, and four methyls. NMR comparison with previously reported phenalenone derivatives has shown similarities with the isolated (+)-scleroderolide (**7**) [32,33], except in the C-2 position. Indeed, the aromatic proton, H-2, of scleroderolide is substituted in **5** by a hydroxyl group in C-2 (δ_C 144.9). This finding is also supported by key HMBC correlations from H-18 (2.61, 3H, s) to C-2 (δ_C 144.9), C-3 (δ_C 120.5), and C-4 (δ_C 109.3). Accordingly, compound **5** has been identified as a new phenalenone derivative and was named (+)-8-hydroxyscleroderolide.

Compound **8** has a molecular formula $C_{18}H_{16}O_7$, deduced from the HRESIMS and NMR data (Tables 1 and 2). Here again, the NRM data of **8** showed the presence of two carbonyl, eight aromatic carbons, one oxymethine, one quaternary carbon, and four methyls. The NMR data of **8** closely resemble those of the previously described and isolated (+)-sclerodin (**10**) [34], except in the C-2 position. The aromatic proton, H-2, of the sclerodin structure is substituted in **8** by a hydroxyl group in C-2 (δ_C 140.4). This finding is supported by key HMBC correlations from H-18 (2.79, 3H, s) to C-2 (δ_C 140.4), C-3 (δ_C 130.3), and C-4 (δ_C 108.9).

The structure of **8**, including the absolute configuration (13*R*), is secured by a single crystal X-ray crystallographic analyses using anomalous scattering of Mo then CuK α radiation through Bijvoet analysis [35], combining maximum likelihood estimation and Bayesian statistics (Figure 9). Therefore, compound **8** was named (+)-8-hydroxyslerodin.

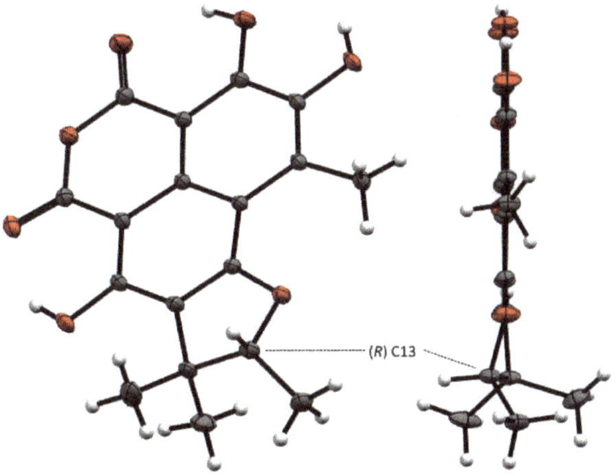

Figure 9. The Oak Ridge Thermal Ellipsoid Plot ORTEP diagram of **8**.

The current study presents the breakthrough advantage of solid-state fermentation coupled with in-situ solid phase extraction (SSF/SSE). Indeed, SSF/SSE leads to a large chemical diversity and higher yields. In addition, the concentration of the target compounds on the resin beads represents an economic and ecofriendly recovery process involving limited quantities of water for medium preparation, limited use of power for static incubation, a limited amount of solvents for the elution of compounds, and reduced waste. We also solved the issue of scale-up on the Platotex technology, offering a reusable 2 m^2 cultivation surface, and more recently on the Unifertex technology.

3. Materials and Methods

3.1. General Experimental Procedures

Optical rotations, $[\alpha]_D$, were measured using an Anton Paar MCP-300 polarimeter at 589 nm (Anton Paar, Les Ulis, France). NMR experiments were performed using a Bruker Avance III 600 MHz spectrometer equipped with a TCi cryo-probe head for compounds **8**, **9**, and **10**, and a Bruker Avance 500 MHz spectrometer for compounds **1** to **7** (Bruker, Vienna, Austria). The spectra were acquired in CD_3OD (δ_H 3.31 ppm and δ_C 49.15 ppm), in CD_2Cl_2 (δ_H 5.32 ppm and δ_C 53.10 ppm) or in Acetone-d_6 (δ_H 2.04 ppm and δ_C 29.8 ppm and 206.5 ppm) at 300K. High-resolution mass spectra were obtained on a Waters LCT Premier XE spectrometer equipped with an electrospray-time of flight (ESI-TOF) by direct infusion of the purified compounds (Waters SAS, Saint-Quentin-en-Yvelines, France). Pre-packed silica gel Redisep columns were used for flash chromatography using a Combiflash-Companion chromatogram (Serlabo, Entraigues-sur-la-Sorgue, France). All other chemicals and solvents were purchased from SDS (SDS, Peypen, France).

The analytical HPLC system consisted of an Alliance Waters 2695 controller coupled with a PhotoDiode Array Waters 2996, an evaporative light-scattering detector ELSD Waters 2424 detector and a mass detector Waters QDa (Waters SAS, Saint-Quentin-en-Yvelines, France). A Sunfire C_{18} column (4.6 × 150 mm, 3.5 μm) was used with a flow rate of 0.7 mL/min. The elution gradient consisted of a linear gradient from 100% solvent A to 100% solvent B in 40 min, then 10 min at 100% B (Solvent A: H_2O + 0,1 HCOOH, Solvent B: ACN + 0,1% HCOOH). Preparative HPLC was performed on a semi-preparative Sunfire C_{18} column (10 × 250 mm, 5 μm) using a Waters autosampler 717, a pump 600, a photodiode array detector 2996, and an ELSD detector 2420 (Waters SAS, Saint-Quentin-en-Yvelines, France). XAD resin (AMBERLITE™ *XAD™16HP* N) was purchased from DOW (DOW France SAS, Saint-Denis, France).

3.2. Invertebrate Collection

The sponge, *Acanthella cavernosa*, was collected by a ROV H800 (ECA, Lannion, France) on the upper mesophotic reef of Eilat at Dekel Beach at 51 m depth in the Gulf of Aqaba, Israel (2 April 2017, 29°32′12.48″N; 34°56′55.656″E). The sponge was identified by Dr. Nicole J. de Voogd from Naturalis, Biodiversity Research Center, Leiden, the Netherlands. Collection of animals complied with a permit issued by the Israel Nature and National Parks Protection Authority.

3.3. Strain Isolation and Identification

Chrysosporium lobatum TM-237-S5 was isolated from a 1 cm^3 sample of *Acanthella cavernosa*. The invertebrate was immediately stored after collection and conserved at −20 °C until lab work processing. Part of the invertebrate (1 cm^3) was ground in sterile sea water and heated at 50 °C for 1 h. The suspension was serially diluted, plated on selective isolation media, and incubated at 28 °C for at least 6 weeks. The strain was isolated from marine agar medium. The colony was purified on PDA and MA media and preserved in 10% glycerol solution.

Genomic DNA of the strain TM237-S5 was isolated using a DNeasy Plant Mini Kit (Qiagen), according to the manufacturer's instructions. The ITS region was amplified with primers ITS1F (5′-CTTGGTCATTTAGAGGAAGTAA -3′) and ITS4 (5′-TCCTCCGCTTATTGATATGC) using described polymerase chain reaction (PCR) conditions [36]. Amplicons were sequenced by Sanger sequencing (GATC, Eurofins genomics), and the sequences were aligned against the non-redundant database of the NCBI using the BLASTn program. Then, phylogeny inference was performed on the Phylogeny.fr platform and comprised the following steps [37]: Sequences from TM237-S5 and representative *Chrysosporium* and *Chrysosporium*-related sequences described by Gurung et al. (2018) were aligned with MUSCLE (v3.8.31) [38]. After alignment, ambiguous regions were removed with Gblocks (v0.91b) [39]. The phylogenetic tree was reconstructed using the maximum likelihood method implemented in the PhyML program (v3.0 aLRT) [40], and reliability for internal branch was assessed using the aLRT test [41]. Graphical representation and edition of the phylogenetic tree were performed with TreeDyn (v198.3) [42]. The strain *Chrysosporium lobatum* TM237-S5 was assigned the GenBank number MN080876.

3.4. Microbial Cultivation

Chrysosporium lobatum TM-237-S5 spores were conserved at −20 °C in 10% glycerol. Before cultivation, the strain was revived for 5 days on a 15 cm petri plate containing potato dextrose agar (PDA). Sterile water (4 × 10 mL) was poured on the plate surface, and the spores were recovered from the plates by gentle scratching of the surface with a scalpel. Three plates offer 100 mL of concentrated spore suspension. Ten bottles were filled with 30 g of XAD Resin (AMBERLITE™ XAD™16HP N) and sterilized. 10 mL of Water and 10 mL of spore suspension were introduced in each resin containing bottle. The mixture was stirred, poured on a 25 × 25 cm petri plate containing PDA medium, homogeneously spread on the surface of the plate, and incubated at 27 °C. Preparative cultures were engaged on 10 25 × 25 cm petri plates.

3.5. Extraction/Purification Procedures

On day 10 of incubation, the resin/mycelium layer was recovered from the surface of the plates and re-suspended three times in 500 mL of Ethyl Acetate. Traces of water were removed on anhydrous sodium sulfate, and the solvent evaporated under reduced pressure. 550 mg of dry extract was recovered and submitted for analytical and structural analysis. The extract was fractionated by flash chromatography using a Combiflash-companion chromatogram, and the compounds were further purified by preparative HPLC to offer 6 to 56 mg of pure compound.

3.6. Structural Elucidation

All the compounds were submitted to one-dimensional and two-dimensional NMR analysis, high resolution mass spectrometry, and, when appropriate, to crystallography.

Peniciphenalenin D (**1**): Red amorphous solid (31 mg); $[\alpha]_D^{25}$: +119.70° (*c* 0.1, MeOH); UV (MeOH) λ_{max} (log ε) 217 (3.83), 279 (3.85), 369 (2.91), 515 (2.90) nm; ^{1}H and ^{13}C NMR data, see Supplementary Information; HRESIMS *m/z* 317.1005 $[M + H]^+$ (calcd. for $C_{17}H_{17}O_6$, 317.1025).

Isoconiolactone (**2**) + Coniolactone (**3**): Orange amorphous powder (40 mg); UV (MeOH) λ_{max} (log ε) 220 (3.52), 254 (2.54), 346 (1.45) nm; ^{1}H and ^{13}C NMR data, Table 1; Table 2; HRESIMS *m/z* 301.1067 $[M + H]^+$ (calcd. for $C_{17}H_{17}O_5$, 301.1076)

(−)-Peniciphenalenin F (**4**): Yellowish amorphous powder (15 mg); $[\alpha]_D$: −36.10° (c 0.1, MeOH); UV (MeOH) λ_{max} (log ε) 221 (4.22), 274 (4.21), 357 (3.51), 393 (3.33) nm; ^{1}H and ^{13}C NMR data, Table 1; Table 2; HRESIMS *m/z* 301.1053 $[M + H]^+$ (calcd. for $C_{17}H_{17}O_5$, 301.1049)

(+)-8-Hydroxyscleroderolide (**5**): Pale yellowish amorphous powder (36 mg); $[\alpha]_D$: +65.01° (c 0.1, MeOH); UV (MeOH) λ_{max} (log ε) 244 (3.56), 448 (1.71) nm; ^{1}H and ^{13}C NMR data, Table 1; Table 2; HRESIMS *m/z* 345.0967 $[M + H]^+$ (calcd. for $C_{18}H_{17}O_7$, 345.0974).

(−)-7,8-Dihydro-3,6-dihydroxy-1,7,7,8-tetramethyl-5H-furo-[2′,3′:5,6]naphtho[1,8-bc]furan-5-one (**6**): Yellowish amorphous powder (5 mg); $[\alpha]_D$: −36.80° (c 0.1, MeOD); UV (MeOH) λ_{max} (log ε) 226 (1.22), 263 (3.65), 359 (3.52) nm; ^{1}H and ^{13}C NMR data, see Supplementary Information; HRESIMS *m/z* 301.1064 $[M + H]^+$ (calcd. for $C_{17}H_{17}O_5$, 301.1076).

(+)-Scleroderolide (**7**): Yellow powder (57 mg); $[\alpha]_D$: +73.0° (c 0.1, MeOD); UV (MeOH) λ_{max} (log ε) 226 (3.88), 250 (2.87), 294 (1.22), 439 (2.12) nm; ^{1}H and ^{13}C NMR data, see Supplementary Information; HRESIMS *m/z* 329.1033 $[M + H]^+$ (calcd. for $C_{18}H_{17}O_6$, 329.1039).

(+)-8-Hydroxysclerodin (**8**): Pale yellow crystal (38 mg); $[\alpha]_D$: +66.01° (c 0.1, MeOH); UV (MeOH) λ_{max} (log ε) 223 (3.38), 308 (1.14), 358 (2.52) nm; ^{1}H and ^{13}C NMR data, Table 1; Table 2; HRESIMS *m/z* 345.0960 $[M + H]^+$ (calcd. for $C_{18}H_{17}O_7$, 345.0961).

Coniosclerodin (**9**): Pale yellow powder (8 mg); UV (MeOH) λ_{max} (log ε) 250 (4.12), 289 (1.14), 351 (3.52) nm; ^{1}H and ^{13}C NMR data, see Supplementary Information; HRESIMS *m/z* 329.1001 $[M + H]^+$ (calcd. for $C_{18}H_{17}O_6$, 329.1025).

(+)-Sclerodin (**10**): Yellowish powder (7 mg); $[\alpha]_D$: +20.01° (c 0.10, CH_2Cl_2); UV (MeOH) λ_{max} (log ε) 216 (3.25), 256 (4.13), 295 (1.24), 359 (3.98) nm; ^{1}H and ^{13}C NMR data, see Supplementary Information; HRESIMS *m/z* 329.1015 $[M + H]^+$ (calcd. for $C_{18}H_{17}O_6$, 329.1025).

3.7. X-ray Crystal Structure Analysis

High-resolution crystallographic data for compound **8** were collected using redundant ω scans on a Rigaku XtaLabPro single-crystal diffractometer using microfocus Mo Kα radiation and a HPAD PILATUS3 R 200K detector. Its structure was readily solved by intrinsic phasing methods (*SHELXT*) and by full-matrix least-squares methods on F2 using *SHELX-L* [43,44]. The non-hydrogen atoms were refined anisotropically, and hydrogen atoms, all identified in difference maps, were positioned geometrically and refined with U_{iso} set to xU_{eq} of the parent atom (x = 1.5 for methyl carbons or hydroxy oxygens and 1.2 for all others). Despite extremely weak anomalous signal and ambiguous Flack parameter [45] obtained with that radiation, the Bijvoet analysis using likelihood methods showed strong probabilities that this characterized enantiopure natural product is (*R*)-2,3,7-trihydroxy-1,8,8,9-tetramethyl-8,9-dihydro-4*H*,6*H*-benzo[*de*]furo[2,3-*g*] isochromene-4,6-dione. Duplicated measurements using a Rigaku mm007 rotating anode consolidated our statement (data not deposited).

Crystallographic data for this structure, **8**, have been deposited in the Cambridge Crystallographic Data Centre database (CCDC) (deposition number CCDC 1963851). Copies of the data can be obtained free of charge from the CCDC at www.ccdc.cam.ac.uk.

Crystal data for **8**: C18H16O7, *M* = 344.31, Orthorhombic, a = 6.6249(2) Å, b = 10.0615(3) Å, c = 22.5473(6) Å a = b = g = 90°, V = 1502.92(8) Å3, T = 293(2) K, space group *P*212121, Z = 4, μ(Mo Kα) = 0.118 mm−1, 47,173 reflections measured, 4370 independent reflections (Rint = 0.0456). The final R1 values were 0.0389 (I > 2σ(I)). The final *wR* (F2) values were 0.1093 (all data). The goodness of fit on F2 was 1.072. Flack parameter = −0.2 (2). Bijvoet Pairs = 1854 (100% coverage): P2 (true) = 1.000. P3 (true) = 0.987, P3 (rac-twin) = 0.013, P3 (false) = $0.8.10^{-6}$. Hooft parameter = −0.1 (2) [35].

Supplementary Materials: The following are available online at http://www.mdpi.com/1660-3397/17/12/678/s1, S1 to S4, spectroscopic characterization of compound **1**; S5 to S11, spectroscopic characterization of compounds **2** + **3**; S12 to S18, spectroscopic characterization of compound **4**; S19 to S25, spectroscopic characterization of compound **5**; S26 to S29, spectroscopic characterization of compound **6**, S30 to S34, spectroscopic characterization of compound **7**; S35 to S42, spectroscopic characterization of compound **8**; S43 to S46, spectroscopic characterization of compound **9**; S47 to S50, spectroscopic characterization of compound **10**; S51 to S57, crystallographic data for compound **8**; S58-S72, crystallographic data for compounds **7** and **10**.

Author Contributions: G.L.G. designed, managed, and implemented the microbial and chemical experiments and elucidated the structures of the reported compounds. She wrote all the technical parts of the paper. P.L. and P.V. participated in the microbial and analytical experiments; P.L. and G.A. participated in compound purification and chromatographic analysis; E.V.E. and P.R. did the crystallographic studies; J.-F.G. recorded the NMR spectra; M.W. and Y.B. collected and identified the sponge *Acanthella cavernosa*; N.F. reviewed and discussed the manuscript; and J.O. coordinated the work and finalized the writing and editing of the manuscript.

Funding: This work was supported and conducted in the frame of the H2020 TASCMAR project, which is funded by the European Union under grant agreement number 634674 (www.tascmar.eu).

Acknowledgments: The photos are the property of CNRS images, they were taken by Cyril Frésillon (© Cyril Frésillon/ICSN/CNRS Photothèque). We thank the Interuniversity Institute for Marine Sciences in Eilat (IUI) for the use of the Sam Rothberg R/V and the professional assistance of its crew members. We are indebted to EcoOcean staff members for operating the ROV. We acknowledge E. Shoham and R. Liberman for their help in the field work. We thank Nicole J. de Voogd from Naturalis, Biodiversity Research Center, Leiden, the Netherlands, for taxonomic identification of the sponge. The Israel Nature and National Parks Protection Authority is acknowledged for issuing collection permits.

Conflicts of Interest: The authors declare no conflict of interest.

References

1. Kiran, G.S.; Sekar, S.; Ramasamy, P.; Thinesh, T.; Hassan, S.; Lipton, A.N.; Ninawe, A.S.; Selvin, J. Marine sponge microbial association: Towards disclosing unique symbiotic interactions. *Mar. Environ. Res.* **2018**, *140*, 169–179. [CrossRef]
2. Brinkmann, C.M.; Marker, A.; Kurtböke, I.D. An Overview on Marine Sponge-Symbiotic Bacteria as Unexhausted Sources for Natural Product Discovery. *Diversity* **2017**, *9*, 40. [CrossRef]
3. Rosenberg, E.; Sharon, G.; Atad, I.; Zilber-Rosenberg, I. The evolution of animals and plants via symbiosis with microorganisms. *Environ. Microbiol. Rep.* **2010**, *2*, 500–506. [CrossRef]
4. Hentschel, U.; Hopke, J.; Horn, M.; Friedrich, A.B.; Wagner, M.; Hacker, J.; Moore, B.S. Molecular evidence for a uniform microbial community in sponges from different oceans. *Appl. Environ. Microbiol.* **2002**, *68*, 4431–4440. [CrossRef]

5. Taylor, M.W.; Radax, R.; Steger, D.; Wagner, M. Sponge-associated microorganisms: Evolution, ecology, and biotechnological potential. *Microbiol. Mol. Biol. Rev.* **2007**, *71*, 295–347. [CrossRef]
6. Slaby, B.M.; Hackl, T.; Horn, H.; Bayer, K.; Hentschel, U. Metagenomic binning of a marine sponge microbiome reveals unity in defense but metabolic specialization. *ISME J.* **2017**, *11*, 2465–2478. [CrossRef]
7. Sacristán-Soriano, O.; Banaigs, B.; Casamayor, E.O.; Becerro, M.A. Exploring the links between natural products and bacterial assemblages in the sponge Aplysina aerophoba. *Appl. Environ. Microbiol.* **2011**, *77*, 862–870. [CrossRef]
8. Wilson, M.C.; Mori, T.; Rückert, C.; Uria, A.R.; Helf, M.J.; Takada, K.; Gerner, C.; Steffens, U.A.; Heycke, N.; Schmitt, S.; et al. An environmental bacterial taxon with a large and distinct metabolic repertoire. *Nature* **2014**, *506*, 58–62. [CrossRef]
9. Hentschel, U.; Usher, K.M.; Taylor, M.W. Marine sponges as microbial fermenters. *FEMS Microbiol. Ecol.* **2006**, *55*, 167–177. [CrossRef]
10. Schippers, K.J.; Sipkema, D.; Osinga, R.; Smidt, H.; Pomponi, S.A.; Martens, D.E.; Wijffels, R.H. Cultivation of sponges, sponge cells and symbionts: Achievements and future prospects. *Adv. Mar. Biol.* **2012**, *62*, 273–337.
11. Maldonado, M.; Ribes, M.; van Duyl, F.C. Nutrient fluxes through sponges: Biology, budgets, and ecological implications. *Adv. Mar. Biol.* **2012**, *62*, 113–182. [PubMed]
12. Gareth Jones, E.B.; Pang, K.-L. *Marine Fungi and Fungal-Like Organisms*; Walter de Gruyter: Göttingen, Germany, 2012.
13. Amend, A.; Burgaud, G.; Cunliffe, M.; Edgcomb, V.P.; Ettinger, C.L.; Gutiérrez, M.H.; Heitman, J.; Hom, E.F.Y.; Ianiri, G.; Jones, A.C.; et al. Fungi in the marine environment: Open questions and unsolved problems. *MBio* **2019**, *10*, e01189-18. [CrossRef] [PubMed]
14. Knoll, A.H. The Multiple Origins of Complex Multicellularity. *Annu. Rev. Earth Planet. Sci.* **2011**, *39*, 217–239. [CrossRef]
15. Hardoim, C.C.; Costa, R. Microbial Communities and Bioactive Compounds in Marine Sponges of the Family Irciniidae—A Review. *Mar. Drugs* **2014**, *12*, 5089–5122. [CrossRef] [PubMed]
16. Calvo, A.M.; Cary, J.W. Association of Fungal Secondary Metabolism and Sclerotial Biology. *Front. Microbiol.* **2015**, *6*, 1–16. [CrossRef] [PubMed]
17. Cary, J.W.; Entwistle, S.; Satterlee, T.; Mack, B.M.; Gilbert, M.K.; Chang, P.K.; Scharfenstein, L.; Yin, Y.; Calvo, A.M. The Transcriptional Regulator Hbx1 Affects the Expression of Thousands of Genes in the Aflatoxin-Producing Fungus *Aspergillus flavus*. *G3 (Bethesda)* **2019**, *9*, 167–178. [CrossRef] [PubMed]
18. Dattenböck, C.; Tisch, D.; Schuster, A.; Monroy, A.A.; Hinterdobler, W.; Schmoll, M. Gene regulation associated with sexual development and female fertility in different isolates of *Trichoderma reesei*. *Fungal Biol. Biotechnol.* **2018**, *5*, 1–11. [CrossRef]
19. Le Goff, G.; Martin, M.-T.; Iorga, B.; Adelin, E.; Servy, C.; Cortial, S.; Ouazzani, J. Isolation and characterization of unusual hydrazides from *Streptomyces* sp. Impact of the cultivation support and extraction procedure. *J. Nat. Prod.* **2013**, *76*, 142–149. [CrossRef]
20. Adelin, E.; Martin, M.-T.; Cortial, S.; Ouazzani, J. New bioactive polyketides isolated from agar-supported fermentation of *Phomopsis* sp. CMU-LMA, taking advantage of the scale-up device, Platotex. *Phytochemistry* **2013**, *93*, 170–175. [CrossRef]
21. Meknaci, R.; Lopes, P.; Servy, C.; Le Caer, J.-P.; Andrieu, J.-P.; Hacène, H.; Ouazzani, J. Agar-supported cultivation of *Halorubrum* sp. SSR, and production of halocin C8 on the scale-up prototype Platotex. *Extremophiles* **2014**, *18*, 1049–1055. [CrossRef]
22. Adelin, E.; Slimani, N.; Cortial, S.; Schmitz-Alfonso, I.; Ouazzani, J. Platotex: An innovative and fully automated device for cell growth scale-up of agar-supported solid-state fermentation. *J. Ind. Microbiol. Biotechnol.* **2010**, *38*, 299–305. [CrossRef] [PubMed]
23. Ouazzani, J.; Sergent, D.; Cortial, S.; Lopes, P. PLATOTEX. PCT/EP2007/054834 2007.
24. Ouazzani, J.; Le Goff, G.; Felezeu, D.; Touron, A.; Allegret-Bourdon, C. UNIFERTEX, UNIversal FERmenTor EXpert. CNRS/PGT, PCT/EP2018/086882 2018.
25. Le Goff, G.; Adelin, E.; Cortial, S.; Servy, C.; Ouazzani, J. Application of solid-phase extraction to agar-supported fermentation. *Bioprocess Biosyst. Eng.* **2013**, *36*, 1285–1290. [CrossRef] [PubMed]
26. Mohanty, S.S.; Prakash, S. Effects of culture media on larvicidal property of secondary metabolites of mosquito pathogenic fungus *Chrysosporium lobatum* (Moniliales: Moniliaceae). *Acta Tropica.* **2009**, *109*, 50–54. [CrossRef] [PubMed]

27. Ivanova, V.B.; Hoshino, Y.; Yazawa, K.; Ando, A.; Mikami, Y. Isolation and Structure Elucidation of Two New Antibacterial Compounds Produced by *Chrysosporium queenslandicum*. *J. Antibiot.* **2002**, *55*, 914–918. [CrossRef] [PubMed]
28. Van der Pyl, D.; Cans, P.; Debernard, J.J.; Herman, F.; Lelievre, Y.; Tahraoui, L.; Vuilhorgne, M.; Leboul, J. RPR113228, a novel farnesyl protein transferase inhibitor produced by *Chrysosporium lobatum*. *J. Antibiot.* **1995**, *48*, 736–737. [PubMed]
29. Kumar, C.G.; Mongolla, P.; Sujitha, P.; Joseph, J.; Babu, K.S.; Suresh, G.; Ramakrishna, K.V.; Purushotham, U.; Sastry, G.N.; Kamal, A. Metabolite profiling and biological activities of bioactive compounds produced by *Chrysosporium lobatum* strain BK-3 isolated from Kaziranga National Park, Assam, India. *SpringerPlus* **2013**, *2*, 122–131. [CrossRef]
30. Li, Q.; Zhu, R.; Yi, W.; Chai, W.; Zhang, Z.; Lian, X.-Y. Peniciphenalenins A–F from the culture of a marine-associated fungus *Penicillium* sp. ZZ901. *Phytochemistry* **2018**, *152*, 53–60. [CrossRef]
31. Elsebai, M.F.; Kehraus, S.; Lindequist, U.; Sasse, F.; Shaaban, S.; Guetschow, M.; Josten, M.; Sahl, H.-G.; Koenig, G.M. Antimicrobial phenalenone derivatives from the marine-derived fungus *Coniothyrium cereale*. *Org. Biomol. Chem.* **2011**, *9*, 802–808. [CrossRef]
32. Ayer, W.A.; Hoyano, Y.; Pedras, M.S.; Clardy, J.; Arnold, E. Metabolites produced by the scleroderris canker fungus, *Gremmeniella abietina*. Part 2. The Structure of scleroderolide. *Can. J. Chem.* **1987**, *65*, 748–753. [CrossRef]
33. Ayer, W.A.; Hoyano, Y.; Pedras, M.S.; Van Altena, I. Metabolites produced by the Scleroderris canker fungus, *Gremmeniella abietina*. *Can. J. Chem.* **1986**, *64*, 1585–1589. [CrossRef]
34. Homma, K.; Fukuyama, K.; Katsube, Y.; Kimura, Y.; Hamasaki, T. Structure and Absolute Configuration of an Atrovenetin-like Metabolite from *Aspergillus silvaticus*. *Agric. Biol. Chem.* **1980**, *44*, 1333–1338. [CrossRef]
35. Hooft, R.W.W.; Straver, L.H.; Spek, A.L. Determination of absolute structure using Bayesian statistics on Bijvoet differences. *J. Appl. Cryst.* **2008**, *41*, 96–103. [CrossRef] [PubMed]
36. Gurung, S.K.; Adhikari, M.; Kim, S.W.; Bazie, S.; Kim, H.S.; Lee, H.G.; Kosol, S.; Lee, H.B.; Lee, Y.S. Discovery of Two *Chrysosporium* Species with Keratinolytic Activity from Field Soil in Korea. *Mycobiology* **2018**, *46*, 260–268. [CrossRef] [PubMed]
37. Dereeper, A.; Guignon, V.; Blanc, G.; Audic, S.; Buffet, S.; Chevenet, F.; Dufayard, J.F.; Guindon, S.; Lefort, V.; Lescot, M.; et al. Phylogeny.fr: Robust phylogenetic analysis for the non-specialist. *Nucleic Acids Res.* **2008**, *36*, 465–469. [CrossRef]
38. Edgar, R.C. MUSCLE: Multiple sequence alignment with high accuracy and high throughput. *Nucleic Acids Res.* **2004**, *32*, 1792–1797. [CrossRef]
39. Castresana, J. Selection of conserved blocks from multiple alignments for their use in phylogenetic analysis. *Mol. Biol. Evol.* **2000**, *17*, 540–552. [CrossRef]
40. Anisimova, M.; Gascuel, O. Approximate likelihood ratio test for branchs: A fast, accurate and powerful alternative. *Syst. Biol.* **2006**, *55*, 539–552. [CrossRef]
41. Guindon, S.; Gascuel, O. A simple, fast, and accurate algorithm to estimate large phylogenies by maximum likelihood. *Syst. Biol.* **2003**, *52*, 696–704. [CrossRef]
42. Chevenet, F.; Brun, C.; Banuls, A.L.; Jacq, B.; Chisten, R. TreeDyn: Towards dynamic graphics and annotations for analyses of trees. *BMC Bioinform.* **2006**, *7*, 439. [CrossRef]
43. Sheldrick, G.M. *SHELXT*-Integrated space-group and crystal-structure determination. *Acta Cryst.* **2015**, *A71*, 3–8. [CrossRef]
44. Sheldrick, G.M. Crystal structure refinement with *SHELXL*. *Acta Cryst.* **2015**, *C71*, 3–8.
45. Flack, H.D. On enantiomorph-polarity estimation. *Acta Cryst.* **1983**, *A39*, 876–881. [CrossRef]

marine drugs

MDPI

Communication

Genome Sequencing of *Streptomyces olivaceus* SCSIO T05 and Activated Production of Lobophorin CR4 via Metabolic Engineering and Genome Mining

Chunyan Zhang [1,2], Wenjuan Ding [1,2], Xiangjing Qin [1] and Jianhua Ju [1,2,*]

1 CAS Key Laboratory of Tropical Marine Bio-resources and Ecology, Guangdong Key Laboratory of Marine Materia Medica, RNAM Center for Marine Microbiology, South China Sea Institute of Oceanology, Chinese Academy of Sciences, 164 West Xingang Road, Guangzhou 510301, China; zhchuny@foxmail.com (C.Z.); 13760785354@163.com (W.D.); xj2005qin@126.com (X.Q.)

2 College of Oceanology, University of Chinese Academy of Sciences, 19 Yuquan Road, Beijing 100049, China

* Correspondence: jju@scsio.ac.cn; Tel./Fax: +86-20-8902-3028

Received: 18 September 2019; Accepted: 16 October 2019; Published: 20 October 2019

Abstract: Marine-sourced actinomycete genus *Streptomyces* continues to be an important source of new natural products. Here we report the complete genome sequence of deep-sea-derived *Streptomyces olivaceus* SCSIO T05, harboring 37 putative biosynthetic gene clusters (BGCs). A cryptic BGC for type I polyketides was activated by metabolic engineering methods, enabling the discovery of a known compound, lobophorin CR4 (**1**). Genome mining yielded a putative lobophorin BGC (*lbp*) that missed the functional FAD-dependent oxidoreductase to generate the D-kijanose, leading to the production of lobophorin CR4 without the attachment of D-kijanose to C17-OH. Using the gene-disruption method, we confirmed that the *lbp* BGC accounts for lobophorin biosynthesis. We conclude that metabolic engineering and genome mining provide an effective approach to activate cryptic BGCs.

Keywords: genome sequencing; gene disruption; lobophorin; metabolic engineering; genome mining

1. Introduction

Microbially produced natural products (NPs) are an important reservoir of therapeutic and agricultural agents [1]. In the previous years, quantities of new bioactive NPs were isolated from marine-derived *Streptomyces* strains, suggesting marine-derived *Streptomyces* as a predominant source of new NPs [2]. In recent years, whole-genome sequencing programs have made it clear that microorganisms have greater biosynthetic potential but are mostly underexplored by virtue that most biosynthetic gene clusters (BGCs) in a single microbial genome are normally silent. Activation of these silent BGCs contributes to new NPs discoveries. Zhang and co-workers activated a cryptic polycyclic tetramate macrolactam (PTM) BGC in *Streptomyces pactum* SCSIO 02999 by promoter engineering and heterologous expression [3], and also promoted the expression of a silent PKS/NRPS hybrid BGC in the same *Streptomyces* strain by the alteration of several regulatory genes [4]. The production of nocardamine [5] and atratumycin [6] in *Streptomyces atratus* SCSIO ZH16 was turned on via metabolic engineering. These genome-based studies exemplify the benefits of genome mining and metabolic engineering used for activating cryptic BGCs and discovering new bioactive NPs.

Lobophorins (Supporting Information (SI), Figure S1) belonging to a large class of spirotetronate antibiotics structurally feature a tetronate moiety *spiro*-linked with a cyclohexene ring, which is called pentacyclic aglycon or kijanolide [7–17]. Almost all of this class of compounds has a broad spectrum of antibacterial activities, as well as antitumor activity. Efforts to produce more spirotetronate antibiotics for drug discovery have thrived. Owing to the structural complexity of this family member, biosynthesis seems to be an effective way to afford the production of spirotetronate antibiotics, providing access to new analogues by pathway engineering and combinatorial biosynthetic approaches. In this paper, we report (i) the complete genome sequence of a deep-sea-derived *Streptomyces olivaceus* SCSIO T05, a talented strain capable of producing an array of putative NPs; (ii) activation of a cryptic lobophorin BGC (*lbp*) by mutagenetic methods and isolation of one known spirotetronate antibiotic lobophorin CR4 (**1**); and (iii) identification of the *lbp* BGC housed in *S. olivaceus* SCSIO T05 by gene-disruption experiment and bioinformatics analysis.

2. Results and Discussion

2.1. Genome Sequencing and Annotation of *Streptomyces olivaceus SCSIO T05*

Whole genome sequence is important when analyzing the potential production of secondary metabolites [5,18]. *S. olivaceus* SCSIO T05, a marine-derived strain, was previously reported to be isolated from the Indian Ocean deep-sea-derived sediment [19]. Its draft genome sequence was first gained by Illumina sequencing technology, but with several gap regions. In order to estimate the biosynthetic potential of *S. olivaceus* SCSIO T05, the complete genome was re-sequenced and acquired by the single-molecule real-time (SMRT) sequencing technology (PacBio). A total of 67156 filtered reads with high-quality data of 432570025 bp were generated, and then they were assembled into a linear contig by the hierarchical genome assembly process (HGAP) [20]. The complete genome revealed that 8458055 base pairs constitute a linear chromosome without a plasmid, with 72.51% of GC content (Figure 1 and Table 1). Totally, 7700 protein-coding genes were predicted, along with 18 rRNA and 65 tRNA. The genome sequence of *S. olivaceus* SCSIO T05 was deposited in GenBank (CP043317).

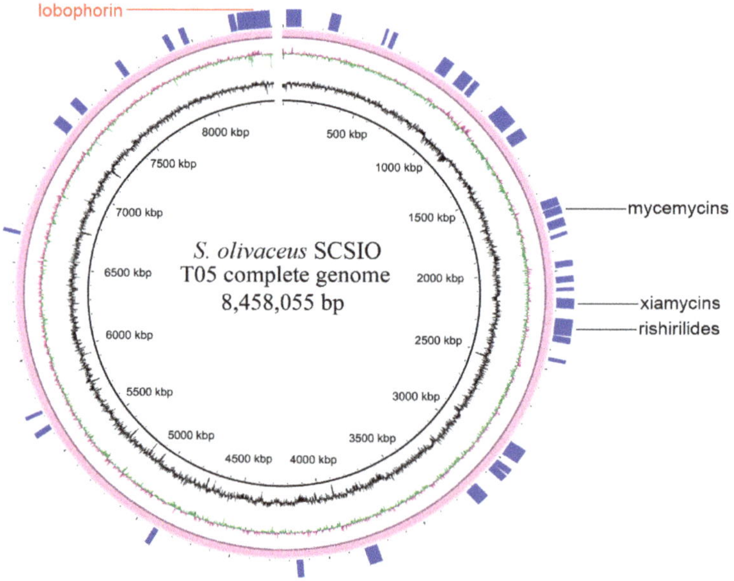

Figure 1. The complete genome of *S. olivaceus* SCSIO T05. The three circles (inner to outer) represent forward GC content, GC skew, and the distribution of putative biosynthetic gene clusters (BGCs) (represented by the bars) generated by antiSMASH 5.0. Clusters 18, 17, and 11 were described as rishirilides, xiamycins, and mycemycins BGCs, respectively. The putative lobophorin BGC with red color was referred to as cluster 37.

Table 1. Genome features of *S. olivaceus* SCSIO T05.

Feature	Value
Genome size (bp)	8,458,055
Average GC content (%)	72.51
Protein-coding genes	7700
Total size of Protein-coding genes (bp)	7,543,173
rRNAs number	18
tRNAs number	65

AntiSMASH analysis by using antiSMASH 5.0 [21] suggested 37 BGCs within the *S. olivaceus* SCSIO T05 genome (Figure 1 and Table 2). The 37 BGCs totally occupy 1.59 Mb, 18.76% of the complete genome. Most of the BGCs distribute in the two subtelomeric regions of the genome of some *Streptomyces* strains [18] and so do the BGCs in *S. olivaceus* SCSIO T05 genome. It is predicted that several BGCs are responsible for the production of polyketide- and nonribosome-peptide-derived secondary metabolites, including four PKS (Type I, Type II and Type III) and six NRPS, and six hybrid BGCs possess genes encoding more than one type of scaffold-synthesizing enzyme. Twenty-one BGCs are predicted to produce terpene, bacteriocin, lanthipeptide, or other categories. This analysis indicates that *S. olivaceus* SCSIO T05 is capable of producing an array of secondary metabolites, serving as a target strain for further metabolic engineering and genome mining.

Table 2. AntiSMASH-predicted BGCs for *S. olivaceus* SCSIO T05.

BGC	Position		Type (Product)
	From	To	
Cluster 1	2725	89768	Type I Polyketide synthase (T1 PKS)
Cluster 2	234616	284137	Non-ribosomal peptide synthetase (NRPS) cluster
Cluster 3	504553	512728	Bacteriocin or other unspecified ribosomally synthesized and post-translationally modified peptide product (RiPP) cluster (Bacteriocin)
Cluster 4	525945	544617	Terpene
Cluster 5	793277	855894	NRPS
Cluster 6	901333	979368	T1 PKS
Cluster 7	980891	1005613	Lanthipeptide cluster (Lanthipeptide)
Cluster 8	1135886	1240760	Other types of PKS cluster (Otherks)-NRPS
Cluster 9	1275164	1347740	NRPS-Terpene
Cluster 10	1651711	1694648	NRPS-Nucleoside cluster (Nucleoside)
Cluster 11	1695020	1734380	Otherks
Cluster 12	1751698	1796277	NRPS
Cluster 13	1840051	1851963	Siderophore cluster (Siderophore)
Cluster 14	1967451	1990613	Lanthipeptide
Cluster 15	2037772	2059400	Terpene
Cluster 16	2090680	2102023	Bacteriocin
Cluster 17	2138860	2187226	T1PKS-NRPS
Cluster 18	2230691	2317060	NRPS-Type II PKS (T2 PKS)-Otherks
Cluster 19	2330735	2352337	Lanthipeptide
Cluster 20	2443907	2456009	Siderophore
Cluster 21	2905748	2978302	T2 PKS
Cluster 22	3029068	3048760	Terpene
Cluster 23	3049806	3075321	Beta-lactone containing protease inhibitor (Betalactone)
Cluster 24	3182776	3235915	NRPS
Cluster 25	3764472	3822515	NRPS
Cluster 26	4131410	4159582	Lanthipeptide
Cluster 27	4881296	4901736	Phenazine cluster (Phenazine)

Table 2. *Cont.*

BGC	Position		Type (Product)
	From	To	
Cluster 28	5633979	5656500	Lasso peptide cluster (Lassopeptide)
Cluster 29	5716930	5727556	Melanin cluster (Melanin)
Cluster 30	6667385	6677783	Ectoine cluster (Ectoine)
Cluster 31	7200930	7253804	NRPS
Cluster 32	7328818	7368924	Type III PKS (T3 PKS)
Cluster 33	7614814	7636052	Aminoglycoside/aminocyclitol cluster (Amglyccycl)
Cluster 34	7882883	7906528	Terpene
Cluster 35	7959695	7980831	Indole cluster (Indole)
Cluster 36	8200560	8221618	Terpene
Cluster 37	8239655	8455702	T1pks-Nrps-T3 PKS-Oligosaccharide cluster (Oligosaccharide)-Other

2.2. Activation of a Cryptic Lobophorin BGC in the Genetically Engineered Mutant

In actuality, only a minority of potential chemicals are produced under standard laboratory culture conditions. Furthermore, the corresponding products are likely to be overlooked for multiple reasons, including low production rates, a large metabolic background, or improper culture conditions [22]. Fermented using modified-RA medium, the secondary metabolites produced by *S. olivaceus* SCSIO T05 were subsequently profiled using HPLC-DAD-UV. Multiple peaks were detected in the fermentation extract (Figure 2, trace i). We previously reported that five known NPs, rishirilides B (**2**) and C (**3**), lupinacidin A (**4**), galvaquinone B (**5**), and xiamycin A (**6**), were produced as major secondary metabolites from the wild-type strain [19,23]. In addition, an orphan dibenzoxazepinone biosynthetic pathway was mutagenically activated, leading to the production of new mycemycins [24], suggesting that *S. olivaceus* SCSIO T05 has a great potential for producing new NPs.

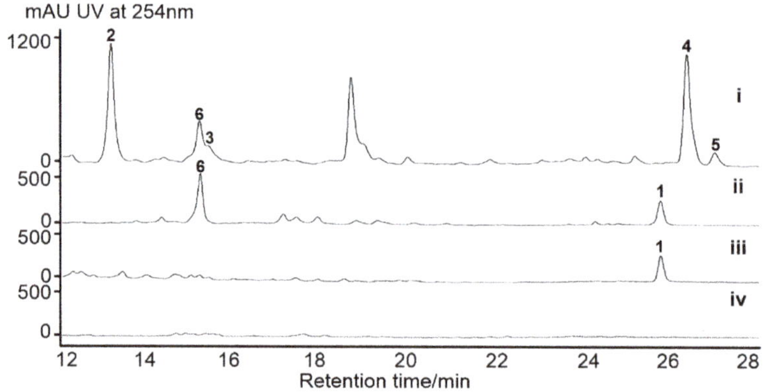

Figure 2. HPLC-based analyses of fermentation broths: (i) *S. olivaceus* SCSIO T05; (ii) *S. olivaceus* SCSIO T05R; (iii) *S. olivaceus* SCSIO T05RX; and (iv) *S. olivaceus* SCSIO T05RXL. Compound **1** is lobophorin CR4. Compounds **2–6** were previously identified as rishirilide B, rishirilide C, lupinacidin A, galvaquinone B, and xiamycin A, respectively.

For exploring other secondary metabolites from the strain, *S. olivaceus* SCSIO T05/Δ*rsdK*$_2$ (*S. olivaceus* SCSIO T05R) was constructed to abolish the production of the anthracenes [19]. The production of the second major secondary metabolites xiamycins was accumulated, along with a new peak around 26 min, distinct from the UV absorption characteristics of xiamycins (Figure 2, trace ii). For further background elimination of xiamycins, a "double-deletion" mutant *S. olivaceus* SCSIO T05/Δ*rsdK*$_2$/Δ*xmcP* (*S. olivaceus* SCSIO T05RX) was constructed [23] in which the new peak (**1**) appeared to be the major product (Figure 2, trace iii). Accordingly, the *S. olivaceus* SCSIO T05RX mutant was fermented at a large scale, enabling the isolation and structure elucidation of this newly generated compound.

It was identified as a known compound designated as lobophorin CR4 (Figure 3), by comparing HRESIMS, ^{1}H, and ^{13}C NMR data (SI, Figures S2–S4) to the reported data of an intermediate isolated from the *Streptomyces* sp. SCSIO 01127/Δ*lobG1* mutant [11]. It is reported that shifting metabolic flux of a wild-type strain by blocking the predominant product pathways may afford new secondary metabolites [5]. During our efforts to acquire new secondary metabolites by shifting the metabolic flux of marine actinomycetes [5,23,24], the production of nocardamine, olimycins, and mycemycins was turned on at the expense of major products by using gene knock-out methods. Similarly, the "double-deletion" mutant (*S. olivaceus* SCSIO T05RX) was constructed to abolish the production of two major secondary metabolites, anthracenes and xiamycins, from the wild-type strain [19,23]. With the engineered shifting of *S. olivaceus* metabolic flux, the newly produced lobophorin CR4 was activated.

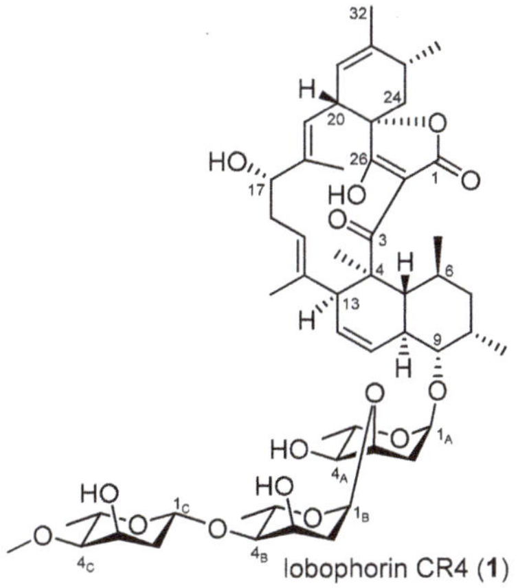
lobophorin CR4 (**1**)

Figure 3. Structure of the isolated lobophorin CR4.

2.3. Identification of a Putative Lobophorin (lbp) BGC via Genome Mining

The antiSMASH analysis of the complete genome of *S. olivaceus* SCSIO T05 revealed a 99.1 kb type I PKS BGC named as lobophorin BGC (*lbp*), showing highly similar traits to the reported *lob* BGCs from *Streptomyces* sp. FXJ7.023 [16] and *Streptomyces* sp. SCSIO 01127 [11]. The complete *lbp* contains 38 open reading frames (ORFs). The genetic organization of *lbp* is shown in Figure 4A, with genes color-coded on the basis of their proposed functions summarized in Table 3. The nucleotide sequences were deposited in GenBank (MN396889). The *lbp* BGC contains six inconsecutive genes *lbpA1–A6*, similar to *lobA1–A5* in *lob* from *S.* sp. SCSIO 01127. Differently, the LobA4 homologue is separated into two polyketide synthases (PKSs), LbpA4 and LbpA5, in *lbp*. The high similarity between the PKS modules in *lbp* and in *lob* enables us to propose that the assembly of the linear polyketide chain catalyzed by LbpA1–A6 utilizes six malonyl CoAs, six methylmalonyl-CoAs, and a 3-carbon glycerol unit (Figure 5) [11]. The *lbp* harbors four putative regulator genes (*lbpR1–R4*) (Figure 4 and Table 3) that are highly similar to *lobR1*, *lobR3*, *lobR4*, and *lobR5* in *lob*, respectively. These four regulators are assumed to be involved in the regulation network of lobophorin CR4 biosynthesis, which seems to be less complex than *lob* but more complex than *kij* [7] and *tca* [8]. In contrast, five regulator genes *lobR1–R5* are identified in *lob*; three regulator genes, *kijA8*, *kijC5*, and *kijD12*, are included in *kij*; *tcaR1* and *tcaR2* both encode regulators in *tca*. There is only one gene, *lbpU2* in *lbp*, with no apparent homologue in *lob* (Figure 4 and Table 3). The other genes included in *lbp* are putatively associated with the biosynthesis of kijanose and L-digitoxose units by virtue of high similarities to corresponding counterparts in *lob* (Figure 4 and Table 3).

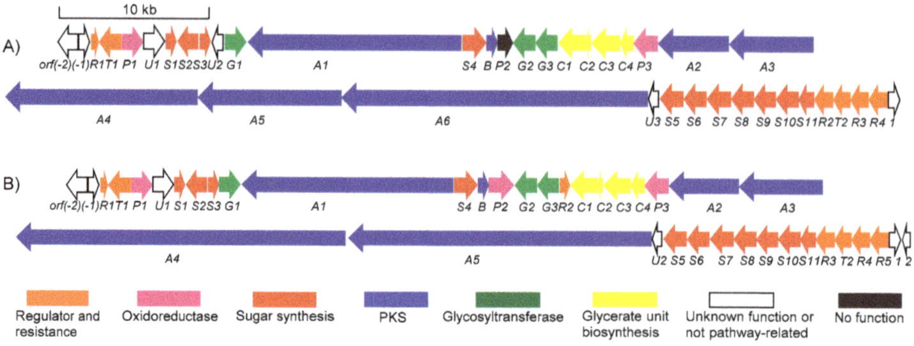

Figure 4. Genetic organizations: (**A**) the *lbp* BGC from *S. olivaceus* SCSIO T05; (**B**) the *lob* BGC from *S.* sp. SCSIO 01127.

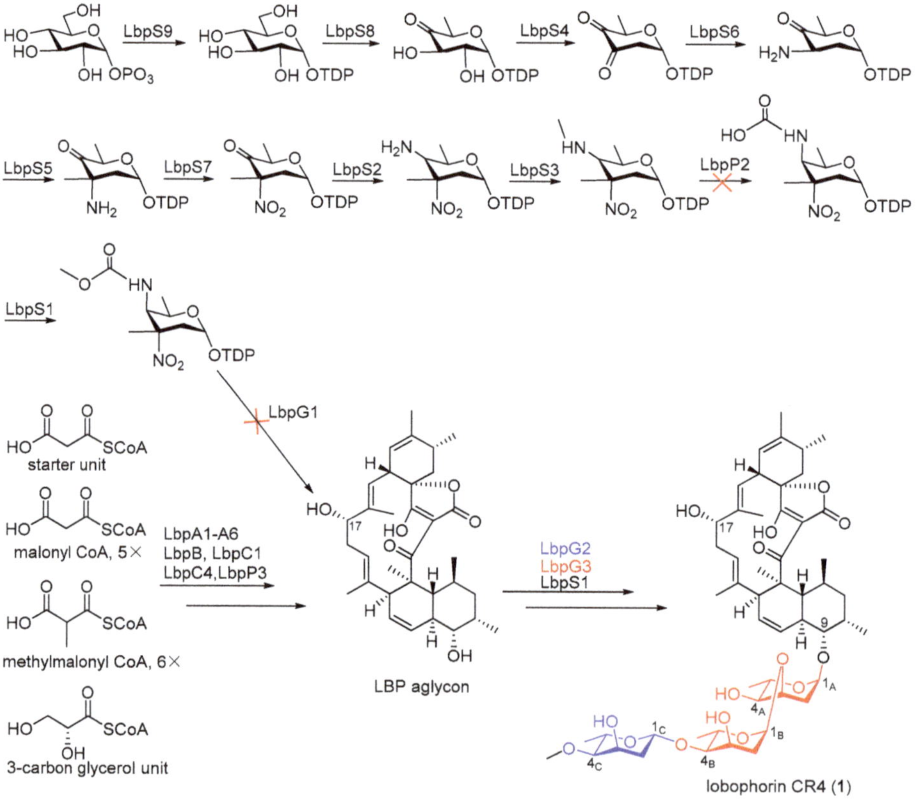

Figure 5. Proposed biosynthetic pathway of lobophorin CR4.

Table 3. Deduced function of open reading frames (ORFs) in the *lbp* BGC.

ORF	Size [a]	Proposed Function	ID/SI [b]	Protein Homologue and Origin
orf(-2)	374	macrolide glycosyltransferase	100/100	Orf(-2) (AGI99472.1); *Streptomyces* sp. SCSIO 01127
orf(-1)	260	FkbM family methyltransferase	100/100	Orf(-1) (AGI99473.1); *Streptomyces* sp. SCSIO 01127
lbpR1	195	TetR type regulatory protein	100/100	lobR1 (AGI99474.1); *Streptomyces* sp. SCSIO 01127
lbpT1	497	efflux permease	100/100	lobT1 (AGI99475.1); *Streptomyces* sp. SCSIO 01127
lbpP1	392	p450 monooxygenase	100/100	lobP1 (AGI99476.1); *Streptomyces* sp. SCSIO 01127
lbpU1	326	aldo/keto reductase	100/100	lobU1 (AGI99477.1); *Streptomyces* sp. SCSIO 01127
lbpS1	271	sugar-O-methyltransferase	99/100	lobS1 (AGI99478.1); *Streptomyces* sp. SCSIO 01127
lbpS2	384	sugar 4-aminotransferase	100/100	lobS2 (AGI99479.1); *Streptomyces* sp. SCSIO 01127
lbpS3	201	SAM-dependent methyltransferase	97/98	lobS3 (AGI99480.1); *Streptomyces* sp. SCSIO 01127
lbpU2	197	hypothetical protein	100/100	hypothetical protein (KMB22099.1); Klebsiella pneumoniae
lbpG1	391	glycosyltransferase	100/100	lobG1 (AGI99481.1); *Streptomyces* sp. SCSIO 01127
lbpA1	3936	PKS (KS-AT-DH-ER-KR-ACP-KS-AT-DH-KR-ACP)	100/100	lobA1 (AGI99482.1); *Streptomyces* sp. SCSIO 01127
lbpS4	483	sugar 2,3-dehydratase	100/100	lobS4 (AGI99483.1); *Streptomyces* sp. SCSIO 01127
lbpB	253	thioesterase	100/100	lobB (AGI99484.1); *Streptomyces* sp. SCSIO 01127
lbpP2	313	FAD-dependent oxidoreductase	100/100	part of lobP2 (AGI99485.1); *Streptomyces* sp. SCSIO 01127
lbpG2	416	glycosyltransferase	99/100	lobG2 (AGI99486.1); *Streptomyces* sp. SCSIO 01127
lbpG3	476	glycosyltransferase	99/100	lobG3 (AGI99487.1); *Streptomyces* sp. SCSIO 01127
lbpC1	680	hydrolase superfamily dihydrolipo-amide acyltransferase-like protein	99/99	lobC1 (AGI99489.1); *Streptomyces* sp. SCSIO 01127
lbpC2	75	ACP	99/100	lobC2 (AGI99490.1); *Streptomyces* sp. SCSIO 01127
lbpC3	621	FkbH-like protein	99/100	lobC3 (AGI99491.1); *Streptomyces* sp. SCSIO 01127
lbpC4	342	ketoacyl acyl carrier protein synthase III	100/100	lobC4 (AGI99492.1); *Streptomyces* sp. SCSIO 01127
lbpP3	492	FAD-dependent oxidoreductase	100/100	lobP3 (AGI99493.1); *Streptomyces* sp. SCSIO 01127
lbpA2	1573	PKS (KS-AT-KR-ACP)	99/100	lobA2 (AGI99494.1); *Streptomyces* sp. SCSIO 01127
lbpA3	1798	PKS (KS-AT-DH-KR-ACP)	99/99	lobA3 (AGI99495.1); *Streptomyces* sp. SCSIO 01127
lbpA4	4376	PKS (KR-ACP-KS-AT-DH-KR-ACP-KS-AT-DH-KR-ACP)	100/100	part of lobA4 (AGI99496.1); *Streptomyces* sp. SCSIO 01127
lbpA5	2881	PKS (KS-AT-DH-KR-ACP-KS-AT-DH)	99/98	part of lobA4 (AGI99496.1); *Streptomyces* sp. SCSIO 01127
lbpA6	6362	PKS (KS-AT-ACP-KS-AT-DH-KR-ACP-KS-AT-DH-KR-ACP-KS-AT-DH-KR-ACP)	99/99	lobA5 (AGI99497.1); *Streptomyces* sp. SCSIO 01127
lbpU3	151	unknown	100/100	lobU2 (AGI99498.1); *Streptomyces* sp. SCSIO 01127
lbpS5	414	sugar 3-C-methyl transferase	100/100	lobS5 (AGI99499.1); *Streptomyces* sp. SCSIO 01127
lbpS6	373	sugar 3-aminotransferase	100/100	lobS6 (AGI99500.1); *Streptomyces* sp. SCSIO 01127
lbpS7	439	acyl-CoA dehydrogenase	100/100	lobS7 (AGI99501.1); *Streptomyces* sp. SCSIO 01127
lbpS8	341	sugar 4,6-dehydratase	100/100	lobS8 (AGI99502.1); *Streptomyces* sp. SCSIO 01127
lbpS9	298	sugar nucleotidyltransferase	99/100	lobS9 (AGI99503.1); *Streptomyces* sp. SCSIO 01127
lbpS10	332	sugar 3-ketoreductase	100/100	lobS10 (AGI99504.1); *Streptomyces* sp. SCSIO 01127
lbpS11	202	sugar 5-epimerase	99/100	lobS11 (AGI99505.1); *Streptomyces* sp. SCSIO 01127
lbpR2	274	TetR type regulatory protein	99/100	lobR3 (AGI99506.1); *Streptomyces* sp. SCSIO 01127
lbpT2	211	forkhead-associated protein	99/100	lobT2 (AGI99507.1); *Streptomyces* sp. SCSIO 01127
lbpR3	298	putative regulatory protein	99/100	lobR4 (AGI99508.1); *Streptomyces* sp. SCSIO 01127
lbpR4	309	LysR family transcriptional regulator	99/100	lobR5 (AGI99509.1); *Streptomyces* sp. SCSIO 01127
orf1	183	acetyltransferase	100/100	Orf1 (AGI99510.1); *Streptomyces* sp. SCSIO 01127

[a] Amino acids. [b] Identity/similarity.

To demonstrate the validity of the putative *lbp* BGC, *lbpC4* coding for ketosynthase-III-like protein, which incorporates a 3-carbon glycerol unit into the biosynthetic precursor LOB aglycon [11], was disrupted by using PCR-targeting methods. As expected, the production of lobophorin CR4 was completely blocked in *S. olivaceus* SCSIO T05/Δ*rsdK*$_2$/Δ*xmcP*/Δ*lbpC4* (*S. olivaceus* SCSIO T05RXL) (Figure 2, trace iv), demonstrating that the *lbp* BGC is indeed responsible for lobophorin biosynthesis. With high similarity to the *lob* BGC, the *lbp* BGC accounts for lobophorin CR4 without the attachment of kijanose to C17-OH, rather than lobophorins A and B in *lob*. Based on bioinformatics analysis, a series of enzymes are proposed to be involved in kijanose biosynthesis (Figure 5) [7]. Among them, the amino acid sequence of the putative FAD-dependent oxidoreductase LbpP2 is far shorter than its homologues LobP2 [11] and KijB3 [7]. KijB3 is proposed to oxidize the methyl group to a carboxylate group, essential for the generation of the kijanose moiety [7]. Multiple protein sequence alignments of LbpP2, LobP2, and KijB3 revealed that the conserved FAD binding domain is missing in LbpP2 (Figure S5). Thus, we speculate that LbpP2 is nonfunctional, failing to catalyze the carboxylation and hinder the generation of kijanose.

Given the high similarity of LbpG3 and LobG3, we envision that LbpG3 has a similar function as LobG3, a glycosyltransferase from *S.* sp. SCSIO 01127, tandemly attaching the first two L-digitoxose at C-9 in lobophorins [11]. LbpG2 has 99% similarity to LobG2, another glycosyltransferase from the same strain, which was established to transfer the terminal L-digitoxose [11]. Both LbpG2 and LbpG3 are likely to be involved in the transfers of three sugar units, sugars A, B, and C, in lobophorin CR4 (Figure 5), consistent with the metabolite profile of Δ*lobG1* in *S.* sp. SCSIO 01127 [11].

3. Experimental Section

3.1. General Experimental Procedures

The plasmids and bacteria used are listed in Table S1. *Streptomyces olivaceus* SCSIO T05 and its mutants were incubated on modified ISP-4 medium [25] with 3% sea salt and fermented in modified RA medium [19]. All cultures for *Streptomyces* were incubated at 28 °C. Luria-Bertani (LB) medium was used for *E. coli*, with appropriate antibiotics added at a final concentration of 100 μg/mL of ampicillin (Amp), 50 μg/mL of kanamycin (Kan), 50 μg/mL of apramycin (Apr), 25 μg/mL of chloroamphenicol (Cml), and 50 μg/mL of trimethoprim (TMP).

A 1260 infinity system (Agilent, Santa Clara, CA, USA), which uses a Phenomenex Prodigy ODS (2) column (150 × 4.6 mm, 5 μm, USA), was used for HPLC-based analyses. Silica gel with the size of 100–200 mesh (Jiangpeng Silica gel development, Inc., Shandong, China) was used for column chromatography (CC). A Primaide 1110 solvent delivery module, which is equipped with a 1430 photodiode array detector (Hitachi, Tokyo, Japan) and uses a YMC-Pack ODS-A column (250 mm × 10 mm, 5 μm), was used for semi-preparative HPLC. A MaXis Q-TOF mass spectrometer (Bruker, Billerica, MA, USA) was used to acquire high-resolution mass spectral data. An MCP-500 polarimeter (Anton Paar, Graz, Austria) was used to record optical rotations. A Bruker Avance 500 was used to record NMR spectra. Carbon signals and the residual proton signals of DMSO-d_6 were used for calibration (δ_C 39.52 and δ_H 2.50).

3.2. Genome Sequencing and Bioinformatic Analysis

Whole genome scanning and annotation of *S. olivaceus* SCSIO T05 were acquired by the single-molecule real-time (SMRT) sequencing technology (PacBio) at Shanghai Majorbio Bio-Pharm Technology Co., Ltd (Shanghai, China). AntiSMASH (AntiSMASH 5.0, available at http://antismash.secondarymetabolites.org/) was used to analyze and assess the potential BGCs. FramePlot (FramePlot 4.0 beta, available at http://nocardia.nih.go.jp/fp4/) was used to analyze ORFs whose functions were predicted based on an online BLAST program (http://blast.ncbi.nlm.nih.gov/).

3.3. Construction of a "Triple-Deletion" Mutant Strain

Gene *lbpC4* from the *lbp* BGC was inactivated by the REDIRECT protocol [26]. All primers used in this study are listed in Table S2. *LbpC4* was replaced by the apramycin resistance gene *oriT/aac(3)IV* fragment in the target cosmids 01-07D or 21-02E. The target mutant clones, *S. olivaceus* SCSIO T05RXL, were accomplished as previously described [19,23,24].

3.4. Fermentation and HPLC-based Analyses of S. olivaceus SCSIO T05 and Its Mutants

The *Streptomyces* used in this study were incubated in modified ISP-4 medium plates for 2–3 d. For fermentation, a portion of mycelium and spores was seeded into 50 mL of modified RA medium in a 250 mL flask and then shaken at 200 rpm and 28 °C for 8 d. The cultures were extracted with an equal volume of butanone. Organic phases were then dissolved in CH_3OH (1 mL) after having been evaporated to dryness, and 40 μL of each relevant sample was injected for HPLC-based analysis. The UV detection was at 254 nm. Solvent A is composed of 85% ddH_2O and 15% CH_3CN, supplemented with 0.1% HOAc. Solvent B is composed of 85% CH_3CN and 15% ddH_2O, supplemented with 0.1% HOAc. Samples were analyzed via the following method: a linear gradient from 0% to 80% solvent B in 20 min, and then, from 80% to 100% solvent B for 1.5 min, finally eluted with 100% solvent B in 6.5 min. The flow rate was 1.0 mL/min.

3.5. Production, Isolation, and Structure Elucidation of Lobophorin CR4

The mycelium of *S. olivaceus* SCSIO T05RX were inoculated into 50 mL of modified-RA medium and then shaken at 200 rpm and 28 °C for 2 d, to gain the seed cultures. After that, the seed cultures were transferred into 150 mL of modified-RA medium and shaken at 200 rpm and 28 °C for 8 d. After the large-scale fermentation was accomplished, a total of 12 L of the growth culture was centrifuged at 4000 g for 10 min to separate the supernatant and mycelium and further extracted by butanone and acetone, respectively. The two organic phases were concentrated (via solvent removal under vacuum), and the residues were combined. The combined sample was subjected to normal phase silica gel CC eluted with $CHCl_3$-CH_3OH (100:0, 98:2, 96:4, 94:6, 92:8, 90:10, 85:15, 80:20, 70:30, 50:50, v/v, each solvent combination in 250 mL volume) to give ten fractions (AFr.1–AFr.10). Fractions A1-A3 were purified to afford the accumulation of compound **1** (98 mg), by preparative HPLC, eluting with 90% solvent B (A: H_2O; B: CH_3CN) over the course of 30 min. The flowrate was 2.5 mL/min and the UV detection was at 254 nm. The purified compound was subjected to MS, ^1H, and ^{13}C NMR spectra measurements and elucidated as a known intermediate **3** during lobophorins A and B biosynthesis [11], and we named it lobophorin CR4 (**1**).

4. Conclusions

In this study, we acquired the complete genome sequence of *S. olivaceus* SCSIO T05. The biosynthetically talented strain harbors 37 putative BGCs analyzed by antiSMASH. To explore the biosynthetic potential of this strain, metabolic engineering and genome mining were performed. The major anthracenes and indolosesquiterpenes biosynthetic pathways were blocked, and an orphan spirotetronate antibiotics BGC (*lbp*) was activated in *S. olivaceus* SCSIO T05, leading to the isolation and identification of one known compound, lobophorin CR4. We have identified the *lbp* BGC accounting for lobophorin biosynthesis by gene-disruption experiments and bioinformatics analysis. The production of lobophorin CR4 without the attachment of D-kijanose to C17-OH was on account that the nonfunctional FAD-dependent oxidoreductase LbpP2 failed to generate D-kijanose. This work highlights that metabolic engineering and genome mining are the effective ways to turn on putative orphan or silent BGCs to acquire new NPs for drugs discovery.

Supplementary Materials: The following are available online at http://www.mdpi.com/1660-3397/17/10/593/s1. This section includes HRESIMS, 1D NMR spectra for compound **1**, construction of Δ*lbpC4*.

Author Contributions: C.Z. performed the experiments and wrote the draft manuscript. W.D. performed the isolation of compound **1**. X.Q. helped to perform the sequence alignments. J.J. supervised the whole work and edited the manuscript. All authors read and approved the final manuscript.

Funding: This research was funded by the National Natural Science Foundation of China (81425022, U1706206, and U1501223), and Natural Science Foundation of Guangdong Province (2016A030312014).

Acknowledgments: We are grateful to Aijun Sun, Xiaohong Zheng, Yun Zhang, Xuan Ma, and Zhihui Xiao, in the analytical facility center of the SCSIO for recording MS and NMR data.

Conflicts of Interest: The authors declare no conflicts of interest.

References

1. Berdy, J. Bioactive microbial metabolites. *J. Antibiot.* **2005**, *58*, 1–26. [CrossRef] [PubMed]
2. Carroll, A.R.; Copp, B.R.; Davis, R.A.; Keyzers, R.A.; Prinsep, M.R. Marine natural products. *Nat. Prod. Rep.* **2019**, *36*, 122–173. [CrossRef] [PubMed]
3. Saha, S.; Zhang, W.; Zhang, G.; Zhu, Y.; Chen, Y.; Liu, W.; Yuan, C.; Zhang, Q.; Zhang, H.; Zhang, L.; et al. Activation and characterization of a cryptic gene cluster reveals a cyclization cascade for polycyclic tetramate macrolactams. *Chem. Sci.* **2017**, *8*, 1607–1612. [CrossRef] [PubMed]
4. Chen, R.; Zhang, Q.; Tan, B.; Zheng, L.; Li, H.; Zhu, Y.; Zhang, C. Genome Mining and Activation of a Silent PKS/NRPS Gene Cluster Direct the Production of Totopotensamides. *Org. Lett.* **2017**, *19*, 5697–5700. [CrossRef]
5. Li, Y.; Zhang, C.; Liu, C.; Ju, J.; Ma, J. Genome sequencing of Streptomyces atratus SCSIO ZH16 and activation production of nocardamine via metabolic engineering. *Front. Microbiol.* **2018**, *9*, 1269. [CrossRef]
6. Sun, C.; Yang, Z.; Zhang, C.; Liu, Z.; He, J.; Liu, Q.; Zhang, T.; Ju, J.; Ma, J. Genome Mining of Streptomyces atratus SCSIO ZH16: Discovery of Atratumycin and Identification of Its Biosynthetic Gene Cluster. *Org. Lett.* **2019**, *21*, 1453–1457. [CrossRef]
7. Zhang, H.; White-Phillip, J.A.; Melançon, C.E.; Kwon, H.J.; Yu, W.L.; Liu, H.W. Elucidation of the Kijanimicin Gene Cluster: Insights into the Biosynthesis of Spirotetronate Antibiotics and Nitrosugars. *J. Am. Chem. Soc.* **2007**, *129*, 14670–14683. [CrossRef]
8. Fang, J.; Zhang, Y.; Huang, L.; Jia, X.; Zhang, Q.; Zhang, X.; Tang, G.; Liu, W. Cloning and Characterization of the Tetrocarcin A Gene Cluster from Micromonospora chalcea NRRL 11289 Reveals a Highly Conserved Strategy for Tetronate Biosynthesis in Spirotetronate Antibiotics. *J. Bacteriol.* **2008**, *190*, 6014–6025. [CrossRef]
9. Wei, R.B.; Xi, T.; Li, J.; Wang, P.; Li, F.C.; Lin, Y.C.; Qin, S. Lobophorin C and D, New Kijanimicin Derivatives from a Marine Sponge-Associated Actinomycetal Strain AZS17. *Mar. Drugs* **2011**, *9*, 359–368. [CrossRef]
10. Niu, S.; Li, S.; Chen, Y.; Tian, X.; Zhang, H.; Zhang, G.; Zhang, W.; Yang, X.; Zhang, S.; Ju, J.; et al. Lobophorins E and F, new spirotetronate antibiotics from a South China Sea-derived Streptomyces sp. SCSIO 01127. *J. Antibiolt.* **2011**, *64*, 711. [CrossRef]
11. Li, S.; Xiao, J.; Zhu, Y.; Zhang, G.; Yang, C.; Zhang, H.; Ma, L.; Zhang, C. Dissecting Glycosylation Steps in Lobophorin Biosynthesis Implies an Iterative Glycosyltransferase. *Org. Lett.* **2013**, *15*, 1374–1377. [CrossRef] [PubMed]
12. Pan, H.Q.; Zhang, S.Y.; Wang, N.; Li, Z.L.; Hua, H.M.; Hu, J.C.; Wang, S.J. New Spirotetronate Antibiotics, Lobophorins H and I, from a South China Sea-Derived Streptomyces sp. 12A35. *Mar. Drugs* **2013**, *11*, 3891–3901. [CrossRef] [PubMed]
13. Chen, C.; Wang, J.; Guo, H.; Hou, W.; Yang, N.; Ren, B.; Liu, M.; Dai, H.; Liu, X.; Song, F.; et al. Three antimycobacterial metabolites identified from a marine-derived Streptomyces sp. MS100061. *Appl. Microbiol. Biotechnol.* **2013**, *97*, 3885–3892. [CrossRef] [PubMed]
14. Cruz, P.G.; Fribley, A.M.; Miller, J.R.; Larsen, M.J.; Schultz, P.J.; Jacob, R.T.; Tamayo-Castillo, G.; Kaufman, R.J.; Sherman, D.H. Novel Lobophorins Inhibit Oral Cancer Cell Growth and Induce Atf4- and Chop-Dependent Cell Death in Murine Fibroblasts. *ACS Med. Chem. Lett.* **2015**, *6*, 877–881. [CrossRef] [PubMed]
15. Song, C.; Pan, H.; Hu, J. Isolation and identification of a new antibiotic, lobophorin J, from a deep sea-derived Streptomyces sp. 12A35. *Chin. J. Antibiot.* **2015**, *40*, 721–727.
16. Yue, C.; Niu, J.; Liu, N.; Lü, Y.; Liu, M.; Li, Y. Cloning and identification of the lobophorin biosynthetic gene cluster from marine Streptomyces olivaceus strain FXJ7.023. *Pak. J. Pharm. Sci.* **2016**, *29*, 287–293. [PubMed]

17. Braña, A.; Sarmiento-Vizcaíno, A.; Osset, M.; Pérez-Victoria, I.; Martín, J.; de Pedro, N.; de la Cruz, M.; Díaz, C.; Vicente, F.; Reyes, F.; et al. Lobophorin K, a new natural product with cytotoxic activity produced by Streptomyces sp. M-207 associated with the deep-sea coral Lophelia pertusa. *Mar. Drugs.* **2017**, *15*, 144. [CrossRef]
18. Low, Z.J.; Pang, L.M.; Ding, Y.; Cheang, Q.W.; Hoang, K.L.M.; Tran, H.T.; Li, J.; Liu, X.-W.; Kanagasundaram, Y.; Yang, L.; et al. Identification of a biosynthetic gene cluster for the polyene macrolactam sceliphrolactam in a Streptomyces strain isolated from mangrove sediment. *Sci. Rep.* **2018**, *8*, 1594. [CrossRef]
19. Zhang, C.; Sun, C.; Huang, H.; Gui, C.; Wang, L.; Li, Q.; Ju, J. Biosynthetic Baeyer–Villiger Chemistry Enables Access to Two Anthracene Scaffolds from a Single Gene Cluster in Deep-Sea-Derived Streptomyces olivaceus SCSIO T05. *J. Nat. Prod.* **2018**, *81*, 1570–1577. [CrossRef]
20. Chin, C.-S.; Alexander, D.H.; Marks, P.; Klammer, A.A.; Drake, J.; Heiner, C.; Clum, A.; Copeland, A.; Huddleston, J.; Eichler, E.E.; et al. Nonhybrid, finished microbial genome assemblies from long-read SMRT sequencing data. *Nat. Methods* **2013**, *10*, 563–569. [CrossRef]
21. Blin, K.; Shaw, S.; Steinke, K.; Villebro, R.; Ziemert, N.; Lee, S.Y.; Medema, M.H.; Weber, T. AntiSMASH 5.0: Updates to the secondary metabolite genome mining pipeline. *Nucleic Acids Res.* **2019**, *47*, W81–W87. [CrossRef] [PubMed]
22. Scherlach, K.; Hertweck, C. Triggering cryptic natural product biosynthesis in microorganisms. *Org. Biomol. Chem.* **2009**, *7*, 1753. [CrossRef] [PubMed]
23. Sun, C.; Zhang, C.; Qin, X.; Wei, X.; Liu, Q.; Li, Q.; Ju, J. Genome mining of Streptomyces olivaceus SCSIO T05: Discovery of olimycins A and B and assignment of absolute configurations. *Tetrahedron* **2018**, *74*, 199–203. [CrossRef]
24. Zhang, C.; Yang, Z.; Qin, X.; Ma, J.; Sun, C.; Huang, H.; Li, Q.; Ju, J. Genome Mining for Mycemycin: Discovery and Elucidation of Related Methylation and Chlorination Biosynthetic Chemistries. *Org. Lett.* **2018**, *20*, 7633–7636. [CrossRef] [PubMed]
25. Liu, W.; Shen, B. Genes for Production of the Enediyne Antitumor Antibiotic C-1027 in Streptomyces globisporus Are Clustered with the cagA Gene That Encodes the C-1027 Apoprotein. *Antimicrob. Agents Chemother.* **2000**, *44*, 382–392. [CrossRef] [PubMed]
26. Gust, B.; Challis, G.L.; Fowler, K.; Kieser, T.; Chater, K.F. PCR-targeted Streptomyces gene replacement identifies a protein domain needed for biosynthesis of the sesquiterpene soil odor geosmin. *Proc. Natl. Acad. Sci. USA* **2003**, *100*, 1541–1546. [CrossRef] [PubMed]

marine drugs

MDPI

Article

Polyketides from the Mangrove-Derived Endophytic Fungus *Cladosporium cladosporioides*

Fan-Zhong Zhang [1,2,3], Xiao-Ming Li [1,2], Xin Li [1,2], Sui-Qun Yang [1,2], Ling-Hong Meng [1,2,*] and Bin-Gui Wang [1,2,3,*]

1 Key Laboratory of Experimental Marine Biology, Center for Ocean Mega-Science, Institute of Oceanology, Chinese Academy of Sciences, Nanhai Road 7, Qingdao 266071, China; fancyzfz@163.com (F.-Z.Z.); lixmqdio@126.com (X.-M.L.); lixin871014@163.com (X.L.); suiqunyang@163.com (S.-Q.Y.)

2 Laboratory of Marine Biology and Biotechnology, Qingdao National Laboratory for Marine Science and Technology, Wenhai Road 1, Qingdao 266237, China

3 University of Chinese Academy of Sciences, Yuquan Road 19A, Beijing 100049, China

* Correspondence: m8545303@163.com (L.-H.M.); wangbg@ms.qdio.ac.cn (B.-G.W.); Tel: +86-532-8289-8553 (B.-G.W.)

Received: 8 April 2019; Accepted: 14 May 2019; Published: 17 May 2019

Abstract: Five new polyketides, namely, 5*R*-hydroxyrecifeiolide (**1**), 5*S*-hydroxyrecifeiolide (**2**), *ent*-cladospolide F (**3**), cladospolide G (**4**), and cladospolide H (**5**), along with two known compounds (**6** and **7**), were isolated from the endophytic fungal strain *Cladosporium cladosporioides* MA-299 that was obtained from the leaves of the mangrove plant *Bruguiera gymnorrhiza*. The structures of these compounds were established by extensive analysis of 1D/2D NMR data, mass spectrometric data, ECDs and optical rotations, and modified Mosher's method. The structures of **3** and **6** were confirmed by single-crystal X-ray diffraction analysis and this is the first time for reporting the crystal structures of these two compounds. All of the isolated compounds were examined for antimicrobial activities against human and aquatic bacteria and plant pathogenic fungi as well as enzymatic inhibitory activities against acetylcholinesterase. Compounds **1–4**, **6**, and **7** exhibited antimicrobial activity against some of the tested strains with MIC values ranging from 1.0 to 64 μg/mL, while **3** exhibited enzymatic inhibitory activity against acetylcholinesterase with the IC_{50} value of 40.26 μM.

Keywords: mangrove plant; endophytic fungus; *Cladosporium cladosporioides*; polyketides; antimicrobial activity; acetylcholinesterase; enzymatic inhibitory activity

1. Introduction

The *Cladosporium* fungi, one of the largest genera of dematiaceous hyphomycetes, have attracted considerable attention of natural products researchers in recent years [1,2]. Versatile bioactive metabolites, such as cladosporin [3], macrolide [4], sulfur-containing diketopiperazines [5], indole alkaloids [6], hybrid polyketides [7], and diterpenes with 5-8-5 ring system [8], have been isolated from the *Cladosporium* strains. As part of our research on discovering structurally novel and biologically active natural products, a series of interesting metabolites have been obtained from marine-derived fungal strains [9,10], including those from *Cladosporium* species [11]. Our current chemical investigation on *C. cladosporioides* MA-299, an endophytic fungus obtained from the fresh inner leaves of the marine mangrove plant *Bruguiera gymnorrhiza*, led to the discovery of five new polyketides, namely, 5*R*-hydroxyrecifeiolide (**1**), 5*S*-hydroxyrecifeiolide (**2**), *ent*-cladospolide F (**3**) [12], cladospolide G (**4**), and cladospolide H (**5**) (Figure 1), as well as two known analogues, including *iso*-cladospolide B (**6**) [13,14], and pandangolide 1 (**7**) [13,15] (Figure 1). Herein, we report the isolation, structure assignment, and biological evaluation of the isolated compounds.

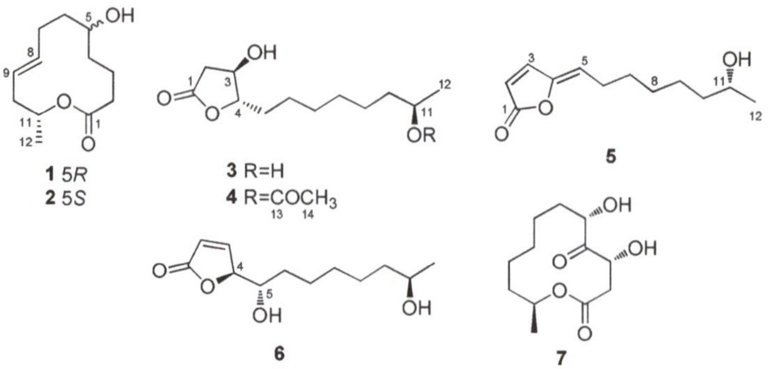

Figure 1. Structures of the isolated compounds **1–7**.

2. Results and Discussion

2.1. Structure Elucidation of the New Compounds

5*R*-Hydroxyrecifeiolide (**1**) was isolated as a colorless oil and the molecular formula $C_{12}H_{20}O_3$ was deduced from the (+)-HRESIMS data, indicating three degrees of unsaturation. The ^{1}H and ^{13}C NMR spectra of **1** showed the signals for one ester/lactone carbonyl, two olefinic and two oxygenated sp^3 methines, six sp^3 methylenes, and one methyl group (Table 1). In addition, the ^{1}H NMR data of **1** were quite similar to those of recifeiolide (11-hydroxy-*trans*-8-dodecenoic acid lactone) [16,17], except that one methylene (δ_H 1.5–2.3 ppm) in recifeiolide was replaced by an oxygenated methine (δ_H 3.51 ppm) in **1**. The key COSY correlations elucidated the connectivity from H-2 through H-12 (Figure 2). Key HMBC correlations from H-2 to C-1 and C-4, from H-3 to C-1 and C-5, and from H-11 to C-1, connected C-1 and C-2 and determined the 12-membered macrolide skeleton of **1** (Figure 2). The relative configuration at C-5 and C-11 for **1** was established by the NOESY experiment (Figure S8). The NOESY correlations (Figure 3) from H-2β to H-5 and H-11 revealed a β orientation of these protons [18]. The coupling constants between H-8 and H-9 ($J_{H\text{-}8/H\text{-}9}$ = 15.3 Hz) suggested the *E*-configuration of the C-8/C-9 double bond. The absolute configuration of C-5 of **1** was assigned by application of the modified Mosher's method [19]. The $\Delta\delta$ values obtained for the (*S*)- and (*R*)-MTPA esters (**1a** and **1b**, respectively) of **1** (Figure 4) suggested that the absolute configuration of C-5 is *R*. Furthermore, the electronic circular dichroism (ECD) spectrum of **1** was recorded and then computed with the time-dependent density function theory (TD-DFT) method at the gas-phase B3LYP/6-31G (d) level [20,21]. The calculated ECD spectra were produced by SpecDis software [22]. The experimental ECD spectrum for **1** matched well with the calculated spectrum for 11*R* (Figure 5). Therefore, the 5*R*, 11*R* configuration of **1** was established, and the trivial name 5*R*-hydroxyrecifeiolide was assigned.

Table 1. ^{1}H and ^{13}C NMR data of **1**, **2**, and **7** (δ in ppm).

Pos.	**1**			**2**		**7**	
	[a] δ_H (*J* in Hz)	[b] δ_H (*J* in Hz)	[d] δ_C	[b] δ_H (*J* in Hz)	[e] δ_C	[c] δ_H (*J* in Hz)	[f] δ_C
1			172.3, C		172.2, C		174.7, C
2	α 2.40, ddd (13.0, 5.6, 3.9) β 1.93, ddd (13.1, 11.0, 4.4)	α 2.40, ddd (13.0, 5.6, 3.9) β 1.93, ddd (13.1, 11.0, 4.4)	35.2, CH_2	α 2.25, m (overlap) β 2.16, m	31.8, CH_2	α 3.23, dd (18.5, 8.5) β 2.90, dd (18.5, 1.7)	43.0, CH_2
3	1.56, m (overlap)	1.56, m (overlap)	18.2, CH_2	α 1.67, m (overlap) β 1.54, m	19.9, CH_2	4.72, dd (8.5, 1.7)	65.7, CH
4	1.43, m (overlap)	1.43, m (overlap)	32.9, CH_2	α 1.41, m β 0.97, m	30.0, CH_2		209.3, C
5	3.51, m	3.51, m	70.2, CH	3.48, m	65.4, CH	4.31, d (5.4)	76.3, CH
6	α 1.60, m (overlap) β 1.35, m (overlap)	α 1.60, m (overlap) β 1.35, m (overlap)	32.6, CH_2	α 1.63, m (overlap) β 1.30, m	33.7, CH_2	α 1.97, m β 1.76, m	30.7, CH_2
7	α 2.17, m β 1.72, m	α 2.17, m β 1.72, m	28.6, CH_2	α 2.05, m β 1.91, m	27.7, CH_2	α 1.45, m (overlap) β 1.18, m (overlap)	20.8, CH_2
8	5.34, ddd (15.3, 10.7, 2.8)	5.34, ddd (15.3, 10.7, 2.8)	135.2, CH	5.26, m	132.7, CH	α 1.60, m (overlap) β 1.31, m (overlap)	26.9, CH_2
9	5.20, ddd (15.3, 10.1, 4.1)	5.20, ddd (15.3, 10.1, 4.1)	125.6, CH	5.11, m	126.7, CH	α 1.51, m (overlap) β 1.10, m (overlap)	22.7, CH_2
10	α 2.25, m β 2.06, m	α 2.25, m β 2.06, m	40.3, CH_2	α 2.29, m (overlap) β 1.99, m (overlap)	40.3, CH_2	α 1.69, m (overlap) β 1.39, m (overlap)	33.5, CH_2
11	4.84, m	4.84, m	68.3, CH	5.02, m	67.8, CH	4.88, m	75.2, CH
12	1.17, d (6.3)	1.17, d (6.3)	20.4, CH_3	1.15, d (6.3)	20.2, CH_3	1.25, d (6.2)	19.3, CH_3
3-OH						3.19, s	
5-OH	4.39, brs	4.39, brs		4.28, brs		3.03, s	

[a] Measured at 600 MHz in DMSO-d_6. [b] Measured at 500 MHz in DMSO-d_6. [c] Measured at 500 MHz in $CDCl_3$. [d] Measured at 150 MHz in DMSO-d_6. [e] Measured at 125 MHz in DMSO-d_6. [f] Measured at 125 MHz in $CDCl_3$.

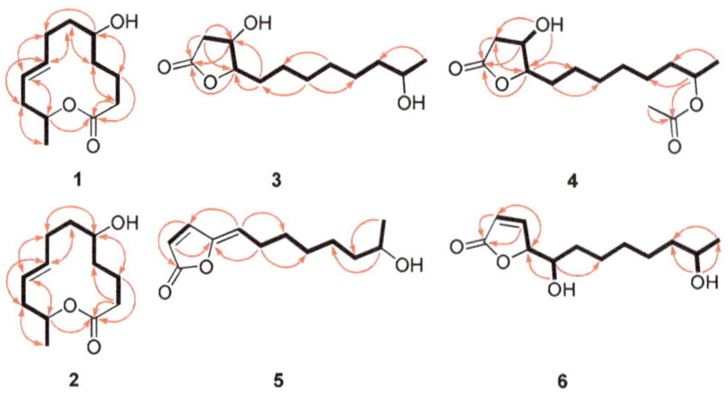

Figure 2. Key COSY (bold lines) and HMBC (red arrows) correlations for **1–6**.

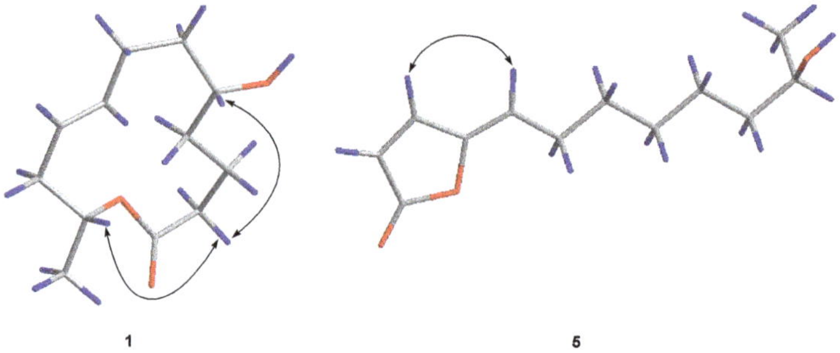

Figure 3. Key NOESY correlations for **1** and **5**.

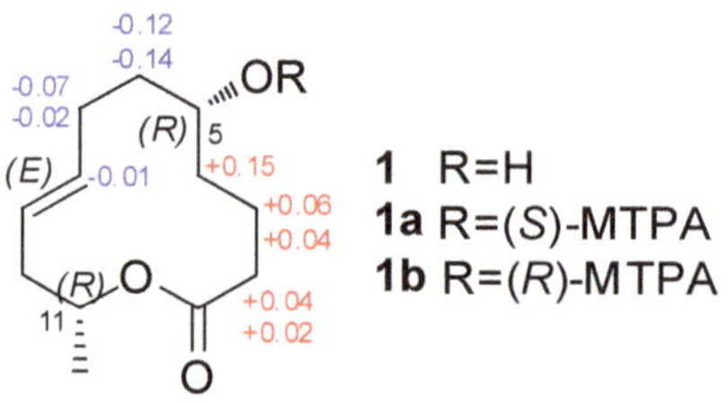

Figure 4. Δδ values (Δδ (in ppm) = $\delta_S - \delta_R$) obtained for the (*S*)-and (*R*)-MTPA esters (**1a** and **1b**, respectively) of **1**.

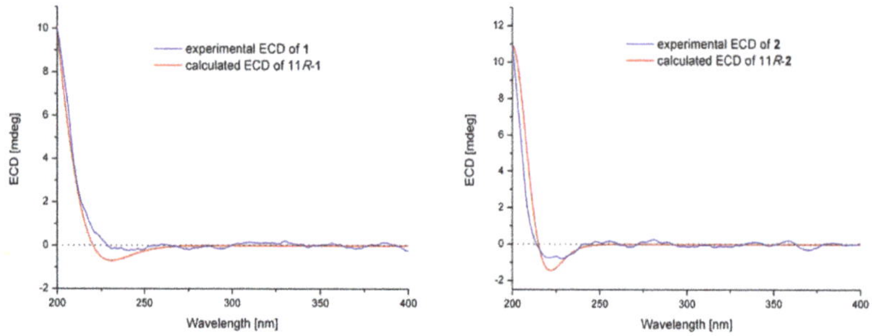

Figure 5. Comparison of experimental and calculated ECD spectra of **1** and **2**.

The molecular formula of **2** was determined as $C_{12}H_{20}O_3$, which was the same as that of **1**, according to its (+)-HRESIMS data. The ^{1}H and ^{13}C NMR spectra (Table 1) of **2** were similar to those of **1**, except for the different ^{13}C chemical shifts at C-5 (δ_C 70.2 in **1**, and δ_C 65.4 in **2**) and its adjacent positions (C-2–C-4 and C-6–C-8), which indicated that compound **2** was the 5-epimer of **1**. The chemical shifts at C-2 and C-8 (γ-position of C-5) exhibited obvious difference in **2** and **1** probably due to the space effect. As expected, the experimental ECD spectrum of **2** matched well with the calculated spectrum of 11*R* (Figure 5). The trivial name 5*S*-hydroxyrecifeiolide was assigned to **2**.

Compound **3** was initially obtained as pale yellow powder and possessed a molecular formula $C_{12}H_{22}O_4$ by (+)-HRESIMS, implying two degrees of unsaturation. The ^{1}H and ^{13}C NMR data (Table 2) exhibited signals attributed to one ester carbonyl, three oxygenated sp^3 methines, seven sp^3 methylenes, and one methyl group. These data were very similar to those of cladospolide F [12], suggesting that they had the same planar structure, which was also confirmed by the COSY and HMBC correlations (Figure 2). However, the signs of the optical rotations of **3** (−29.41, MeOH) and cladospolide F (+15.7, MeOH) were opposite, indicating that the absolute configurations of their stereogenic carbons were different. The relative configuration at C-3, C-4, and C-11 could not be concluded by NOESY experiment. Nevertheless, suitable crystals were obtained for X-ray diffraction analysis using Cu Kα radiation which confirmed the absolute configuration of C-3, C-4 and C-11 as 3*R*, 4*S*, and 11*R* (Figure 6). The *ent*-cladospolide F was therefore assigned as a trivial name for **3**.

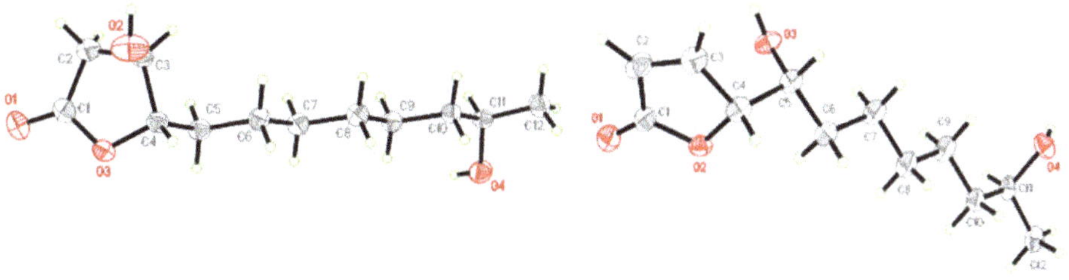

3 **6**

Figure 6. Ortep diagrams of *ent*-cladospolide F (**3**) and *iso*-cladospolide B (**6**).

Compound **4** was obtained as a pale yellow oil and its molecular formula was determined as $C_{14}H_{24}O_5$ on the basis of (+)-HRESIMS, requiring three degrees of unsaturation. The ^{1}H and ^{13}C NMR data for **4** (Table 2) were quite similar to those of **3**, except for the presence of additional ester carbonyl (C-13) and methyl (C-14) groups, which indicated the replacement of 11-OH group in **3** by an OAc group in **4**, and thus caused the down-field shift of 11-H from δ_H 3.55 in **3** to δ_H 4.78 in **4**. Detailed interpretation of the COSY and HMBC spectra revealed that **4** was an analogue of **3**, with the hydroxyl group at C-11 in **3** being replaced by an acetoxyl group in **4**. The HMBC correlation from H-11 to C-13 established the presence of an acetoxyl group at C-11, and the planar structure of **4** was hence confirmed as shown (Figure 2). In a biogenetic perspective, it was tentatively assigned the same relative configuration as that of **3**. The similar optical rotations of **4** (−24.56, MeOH) and **3** (−29.41, MeOH) also supported that the absolute configurations of the stereogenic carbons in **4** were the same as those in **3**. Therefore, the absolute configurations of the stereogenic carbons in **4** were tentatively assigned as 3*R*, 4*S*, and 11*R*, and the trivial name cladospolide G was assigned. Acetylation of compounds **3** and **4** using acetyl chloride yielded the same diacetylated derivative, which further correlated the structure relationship of compounds **3** and **4**.

Table 2. ^1H and ^{13}C NMR data of **3–6** (δ in ppm).

Pos.	3				4		5		6	
	$^a\ \delta_H$ (*J* in Hz)	$^b\ \delta_H$ (*J* in Hz)	$^d\ \delta_C$	$^e\ \delta_C$	$^c\ \delta_H$ (*J* in Hz)	$^f\ \delta_C$	$^a\ \delta_H$ (*J* in Hz)	$^d\ \delta_C$	$^a\ \delta_H$ (*J* in Hz)	$^d\ \delta_C$
1			175.5, C	175.8, C		175.5, C		169.7, C		173.2, C
2	α 2.85, dd (17.7, 6.4) β 2.25, dd (17.7, 3.2)	α 2.78, dd (18.0, 6.7) β 2.47, dd (18.0, 3.7)	37.0, CH_2	37.8, CH_2	α 2.85, dd (17.7, 6.4) β 2.25, dd (17.7, 3.2)	37.0, CH_2	6.37, d (5.4)	118.4, CH	6.21, d (5.6)	121.1, CH
3	4.09, m	4.22, m	70.1, CH	71.7, CH	4.09, m	70.1, CH	7.80, d (5.4)	145.1, CH	7.71, d (5.6)	156.6, CH
4	4.18, m	4.31, ddd (8.3, 5.3, 3.0)	87.5, CH	88.2, CH	4.18, ddd (8.1, 5.5, 2.5)	87.5, CH		149.4, C	5.04, d (1.5)	86.2, CH
5	α 1.56, m β 1.48, m	1.57, m	32.1, CH_2	33.2, CH_2	α 1.57, m β 1.48, m (overlap)	32.0, CH_2	5.53, t (7.9)	117.1, CH	3.66, m	69.4, CH
6	1.26, m (overlap)	1.34, m (overlap)	25.2, CH_2	25.7, CH_2	1.25, m (overlap)	24.7, CH_2	2.30, m	25.8, CH_2	1.44, m (overlap)	40.0, CH_2
7	1.33, m (overlap)	1.41, m (overlap)	29.0, CH_2	29.5, CH_2	1.33, m (overlap)	28.6, CH_2	1.44, m	28.3, CH_2	1.34, m (overlap)	32.8, CH_2
8	1.31, m (overlap)	1.28, m (overlap)	28.8, CH_2	29.3, CH_2	1.31, m (overlap)	28.5, CH_2	1.23, m (overlap)	28.7, CH_2	1.29, m (overlap)	29.1, CH_2
9	1.24, m (overlap)	1.26, m (overlap)	24.8, CH_2	25.3, CH_2	1.24, m (overlap)	24.6, CH_2	1.27, m (overlap)	25.0, CH_2	1.25, m (overlap)	25.3, CH_2
10	1.36, m (overlap)	1.45, m (overlap)	39.0, CH_2	39.3, CH_2	1.45, m (overlap)	35.2, CH_2	1.32, m (overlap)	38.9, CH_2	1.39, m (overlap)	39.0, CH_2
11	3.55, m	3.75, m	65.7, CH	68.3, CH	4.78, m	70.1, CH	3.55, m (overlap)	65.6, CH	3.55, m	65.7, CH
12	1.02, d (6.1)	1.15, d (6.2)	23.6, CH_3	23.7, CH_3	1.15, d (6.3)	19.7, CH_3	1.02, d (6.1)	23.6, CH_3	1.02, d (6.2)	23.6, CH_3
13						169.9, C				
14					1.97, s	21.0, CH_3				
3-OH	5.49, s				5.50, d (4.0)					
5-OH									4.95, d (6.3)	
11-OH	4.27, d (4.2)						3.41, brs		4.29, d (4.7)	

^{a} Measured at 500 MHz in DMSO-d_6. ^{b} Measured at 500 MHz in $CDCl_3$. ^{c} Measured at 600 MHz in DMSO-d_6. ^{d} Measured at 125 MHz in DMSO-d_6. ^{e} Measured at 125 MHz in $CDCl_3$. ^{f} Measured at 150 MHz in DMSO-d_6.

Compound **6** was isolated as colorless crystals and gave ion peaks at *m/z* 229.1432 [M + H]$^+$ and 246.1699 [M + NH_4]$^+$ in the (+)-HRESIMS, corresponding to a molecular formula $C_{12}H_{20}O_4$, indicating three degrees of unsaturation. All the ^1H and ^{13}C NMR data of **6** were quite similar to those of the previously reported polyketide metabolite *iso*-cladospolide B [13]. The COSY and HMBC correlations (Figure 2) confirmed that the planar structure of **6** was the same as that of *iso*-cladospolide B. The high similarity of specific rotations of **6** ($[\alpha]_D^{25}$ = −90.91 (*c* 0.11, MeOH)) and *iso*-cladospolide B ($[\alpha]_D^{25}$= −90 (*c* 0.23, MeOH)) [13] suggested that they may have the same relative and absolute stereochemistry. However, neither the relative nor the absolute configuration was determined [13]. In 2001, Franck et al. carried out the first synthesis of *iso*-cladospolide B and proposed that it has the 4*S*, 5*S*, and 11*R* configuration [14]. Later, in 2005, the absolute configuration of *iso*-cladospolide B, isolated from *Cladosporium sp.* isolated from the Red Sea sponge *Niphates rowi*, was assigned to be 4*S*, 5*S*, and 11*S* ($[\alpha]_D^{28}$ = −61 (*c* 16.6, MeOH)) [15]. It was later stated that both diastereomers appear to be natural products and (4*S*, 5*S*, 11*S*)-isomer referred to as 11-*epi*-*iso*-cladospolide B [23,24]. The relative configuration of **6** could not be assigned by NOESY experiments but the coupling constant for C-4 (*J* = 1.5 Hz) confirmed the *threo* relative configuration [14]. Upon slow evaporation of the solvent (MeOH-H_2O), compound **6** was crystallized and the X-ray analysis was carried out, which was first reported for *iso*-cladospolide B (Figure 4). The Cu Kα Flack parameter 0.5 (7) allowed preliminary confirmation of the relative configurations of **6** as 4*S**, 5*S**, 11*R**.

Compound **5** was obtained as a pale yellow oil and possessed a molecular formula of $C_{12}H_{18}O_3$ by (+)-HRESIMS, implying four degrees of unsaturation. The 1D NMR data (Table 2) and HSQC spectrum (Figure S38) suggested signals attributed to one ester and one olefinic quaternary carbons, one oxygenated and three olefinic methines, five sp^3 methylenes, and one methyl group. These NMR data were similar to those of *iso*-cladospolide B (**6**) [13]. However, resonances for two oxygenated methines (C-4 and C-5) in **6** were not detected in the NMR spectra of **5**. Instead, two additional olefinic signals including one quaternary sp^2 (C-4, δ_C 149.4) and one methine sp^2 (C-5, δ_C 117.1/δ_H 5.53) carbons were observed in the NMR spectra of **5** (Table 2). These data indicated that **5** was a reduced analogue of **6**, and this deduction was supported by the molecular formula. The COSY and HMBC spectra established the structure of **5** as shown in Figure 1. In the NOESY experiment, the correlation between H-3 and H-5 indicated the *Z*-conformation of the double bond between C-4 and C-5 (Figure 3). The absolute stereochemistry of **5** could not be determined by Mosher's method because of the limited amount of material available. From a biogenetic point of view, **5** was putatively produced by reduction of **6**. Therefore, it was tentatively assigned the absolute configuration of C-11 of **5** as 11*R*. From these data, the name cladospolide H was assigned for **5**.

Compound **7** was acquired as white powder and showed ion peaks at *m/z* 267.1197 [M + Na]$^+$ in the positive HRESIMS, corresponding to a molecular formula of $C_{12}H_{20}O_5$. A literature search indicated that all the ^1H and ^{13}C NMR data of **7** were almost the same as those of previously reported compound pandangolide 1 [13,15]. The almost exactly the same specific rotations of **7** ($[\alpha]_D^{25}$ = −30.16 (c 1.22, MeOH)) and pandangolide 1 ($[\alpha]_D^{25}$= −30 (c 2.3, MeOH)) [15] revealed that they may have the same relative and absolute configurations.

2.2. Biological Activities of the Isolated Compounds

Compounds **1**–**7** were tested for antimicrobial activities against two human pathogens (*Escherichia coli, Staphylococcus aureus*), ten aquatic bacteria (*Aeromonas hydrophilia, Edwardsiella ictarda, E. tarda, Micrococcus luteus, Pseudomonas aeruginosa, Vibrio alginolyticus, V. anguillarum, V. harveyi, V. parahaemolyticus,* and *V. vulnificus*), and 15 plant pathogenic fungi (*Alternaria solani, Bipolaris sorokiniana, Ceratobasidium cornigerum, Colletotrichum glecosporioides, Coniothyrium diplodiella, Fusarium graminearum, F. oxysporum* f. sp. *cucumerinum, F. oxysporum* f. sp. *momodicae, F. oxysporum* f. sp. *radicis lycopersici, F. solani, Glomerella cingulate, Helminthosporium maydis, Penicillium digitatum, Physalospora piricola Nose,* and *Valsa mali*). As shown in Table 3, **3** exhibited moderate inhibitory activities against human pathogenic bacteria S. aureus with MIC value of 8.0 μg/mL. Compound **4** showed potent inhibitory activities against plant-pathogenic fungi (*G. cingulate* and *F. oxysporum* f. sp. *cucumerinum*), each with an MIC value of 1.0 μg/mL, while **7** showed activity against aquatic bacterium (E. ictarda) and plant-pathogenic fungus (*G. cingulate*), with MIC values of 4.0 and 1.0 μg/mL, respectively.

Table 3. Antimicrobial Activities of **1–7** (MIC, μg/mL) [a].

Strains	Compounds						
	1	**2**	**3**	**4**	**6**	**7**	**Positive control**
E. coli [b]	–	–	–	32	32	–	2.0
S. aureus [b]	–	–	8.0	–	–	32	1.0
E. tarda [b]	–	–	–	–	32	–	0.5
E. ictarda [b]	32	–	16	–	16	4.0	0.5
G. cingulate [c]	–	16	–	1.0	64	1.0	0.5
B. sorokiniana [c]	–	–	–	32	–	–	0.5
P. aeruginosa [c]	32	–	64	–	–	32	2.0
F.oxysporum* f. sp. *Cucumerinum [c]	–	–	–	1.0	–	–	0.5

[a] (–) = MIC > 64 μg/mL, [b] Chloramphenicol as positive control, [c] Amphotericin B as positive control.

Compounds **1–7** were also evaluated for acetylcholinesterase inhibitory activity. Compound **3** exhibited potent activity against acetylcholinesterase with the IC_{50} value of 40.26 μM. The other compounds have a weak activity (IC_{50} > 50 μM).

3. Experimental Section

3.1. General Experimental Procedures

Melting points were determined by an SGW X-4 micro-melting-point apparatus (Shanghai Shenguang Instrument Co. Ltd, Shanghai, China). Optical rotations were measured on an Optical Activity AA-55 polarimeter (Optical Activity Ltd., Cambridgeshire, UK). UV spectra were measured on a PuXi TU-1810 UV-visible spectrophotometer (Shanghai Lengguang Technology Co. Ltd., Shanghai, China). ECD spectra were acquired on a Chirascan spectropolarimeter (Applied Photophysics Ltd., Leatherhead, UK). The ^{1}H, ^{13}C, and 2D NMR spectra were acquired using a Bruker Avance 500 or 600 M spectrometer (Bruker Biospin Group, Karlsruhe, Germany). Chemical shifts (δ) were expressed in ppm with reference to the solvent peaks (^{13}C, $CDCl_3$: 77.16 ppm, DMSO-d_6: 39.52 ppm; ^{1}H, $CDCl_3$: 7.26 ppm, DMSO-d_6: 2.50 ppm). Mass spectra were obtained from an API QSTAR Pulsar 1 mass spectrometer (Applied Biosystems, Foster, Waltham, MA, USA). Analytical HPLC analyses were performed using a Dionex HPLC system (Dionex, Sunnyvale, CA, USA) equipped with P680 pump, ASI-100 automated sample injector, and UVD340U multiple wavelength detector controlled by Chromeleon software (version 6.80). Column chromatography (CC) was performed with silica gel (200–300 mesh, Qingdao Haiyang Chemical Factory, Qingdao, China), Lobar LiChroprep RP-18 (40–60 μm, Merck, Darmstadt, Germany), and Sephadex LH-20 (18–110 μm, Merck).

3.2. Fungal Material

The fungal strain *Cladosporium cladosporioides* MA-299 was isolated from the leaves of the mangrove plant *Bruguiera gymnorrhiza*, collected in Hainan Island, China, in March 2015. The strain was identified as *Cladosporium cladosporioides* by analysis of its ITS region of the rDNA, which is the same (100%) as that of *C. cladosporioides* DCF-1 (accession no. MG208055). The sequence data were deposited in GenBank with the accession number MH822624. The strain is preserved at Key Laboratory of Experimental Marine Biology, Institute of Oceanology of the Chinese Academy of Sciences (IOCAS).

3.3. Fermentation

For chemical investigations, the strain of *C. cladosporioides* MA-299 was cultured on PDA (Potato Dextrose Agar) medium at 28 °C for six days and then inoculated into 100 × 1 L flasks, each containing 70 g of rice, 0.1 g corn syrup, 0.3 g peptone, 0.1 g methionine and 100 mL seawater that was obtained from the Huiquan Gulf of the Yellow Sea near the campus of IOCAS, statically cultured for 48 days at room temperature.

3.4. Extraction and Isolation

After 48 days, the fermented rice substrate was mechanically fragmented and then extracted three times with 300 mL EtOAc every flask. All of the EtOAc extracts were filtered and evaporated under reduced pressure to yield a crude extract (52.3 g).

The crude extract was subjected to a silica gel vacuum liquid chromatography (VLC), eluting with different solvents of increasing polarity from petroleum ether (PE) to MeOH to yield ten fractions (Frs. 1–10) based on TLC and HPLC analysis. Fr. 5 (2.1 g) was further purified by reversed-phase column chromatography (CC) over Lobar LiChroprep RP-18 with a MeOH-H_2O gradient (from 10: 90 to 100: 0) to afford four subfractions (Frs. 5.1–5.4). Fr. 5.2 was further purified by CC on Sephadex LH–20 (MeOH) and then by preparative TLC (plate: 20 × 20 cm, developing solvents: CH_2Cl_2/MeOH, 30: 1) to obtain **5** (2.6 mg). Fr. 5.3 was subjected to CC on silica gel eluted with CH_2Cl_2-MeOH (100:1 to 5:1) to obtain **1** (4.1 mg) and **2** (3.0 mg). Fr. 6 (1.7 g) was further fractionated by CC over Lobar LiChroprep RP-18 with a MeOH/H_2O gradient (from 10:90 to 100:0) to yield six subfractions (Frs. 6.1–6.6). Fr. 6.1 (112.4 mg) was further purified by prep. TLC (plate: 20 × 20 cm, developing solvents: petroleum ether/acetone, 2:1) and then on Sephadex LH–20 (MeOH) to obtain **7** (3.2 mg). Fr. 6.5 was subjected to CC on silica gel eluted with CH_2Cl_2-MeOH (150:1 to 70:1) to obtain **4** (5.7 mg). Further purification of Fr. 7 (3.6 g) by CC over Lobar LiChroprep RP-18 with a MeOH/H_2O gradient (from 10:90 to 100:0) yielded seven subfractions (Frs. 7.1–7.7). Fr. 7.1 (736.2 mg) was purified by CC on silica gel eluting with a petroleum ether-acetone gradient (from 10:1 to 2:1), and further fractionated by Sephadex LH-20 (MeOH) to afford **3** (91.6 mg). Fr. 7.2 (960.7 mg) was further separated by CC on silica gel eluting with a petroleum ether-acetone gradient (from 10:1 to 1:1) purification, to afford **6** (23.4 mg).

5*R*-Hydroxyrecifeiolide (**1**): Colourless oil; $[\alpha]_D^{25}$ +33.33 (*c* 0.09, MeOH); UV (MeOH) λ_{max} (log ε) 205 (3.06), 220 (3.01); ECD (7.55 mM, MeOH) λ_{max} ($\Delta\varepsilon$) 233 (−0.01) nm; ^{1}H and ^{13}C NMR data, see Table 1; ESIMS *m/z* 235 $[M + Na]^+$; (+)-HRESIMS at *m/z* 235.1298 $[M + Na]^+$ (calcd for $C_{12}H_{20}O_3Na$, 235.1305).

5*S*-hydroxyrecifeiolide (**2**): Colourless oil; $[\alpha]_D^{25}$ +23.07 (*c* 0.13, MeOH); UV (MeOH) λ_{max} (log ε) 205 (3.01), 220 (3.06); ECD (8.49 mM, MeOH) λ_{max} ($\Delta\varepsilon$) 230 (−0.03) nm; ^{1}H and ^{13}C NMR data, see Table 1; ESIMS *m/z* 235 $[M + Na]^+$; (+)-HRESIMS at *m/z* 235.1299 $[M + Na]^+$ (calcd for $C_{12}H_{20}O_3Na$, 235.1305).

ent-Cladospolide F (**3**): Colorless crystal (MeOH); mp 59–62 °C; $[\alpha]_D^{25}$ −29.41 (*c* 0.17, MeOH); UV (MeOH) λ_{max} (log ε) 206 (3.42); ECD (7.82 mM, MeOH) λ_{max} ($\Delta\varepsilon$) 210 (+0.28) nm, 267 (+0.03) nm; ^{1}H and ^{13}C NMR data, see Table 2; ESIMS *m/z* 231 $[M + H]^+$, *m/z* 253 $[M + Na]^+$; (+)-HRESIMS at *m/z* 231.1589 $[M + H]^+$ (calcd for $C_{12}H_{23}O_4$, *m/z* 231.1591), at *m/z* 253.1407 $[M + Na]^+$ (calcd for $C_{12}H_{22}O_4Na$, *m/z* 253.1410).

Cladospolide G (**4**): Yellow oil; $[\alpha]_D^{25}$ −24.56 (*c* 0.57, MeOH); UV (MeOH) λ_{max} (log ε) 206 (3.49), 220 (3.27), 275 (2.62); ECD (4.04 mM, MeOH) λ_{max} ($\Delta\varepsilon$) 207 (+0.80) nm, 323 (−0.10) nm; ^{1}H and ^{13}C NMR data, see Table 2; ESIMS *m/z* 273 $[M + H]^+$, *m/z* 295 $[M + Na]^+$; (+)-HRESIMS at *m/z* 273.1700 $[M + H]^+$ (calcd for $C_{14}H_{25}O_5$, *m/z* 273.1697), at *m/z* 290.1970 $[M + NH_4]^+$ (calcd for $C_{14}H_{28}O_5N$, *m/z* 290.1962), at *m/z* 295.1515 $[M + Na]^+$ (calcd for $C_{14}H_{24}O_5Na$, *m/z* 295.1516).

Cladospolide H (**5**): pale yellow oil; ^{1}H and ^{13}C NMR data, see Table 2; ESIMS *m/z* 233 $[M + Na]^+$; (+)-HRESIMS at *m/z* 233.1151 $[M + Na]^+$ (calcd for $C_{12}H_{18}O_3Na$, *m/z* 233.1148). (The optical rotation and ECD of **5** could not be detected due to the limited quantity).

Iso-cladospolide B (**6**): colorless crystal (MeOH); mp 105–112 °C; $[\alpha]_D^{25}$ −90.91 (*c* 0.11, MeOH); UV (MeOH) λ_{max} (log ε); ECD (9.21 mM, MeOH) λ_{max} ($\Delta\varepsilon$) 213 (−5.69) nm; ^{1}H and ^{13}C NMR data, see Table 2; (+)-HRESIMS at *m/z* 229.1432 $[M + H]^+$ (calcd for $C_{12}H_{21}O_4$, 229.1434), at *m/z* 246.1699 $[M + NH_4]^+$ (calcd for $C_{12}H_{24}O_4N$, 246.1700).

3.5. X-Ray Crystallographic Analysis of Compounds 3 and 6

All crystallographic data were collected on an Agilent Xcalibur Eos Gemini CCD plate diffractometer, using graphite monochromatized Cu/Kα radiation (λ= 1.54178 Å) [25]. The data were corrected for absorption by using the program SADABS [26]. The structures were solved by direct methods with the SHELXTL software package [27]. All nonhydrogen atoms were refined anisotropically. The H atoms were located by geometrical calculations, and their positions and thermal parameters were fixed during the structure refinement. The structure was refined by full-matrix least-squares techniques [28].

Crystal data for compound **3**: $C_{12}H_{22}O_4$, F.W. = 230.30, Orthorhombic space group P2(1)2(1)2(1), unit cell dimensions a = 5.4655(4) Å, b = 5.5812(6) Å, c = 41.275(3) Å, V = 1259.06(19) Å^3, $\alpha = \beta = \gamma = 90°$, Z = 4, d_{calcd} = 1.215 mg/m^3, crystal dimensions 0.40 × 0.28 × 0.10 mm^3, μ = 0.734 mm^{-1}, F(000) = 504. The 2385 measurements yielded 1827 independent reflections after equivalent data were averaged, and Lorentz and polarization corrections were applied. The final refinement gave R_1 = 0.0487 and wR_2 = 0.0970 ($I > 2\sigma(I)$). The Flack parameter was 0.0 (5) in the final refinement for all 1827 reflections with 147 Friedel pairs.

Crystal data for compound **6**: $C_{12}H_{20}O_4$, F.W. = 228.13, Orthorhombic space group P2(1)2(1)2(1), unit cell dimensions a = 5.5217(5) Å, b = 7.6778(7) Å, c = 28.947(2) Å, V = 1227.17(19) Å^3, $\alpha = \beta = \gamma = 90°$, Z = 6, d_{calcd} = 1.236 mg/m^3, crystal dimensions 0.35 × 0.24 × 0.16 mm^3, μ = 0.752 mm^{-1}, F(000) = 496. The 5282 measurements yielded 2081 independent reflections after equivalent data were averaged, and Lorentz and polarization corrections were applied. The final refinement gave R_1 = 0.0727 and wR_2 = 0.1620 ($I > 2\sigma(I)$). The Flack parameter was 0.5 (7) in the final refinement for all 2081 reflections with 150 Friedel pairs.

3.6. Acetylation of Compounds 3 and 4

To 5 μmol samples of compound **3** or **4** in glass-stoppered flask were added 400 μL dichloromethane, then excess amount of triethylamine was added. Drip 20 μmol of acetylchloride slowly into the flask in ice bath and keeping the reaction for 12 h. Then stop the reaction by adding 20 μL of water into the flask. The progress of the reaction was monitored by TLC analysis. The resulting reaction mixture was extracted with dichloromethane (2 × 400 μL), dried with Na_2SO_4, and concentrated in vacuo to obtain the product.

3.7. Antimicrobial Assay

Antimicrobial evaluation against two human pathogens (*Escherichia coli* EMBLC-1, *Staphylococcus aureus* EMBLC-2) and ten aquatic pathogens (*Aeromonas hydrophilia* QDIO-1, *Edwardsiella ictarda* QDIO-9, *E. tarda* QDIO-2, *Micrococcus luteus* QDIO-3, *Pseudomonas aeruginosa* QDIO-4, *Vibrio alginolyticus* QDIO-5, *V. anguillarum* QDIO-6, *V. harveyi* QDIO-7, *V. parahaemolyticus* QDIO-8, and *V. vulnificus* QDIO-10), as well as 15 plant-pathogenic fungi (*Alternaria solani* QDAU-1, *Bipolaris sorokiniana* QDAU-5, *Ceratobasidium cornigerum* QDAU-6, *Colletotrichum glecosporioides* QDAU-2, *Coniothyrium diplodiella* QDAU-7, *Fusarium graminearum* QDAU-4, *F. oxysporum* f. sp. *cucumerinum* QDAU-8, *F. oxysporum* f. sp. *momodicae* QDAU-9, *F. oxysporum* f. sp. *radicis lycopersici* QDAU-10, *F. solani* QDAU-11, *Glomerella cingulate* QDAU-12, *Helminthosporium maydis* QDAU-15, *Penicillium digitatum* QDAU-14, *Physalospora piricola* Nose QDAU-15, and *Valsa mali* QDAU-16), was carried out by the 96-well microtiter plates assay [29]. The pathogens were obtained from the Institute of Oceanology, Chinese Academy of Sciences. Chloramphenicol and amphotericin were used as positive controls for bacteria and fungi, respectively. All of the tested compounds and controls were dissolved in DMSO.

3.8. Enzyme inhibitory Assay

A modified Ellman's method [30] was used to evaluate AChE inhibitory activities of compounds **1–7** in 96-well microplates. Tacrine was used as the standard inhibitor, and control test was performed without the presence of AChE inhibitors. All the inhibitors, solubilized in MeOH, were diluted stepwise from initial concentration of 32 μM. Every experiment was performed in triplicate. 5 μL inhibitor was added to each well and dried, then 50 μL phosphate buffer (PBS, 10 × 0.01 M, pH 7.2–7.4) was dispensed followed by 10 μL AChE (2 U/mL) and 20 μL 5,5-dithiobis 2-nitrobenzoic acid (DTNB, 5 mM). After 10 min culturing at 37 °C, 20 μL acetylthiocholine iodide (ATCh, 10 mM) was added and then OD was read at 405 nm over another period of 10 min culturing at 37 °C. The enzymatic inhibitory activity was calculated according to the following equation: Inhibition % = $((C - C_{backgroud}) - (A - A_{backgroud}))/(C - C_{backgroud}) \times 100\%$, where C is the OD value of the control and A is the OD value in the presence of the inhibitor. As for the background, ATCh was replaced by PBS in A and C and bovine albumin (BSA, 1mg/mL) took the place of AChE in C.

4. Conclusions

In summary, five new compounds (**1–5**) and two previously reported metabolites (**6** and **7**) were isolated from the mangrove-derived endophytic fungus *C. cladosporioides* MA-299. The structures of **3** and **6** were confirmed by single-crystal X-ray diffraction analysis and this is the first time for reporting the crystal structures of the two compounds. Compound **4** showed potent inhibitory activity against plant-pathogenic fungi (*G. cingulate* and *F.oxysporum* f. sp. *cucumerinum*), each with MIC value of 1.0 μg/mL, while **7** showed potent inhibitory activity against aquatic bacterium (*E. ictarda*) and plant-pathogenic fungus (*G. cingulate*), with MIC values of 4.0 and 1.0 μg/mL respectively. Compound **3** exhibited moderate inhibitory activity against human pathogenic bacterium *S. aureus* with MIC value of 8.0 μg/mL and acetylcholinesterase inhibitory activity with IC_{50} value of 40.26 μM.

Supplementary Materials: The following are available online at http://www.mdpi.com/1660-3397/17/5/296/s1, 1D and 2D NMR spectra and ECDs of compounds **1–5** as well as crystal packing of compounds **3** and **6**.

Author Contributions: F.-Z.Z. performed the experiments for the isolation, structure elucidation, and antimicrobial evaluation; and prepared the manuscript; X.-M.L. performed the 1D and 2D NMR experiments; X.L. contributed to part of the structure determination; S.-Q.Y. contributed the optimization of fermentation; L.-H.M contributed to part of the structure determination and jointly supervised the research; B.-G.W. supervised the research work and revised the manuscript.

Funding: Financial support from the Natural Science Foundation of China (81673351 and 31600267) and from the Natural Science Foundation of Shandong Province, China (ZR2016BQ17), is gratefully acknowledged. Bin-Gui Wang acknowledges the support of Taishan Scholar project from Shandong province.

Conflicts of Interest: The authors declare no conflict of interest.

References

1. Bensch, K.; Groenewald, J.Z.; Braun, U.; Dijksterhuis, J.; de Jesus Yáñez-Morales, M.; Crous, P.W. Common but different: The expanding realm of *Cladosporium*. *Stud. Mycol.* **2015**, *82*, 23–74. [CrossRef]
2. Imhoff, J.F. Natural products from marine fungi—still an underrepresented resource. *Mar. Drugs* **2016**, *14*, 19. [CrossRef] [PubMed]
3. Jacyno, J.M.; Harwood, J.S.; Cutler, H.G.; Lee, M.K. Isocladosporin, a biologically active isomer of cladosporin from *Cladosporium cladosporioides*. *J. Nat. Prod.* **1993**, *56*, 1397–1401. [CrossRef]
4. Shigemori, H.; Kasai, Y.; Komatsu, K.; Tsuda, M.; Mikami, Y.; Kobayashi, J. Sporiolides A and B, new cytotoxic twelve-membered macrolides from a marine-derived fungus *Cladosporium* species. *Mar. Drugs* **2004**, *2*, 164–169. [CrossRef]
5. Gu, B.B.; Zhang, Y.Y.; Ding, L.J.; He, S.; Wu, B.; Dong, J.D.; Zhu, P.; Chen, J.J.; Zhang, J.R.; Yan, X.J. Preparative separation of sulfur-containing diketopiperazines from marine fungus *Cladosporium* sp. using high-speed counter-current chromatography in stepwise elution mode. *Mar. Drugs* **2015**, *13*, 354–365. [CrossRef] [PubMed]

6. Peng, J.X.; Lin, T.; Wang, W.; Xin, Z.H.; Zhu, T.J.; Gu, Q.Q.; Li, D.H. Antiviral alkaloids produced by the mangrove-derived fungus *Cladosporium* sp. PJX-41. *J. Nat. Prod.* **2013**, *76*, 1133–1140. [CrossRef]
7. Wu, G.W.; Sun, X.H.; Yu, G.H.; Wang, W.; Zhu, T.J.; Gu, Q.Q.; Li, D.H. Cladosins A–E, hybrid polyketides from a deep-sea-derived fungus, *Cladosporium sphaerospermum*. *J. Nat. Prod.* **2014**, *77*, 270–275. [CrossRef]
8. Sassa, T.; Ooi, T.; Nukina, M.; Ikeda, M.; Kato, N. Structural confirmation of cotylenin A, a novel fusicoccane-diterpene glycoside with potent plant growth-regulating activity from *Cladosporium* fungus sp. 501-7w. *Biosci. Biotechnol. Biochem.* **1998**, *62*, 1815–1818. [CrossRef]
9. Li, X.D.; Li, X.; Li, X.M.; Xu, G.M.; Liu, Y.; Wang, B.G. 20-Nor-isopimarane epimers produced by *Aspergillus wentii* SD-310, a fungal strain obtained from deep sea sediment. *Mar. Drugs* **2018**, *16*, 440. [CrossRef]
10. Yang, S.Q.; Li, X.M.; Li, X.; Chi, L.P.; Wang, B.G. Two New Diketomorpholine Derivatives and a New Highly Conjugated Ergostane-Type Steroid from the Marine Algal-Derived Endophytic Fungus *Aspergillus alabamensis* EN-547. *Mar. Drugs* **2018**, *16*, 114. [CrossRef]
11. Li, H.L.; Li, X.M.; Mándi, A.; Antus, S.; Li, X.; Zhang, P.; Liu, Y.; Kurtán, T.; Wang, B.G. Characterization of cladosporols from the marine algal-derived endophytic fungus *Cladosporium cladosporioides* EN-399 and configurational revision of the previously reported cladosporol derivatives. *J. Org. Chem.* **2017**, *82*, 9946–9954. [CrossRef] [PubMed]
12. Zhu, M.L.; Gao, H.Q.; Wu, C.M.; Zhu, T.J.; Che, Q.; Gu, Q.Q.; Guo, P.; Li, D.H. Lipid-lowering polyketides from a soft coral-derived fungus *Cladosporium* sp. TZP29. *Bioorg. Med. Chem. Lett.* **2015**, *25*, 3606–3609. [CrossRef]
13. Smith, C.J.; Abbanat, D.; Bernan, V.S.; Maiese, W.M.; Greenstein, M.; Jompa, J.; Tahir, A.; Ireland, C.M. Novel polyketide metabolites from a species of marine fungi. *J. Nat. Prod.* **2000**, *63*, 142–145. [CrossRef]
14. Franck, X.; Araujo, M.E.V.; Jullian, J.C.; Hocquemiller, R.; Figadère, B. Synthesis and structure determination of *iso*-cladospolide B. *Tetrahedron Lett.* **2001**, *42*, 2801–2803. [CrossRef]
15. Gesner, S.; Cohen, N.; Ilan, M.; Yarden, O.; Carmeli, S. Pandangolide 1a, a metabolite of the sponge-associated fungus *Cladosporium* sp., and the absolute stereochemistry of pandangolide 1 and *iso*-cladospolide B. *J. Nat. Prod.* **2005**, *68*, 1350–1353. [CrossRef]
16. Corey, E.J.; Ulrich, P.; Fitzpatrick, J.M. A stereoselective synthesis of (±)-11-Hydroxy-*trans*-8-dodecenoic acid lactone, a naturally occurring macrolide from *Cephalosporium recifei*. *J. Am. Chem. Soc.* **1976**, *98*, 222–224. [CrossRef]
17. Rodphaya, D.; Sekiguchi, J.; Yamada, Y. New macrolides from *Penicillium Urticae* mutant S11R59. *J. Antibiot.* **1986**, *39*, 629–635. [CrossRef]
18. Sun, P.; Xu, D.X.; Mándi, A.; Kurtán, T.; Li, T.J.; Schulz, B.; Zhang, W. Structure, absolute configuration, and conformational study of 12-membered macrolides from the fungus *Dendrodochium* sp. associated with the sea cucumber *Holothuria nobilis* selenka. *J. Org. Chem.* **2013**, *78*, 7030–7047. [CrossRef]
19. Ohtani, I.; Kusumi, T.; Kashman, Y.; Kakisawa, H. High-field FT NMR application of Mosher's method. The absolute configurations of marine terpenoids. *J. Am. Chem. Soc.* **1991**, *113*, 4092–4096. [CrossRef]
20. Calculator Plugins Were Used for Structure Property Prediction and Calculation, Marvin 5.9.2, 2012, ChemAxon. Available online: http://www.chemaxon.com (accessed on 31 August 2018).
21. Frisch, M.J.; Trucks, G.W.; Schlegel, H.B.; Scuseria, G.E.; Robb, M.A.; Cheeseman, J.R.; Scalmani, G.; Barone, V.; Mennucci, B.; Petersson, G.A.; et al. *Gaussian 09, Revision, C.01*; Gaussian, Inc.: Wallingford, CT, USA, 2010.
22. Bruhn, T.; Hemberger, Y.; Schaumloffel, A.; Bringmann, G. *SpecDis, Version 1.51*; University of Wuerzburg: Würzburg, Germany, 2011.
23. Trost, B.M.; Aponick, A. Palladium-catalyzed asymmetric allylic alkylation of *meso*- and *dl*-1,2-divinylethylene carbonate. *J. Am. Chem. Soc.* **2006**, *128*, 3931–3933. [CrossRef]
24. Reddy, C.R.; Rao, N.N.; Sujitha, P.; Kumar, C.G. Protecting group-free syntheses of (4*S*,5*S*,11*R*)- and (4*S*,5*S*,11*S*)-*iso*-Cladospolide B and their biological evaluation. *Synthesis* **2012**, *44*, 1663–1666. [CrossRef]
25. Crystallographic data of compounds **3** and **6** have been deposited in the Cambridge Crystallographic Data Centre as CCDC 1889697 and 1889726, respectively. 2019. Available online: http://www.ccdc.cam.ac.uk/datarequest/cif (accessed on 31 March 2019).
26. Sheldrick, G.M. *SADABS, Software for Empirical Absorption Correction*; University of Gottingen: Gottingen, Germany, 1996.
27. Sheldrick, G.M. *SHELXTL, Structure Determination Software Programs*; Bruker Analytical X-ray System Inc.: Madison, WI, USA, 1997.

28. Sheldrick, G.M. *SHELXL-97 and SHELXS-97, Program for X-ray Crystal Structure Solution and Refinement*; University of Göttingen: Göttingen, Germany, 1997.
29. Ellman, G.L.; Courtney, K.D.; Andres Jr, V.; Featherstone, R.M. A new and rapid colorimetric determination of acetylcholinesterase activity. *Biochem. Pharmacol.* **1961**, *7*, 88–95. [CrossRef]
30. Pierce, C.G.; Uppuluri, P.; Tristan, A.R.; Wormley Jr, F.L.; Mowat, E.; Ramage, G.; Lopez-Ribot, J.L. A simple and reproducible 96-well plate-based method for the formation of fungal biofilms and its application to antifungal susceptibility testing. *Nat. Protoc.* **2008**, *3*, 1494–1500. [CrossRef]

marine drugs

MDPI

Article

Altercrasins A–E, Decalin Derivatives, from a Sea-Urchin-Derived *Alternaria* sp.: Isolation and Structural Analysis Including Stereochemistry

Takeshi Yamada [1,*], Asumi Tanaka [1], Tatsuo Nehira [2], Takumi Nishii [1] and Takashi Kikuchi [1]

1 Department of Medicinal Molecular Chemistry, Osaka University of Pharmaceutical Sciences, 4-20-1, Nasahara, Takatsuki, Osaka 569-1094, Japan; ichigo-ame.xxx@ezweb.ne.jp (A.T.); n.t.rokusyo@i.softbank.jp (T.N.); t.kikuchi@gly.oups.ac.jp (T.K.)

2 Graduate School of Integrated Arts and Sciences, Hiroshima University, 1-7-1 Kagamiyama, Higashi-Hiroshima 739-8521, Japan; tnehira@hiroshima-u.ac.jp

* Correspondence: yamada@gly.oups.ac.jp; Tel./Fax: +81-726-90-1085

Received: 25 March 2019; Accepted: 9 April 2019; Published: 11 April 2019

Abstract: In order to find out the seeds of antitumor agents, we focused on potential bioactive materials from marine-derived microorganisms. Marine products include a number of compounds with unique structures, some of which may exhibit unusual bioactivities. As a part of this study, we studied metabolites of a strain of *Alternaria* sp. OUPS-117D-1 originally derived from the sea urchin *Anthocidaris crassispina*, and isolated five new decalin derivatives, altercrasins A–E (**1**–**5**). The absolute stereostructure of altercrasins A (**1**) had been decided by chemical transformation and the modified Mosher's method. In this study, four decalin derivatives, altercrasins B–E (**2**–**5**) were purified by silica gel chromatography, and reversed phase high-performance liquid chromatography (RP HPLC), and their structures were elucidated on the basis of 1D and 2D nuclear magnetic resonance (NMR) spectroscopic analyses. The absolute configuration of them were deduced by the comparison with **1** in the NMR chemical shifts, NOESY correlations, and electronic circular dichroism (ECD) spectral analyses. As a result, we found out that compound pairs of **1**/**2** and **4**/**5** were respective stereoisomers. In addition, their cytotoxic activities using murine P388 leukemia, human HL-60 leukemia, and murine L1210 leukemia cell lines showed that **4** and **5** exhibit potent cytotoxicity, in especially, the activity of **4** was equal to that of 5-fluorouracil.

Keywords: altercrasins; *Alternaria* sp.; *Anthocidaris crassispina*; decalin derivatives; cytotoxicity

1. Introduction

Marine organisms are a potential prolific source of highly bioactive secondary metabolites with unique structures that may serve as useful seeds for the development of new chemotherapy agents [1,2]. Previously, our group has focused on potential new antitumor materials from marine-derived microorganisms that produce several compounds bearing unique structures [3–5]. As a part of this study, metabolites from the fungus *Alternaria* sp. OUPS-117D-1 originally obtained from the sea urchin *Anthocidaris crassispina* were examined, and a new compound designated as altercrasin A (**1**) (Figure 1) was isolated. As has been reported previously, **1** was a cytochalasin-like decalin derivative with spirotetramic acid [6]. Previous reports have also introduced delaminomycins [7] isolated from *Streptomyces albulus*; lucensimycins [8–10] isolated from *Streptomyces lusensis*, fusarisetin A [11–13] isolated from *Fusarium* sp., and diaporthichalasin [14,15] isolated from *Diaporte* sp. as metabolites with a similar decalin derivative. The absolute configuration of this class with a spiro-lactam or -lactone cannot be experimentally determined unless a good single crystal is obtained [11]. However, in a previously reported study for the absolute stereostructure of **1**, our group has successfully determined it by experiments via a chemical transformation [6]. Our continuous search for cytotoxic metabolites from this fungal strain afforded four new decalin derivatives designated as altercrasins B–E (2–5), respectively (Figure 1). As these were minor components, the above-mentioned method was not used to elucidate the stereostructures. In this study, the chiral centers in these metabolites were assigned by NMR and ECD spectral analyses.

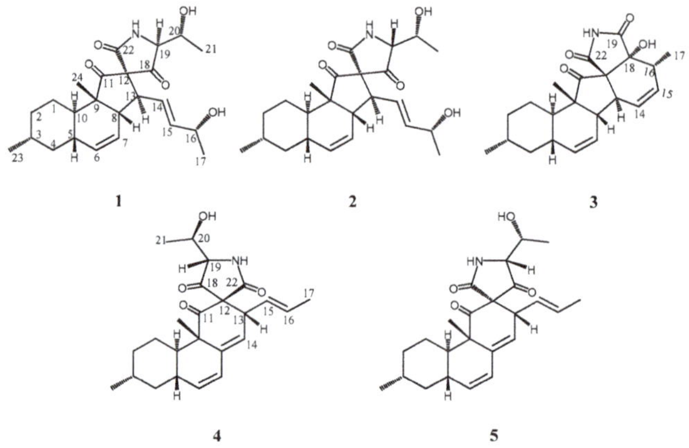

Figure 1. Structures of altercrasins A–E (**1–5**).

2. Results and Discussion

Alternaria sp., a microorganism from *A. crassispina*, was cultured at 27 °C for 6 weeks in a medium (70 L) containing 1% glucose, 1% malt extract, and 0.05% peptone in artificial seawater adjusted to pH 7.5. After incubation, the EtOAc extract of the culture filtrate was purified via bioassay-directed fractionation by using a stepwise combination of silica-gel column and Sephadex LH-20 chromatography, followed by reverse-phase HPLC, affording altercrasins A (**1**) (10.3 mg, 0.020%), B (**2**) (6.5 mg, 0.012%), C (**3**) (4.6 mg, 0.009%), D (**4**) (1.3 mg, 0.002%), and E (**5**) (5.3 mg, 0.010%) as pale yellow oils.

As it has been observed for previously reported **1** [6], altercrasin B (**2**) also exhibited the molecular formula $C_{24}H_{33}NO_5$ as established by the $[M + Na]^+$ peak in HRFABMS. The IR spectrum exhibited absorption bands at 3478, 1720, and 1710 cm^{-1} characteristic of hydroxyl and carbonyl groups. The close inspection of the ^1H and ^{13}C NMR spectra of **2** (Table 1 and Table S1) by using distortionless enhancement by polarization transfer (DEPT) and ^1H–^{13}C correlation spectroscopy (HMQC) revealed the presence of two secondary methyl groups (C-17 and C-23, respectively); a tertiary methyl (C-24) group; three sp^3-hybridized methylene groups (C-1, C-2, and C-4, respectively); six sp^3-methine groups (C-3, C-5, C-8, C-10, C-13, and C-16, respectively); two quaternary sp^3-carbon groups (C-9 and C-12, respectively); four sp^2-methine groups (C-6, C-7, C-14, and C-15, respectively); and three carbonyl groups (C-11, C-18, and C-22, respectively), including an amide carbonyl (C-22). The ^1H–^1H COSY analysis of **2** led to three partial structures, including a hydroxy butylene group (H-13/H-14, H-14/H-15, H-15/H-16, H-16/16-OH, and H-16/H-17) and a hydroxyethyl group (H-19/H-20, H-20/20-OH, and H-20/H-21), as indicated by the bold-faced lines shown in Figure 2. The key HMBC correlations shown in Figure 2 verified the connection of these three units and the remaining functional groups, indicating that the planar structure of **2** is the same as that of **1**.

Table 1. NMR spectral data for **1–3** in acetone-d_6.

Position	1					2					3				
	$^1H^a$ (*J*,Hz)			$^{13}C^b$		$^1H^a$ (*J*,Hz)			$^{13}C^b$		$^1H^a$ (*J*,Hz)			$^{13}C^b$	
1a	1.55	dq	13.2, 3.6	25.9	(t)	1.52	dq	13.2, 3.6	25.9	(t)	1.80	dq	12.6, 3.6	26.0	(t)
1b	1.12	qd	13.2, 3.6			1.13	qd	13.2, 3.6			1.20	qd	12.6, 3.6		
2a	0.91	m		36.0	(t)	0.90	m		36.0	(t)	0.87	qd	12.6, 3.6	36.2	(t)
2b	1.74	ddt	12.6, 5.4, 3.6			1.75	ddt	12.6, 5.4, 3.6			1.74	ddt	12.6, 5.4, 3.6		
3	1.48	m		33.5	(d)	1.49	m		33.5	(d)	1.49	m		33.7	(d)
4a	0.82	q	12.6	42.6	(t)	0.83	q	12	42.7	(t)	0.79	q	12.6	43.0	(t)
4b	1.87	ddd	12.6, 5.8, 3.5			1.88	ddd	12.0, 5.4, 3.5			1.87	ddd	12.6, 5.4, 3.6		
5	1.92	br t	12.6	37.4	(d)	1.93	m		37.5	(d)	1.95	br t	12.6	37.5	(d)
6	5.55	d	10.2	133.2	(d)	5.54	d	10.2	132.9	(d)	5.57	d	9.6	133.1	(d)
7	5.70	ddd	10.2, 5.0, 2.2	125.3	(d)	5.69	ddd	10.2, 4.8, 2.4	125.7	(d)	5.97	ddd	9.6, 4.8, 3.0	126.1	(d)
8	2.65	ddt	11.8, 5.0, 1.8	49.9	(d)	2.74	ddt	12.0, 4.8, 1.8	49.7	(d)	3.34	ddt	12.6, 4.8, 0.9	45.3	(d)
9				52.9	(s)				52.9	(s)				53.4	(s)
10	1.49	m		38.7	(d)	1.40	td	13.2, 3.0	39.0	(d)	1.35	td	12.6, 3.6	40.4	(d)
11				211.6	(s)				211.7	(s)				211.3	(s)
12				74.0	(s)				74.2	(s)				74.7	(s)
13	3.16	dd	11.8, 9.0	52.8	(d)	3.01	dd	12.0, 9.0	52.5	(d)	2.83	ddd	12.6, 5.4, 2.4	45.5	(d)
14	5.62	ddd	15.5, 9.0, 1.8	124.3	(d)	5.82	ddd	15.0, 9.0, 1.8	125.5	(d)	6.42	ddq	8.8, 5.4, 2.4	133.6	(d)
15	5.73	dd	15.5, 5.5	141.9	(d)	5.59	ddd	15.0, 5.4, 0.6	140.8	(d)	5.83	ddq	8.8, 5.4, 2.4	134.3	(d)
16	4.21	m		67.8	(d)	4.17	m		68.0	(d)	2.48	m		43.7	(d)
17	1.16	d	6.6	24.2	(q)	1.14	d	6.6	23.9	(q)	1.20	d	7.2	15.3	(q)
18				207.1	(s)				207.8	(s)				81.2	(s)
19	3.66	d	6.8	70.4	(d)	3.93	d	4.2	69.7	(d)				173.3	(d)
20	3.99	m		67.9	(d)	3.98	m		67.4	(d)					
21	1.25	d	6.0	20.4	(q)	1.27	d	6.0	20.7	(q)					
22				170.7	(s)				170.2	(s)				177.5	(s)
23	0.91	d	6.6	22.6	(q)	0.92	d	6.6	22.6	(q)	0.89	d	6.6	22.8	(q)
24	0.99	s		16.0	(q)	0.99	s		16.1	(q)	1.05	s		17.3	(q)
16-OH	3.79	d	5.0			3.47	br s								
20-OH	4.17	d	6.0			4.02	br s								
NH	8.01	br s				8.02	br s								

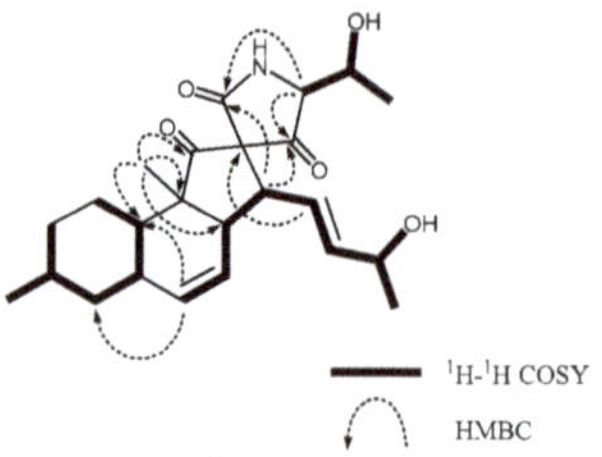

2

Figure 2. Typical 2D NMR correlations in **2**.

The stereochemistry of **2** was deduced from NOESY experiments and the comparison of NMR and ECD spectral data with **1**, where the absolute configuration of **1** was determined by the application of the modified Mosher's method after the NOESY experiment of the acetonide derivative following the stereoselective reduction at the carbonyl C-18 group in **1**.[4] The observed NOESY correlations of **2** (H-1β/H-3, H-1β/H-5, H-1β/H-24, H-5/H-24, H-8/H-14, H-8/H-24, and H-10/H-13) revealed that the relative configuration of the decalin moiety is the same as that of **1**; i.e., **2** was a diastereomer of **1** at C-12, C-16, C-19, or C-20. In ^{1}H NMR spectrum of **2** (Table 1 and Table S1), the general features closely resembled those of **1**, except for the ^{1}H NMR signals for H-19 (**1**; δ_H 3.66 and **2**; δ_H 3.93)). In addition, the coupling constant for the H-19 signal was different (**1**; $J_{19,20}$ = 6.8 Hz and **2**; $J_{19,20}$ = 4.2 Hz). These differences were supposedly related to the magnetic anisotropic effect of the carbonyl group (C-18) that reflected the change of a dihedral angle between H-19 and H-20, indicating that the absolute configuration at C-19 in **2** is opposite to that of **1**. The chemical shifts for the ^{1}H and ^{13}C NMR signals at C-16 and C-20 in **2** resembled those of **1**, indicative of identical chirality at C-16 and C-20 between **1** and **2** (Table 1). On the other hand, the ECD Cotton effects were expected to be induced by the carbonyl groups (C-11, C-18, and C22) around C-12. Hence, the experimental observation that the ECD spectrum of **2** shows good agreement with that of **1** revealed identical chirality at C-12 between **1** and **2** (Figure 3). The above evidence suggested that **2** is an epimer of **1** at C-19.

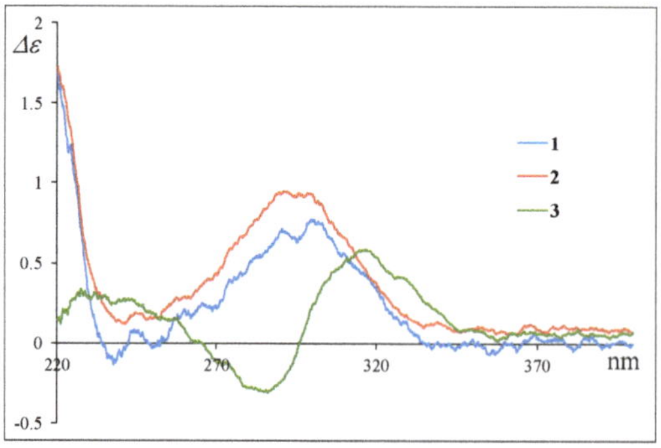

Figure 3. Experimental ECD spectra of **1**, **2**, and **3**.

According to HRFABMS data, altercrasin C (**3**) was assigned the molecular formula $C_{22}H_{27}NO_4$. The general features of its IR spectrum matched those of **1** and **2**. By the accurate inspection of the NMR spectrum of **3**, the signals corresponding to the hydroxyethyl moiety (C-20–C-21) and the carbonyl (C-18) group observed in **1** and **2** were replaced by amide carbonyl (C-19 (δ_C 173.3)) and a quaternary sp^3 carbon groups with a hydroxyl group (C-18 (δ_C 81.2)) (Table 1 and Table S2). In addition, the geometrical configuration of the side-chain olefin moiety (C-14 to C-15) as *cis* from the ^{1}H NMR coupling constant ($J_{14,\,15}$ 8.8 Hz) was revealed to be less than that of **1** ($J_{14,\,15}$ 15.5 Hz). The above evidences and the ^{1}H–^{1}H COSY and HMBC correlation shown in Figure 4 and Table S3 led to the planar structure of **3**, which had a cyclic imide. For the stereochemistry of **3**, the NOESY correlations (H-1/H-3, H-1/H-5, H-1/H-24, H-4/H-10, H-5/H-24, H-8/H-24, and H-10/H-13) for the decalin moiety revealed that the relative configurations among C-3, C-5, C8, C-9, C-10, and C-13 are the same as **1** and **2**. In addition, the NOESY correlation between H-13 and H-17 revealed that the 16-methyl group is oriented *cis* to H-13 (Figure 5). The absolute configurations in the decalin moiety were hypothesized as those of the above compounds in terms of the biosynthetic pathway. To determine the absolute configuration of the remaining chiral centers (C-12 and C-18), the ECD spectrum of **3** following a conformational consideration by the NOESY experiment and the building of an HGS molecular model was recorded. For all possible combinations, **3a** (12*S*, 18*R*), **3b** (12*S*, 18*S*), **3c** (12*R*, 18*R*), and **3d** (12*R*, 18*S*) (Figure 6), the *trans* ring junction at C-12 and C-18 such as **3a** and **3d** led to a large distortion of the five-membered cyclic imide; hence, the possibility of **3** exhibiting the **3a** and **3d** stereostructures is excluded in addition to some contradiction of NOESY correlation; i.e., the correlation between H-17 and H-13 should not be observed in **3a**. In ECD spectra of **1**, **2**, and **3**, the Cotton effect at 285 nm corresponded to the carbonyl groups ($n \rightarrow \pi^*$ interaction); hence, the absolute configuration at C-12 is assigned (Figure 3). The ECD spectra of **3** showed a negative Cotton effect at 285 nm; hence, the absolute configuration at C-12 in **3** is deduced to be 12*R*, i.e., **3** exhibited the stereostructure of **3c**.

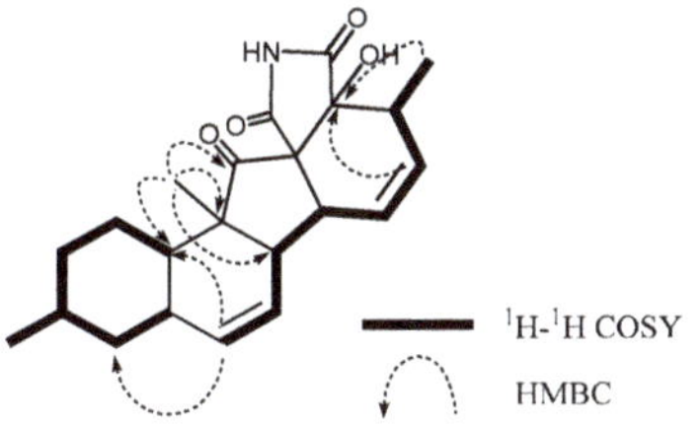

3

Figure 4. Typical 2D NMR correlations in **3**.

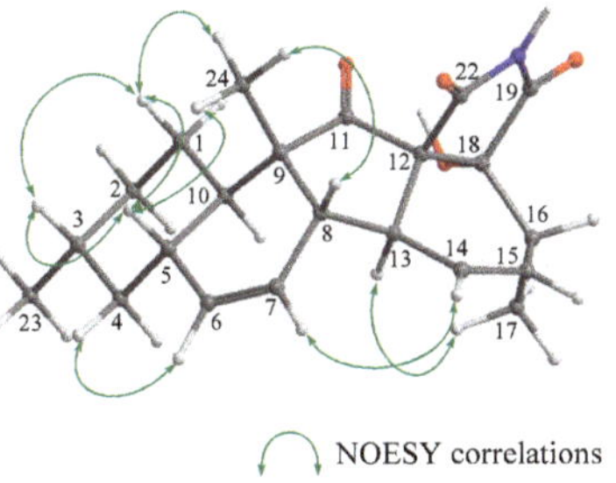

Figure 5. Key NOESY correlations in **3**.

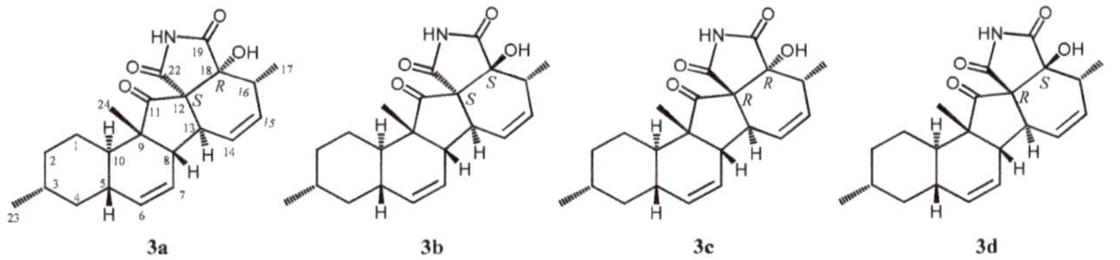

3a **3b** **3c** **3d**

Figure 6. Four plausible structures of **3**.

Altercrasins D (**4**) and E (**5**) were assigned the same molecular formula $C_{24}H_{31}NO_4$ based on the deduction according to HRFABMS data. ^{1}H and ^{13}C NMR spectra of **4** and **5** revealed similar features except that the differences for the chemical shift between **4** (proton signals: H-1α (δ_H 1.67), H-10 (δ_H 1.70), H-13 (δ_H 3.71), H-14 (δ_H 5.52), and H-19 (δ_H 3.49); carbon signals: C-11 (δ_C 208.4), C-12 (δ_C 70.5), C-13 (δ_C 43.6), C-14 (δ_C 124.6), C-18 (δ_C 208.4), and C-22 (δ_C 168.1)) and **5** (proton signals: H-1α (δ_H 1.91), H-10 (δ_H 1.37), H-13 (δ_H 3.96), H-14 (δ_H 5.70), and H-19 (δ_H 3.81); carbon signals: C-11 (δ_C 205.2), C-12 (δ_C 72.7), C-13 (δ_C 41.5), C-14 (δ_C 126.9), C-18 (δ_C 204.7), and C-22 (δ_C 170.7)) were observed (Table 2, Tables S3 and S4). Analyses of HMBC correlations confirmed that **4** and **5** have the same planar structure (Figure 7). In the NOESY experiments of **4** and **5** (Table 2, Tables S3 and S4), the observed correlations clearly indicated their homologous stereochemistry except for the spiro γ-lactam moiety; i.e., diastereomeric relationship at C-12, C-19, or C-20 between **4** and **5** was revealed.

Table 2. NMR spectral data for **4** and **5** in acetone-d_6.

Position	4					5				
	$^1H^a$ (J,Hz)			$^{13}C^b$		$^1H^a$ (J,Hz)			$^{13}C^b$	
1α	1.67	m		27.6	(t)	1.91	dq	12.6, 3.6	28.0	(t)
1β	1.20	qd	12.6, 3.6			1.20	qd	12.6, 3.6		
2α	0.85	qd	12.6, 3.6	36.1	(t)	0.90	m		36.2	(t)
2β	1.72	m				1.73	ddt	11.4, 5.4, 3.6		
3	1.49	m		33.5	(d)	1.49	m		33.5	(d)
4α	0.79	q	12.6	42.6	(t)	0.80	q	12	42.9	(t)
4β	1.85	ddd	12.6, 5.4, 3.6			1.87	ddd	12.0, 5.8, 3.5		
5	2.08	m		39.1	(d)	2.09	m		38.6	(d)
6	5.48	d	10.2	133.3	(d)	5.49	d	10.2	133.5	(d)
7	6.04	dd	10.2, 3.0	127.7	(d)	6.07	dd	10.2, 3.0	127.4	(d)
8				141.5	(s)				140.1	(s)
9				50.7	(s)				50.6	(s)
10	1.70	m		44.7	(d)	1.37	td	12.6, 3.6	45.3	(d)
11				208.4	(s)				205.2	(s)
12				70.5	(s)				72.7	(s)
13	3.71	d	9.6	43.6	(d)	3.96	d	9	41.5	(d)
14	5.52	d	1.8	124.6	(d)	5.70	d	1.8	126.9	(d)
15	5.37	ddq	16.8, 9.6, 1.8	128.4	(d)	5.37	ddq	16.8, 9.0, 1.8	129.4	(d)
16	5.57	dq	16.8, 6.6	131.0	(d)	5.62	dq	16.8, 6.6	129.9	(d)
17	1.62	d	6.6	18.0	(q)	1.59	d	6.6	17.9	(q)
18				208.4	(s)				204.7	(s)
19	3.49	d	7.2	69.9	(d)	3.81	d	4.8	68.9	(d)
20	3.99	m		68.1	(d)	3.90	m		67.0	(d)
21	1.28	d	6.6	20.2	(q)	1.29	d	6.0	20.8	(q)
22				168.1	(s)				170.7	(s)
23	0.89	d	6.6	22.6	(q)	0.89	d	6.6	22.6	(q)
24	1.12	s		17.4	(q)	1.12	s		16.6	(q)
20-OH	4.06	br s				4.02	d	6.0		
NH	7.88	br s				7.86	br s			

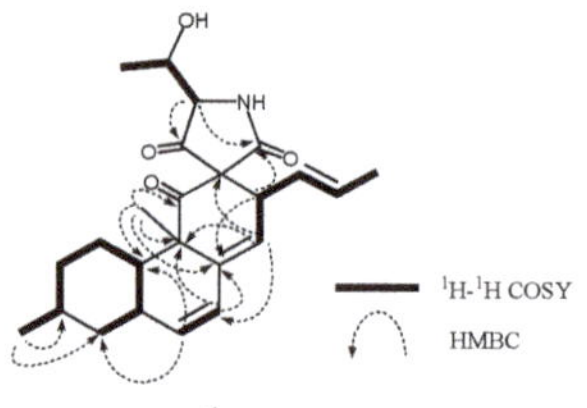

4

Figure 7. Typical 2D NMR correlations in **4**.

Their absolute stereostructure was considered to be based on the relationship between the ECD Cotton effects and the absolute configuration at C-12 as described above. The Cotton effects at 285 nm in the CD spectra of **4** and **5** clearly revealed the absolute configuration at C-12, i.e., **4** possessed 12*S*, and **5** possessed 12*R* (Figure 8). For the ^{1}H and ^{13}C NMR signals at C-20 in **4** and **5**, the chemical shifts were in good agreement with those of **1** and **2**. Based on this evidence and the fact that these were isolated from the same fungal metabolites, we guessed that **4** and **5** exhibit a 20*R* configuration as **1** and **2**. On the other hand, the ^{1}H NMR signals for H-19 in **4** and **5** demonstrated the same difference in the chemical shifts and spin–spin coupling constants (**4**: δ_H 3.49 (7.2 Hz) and **5**: δ_H 3.81 (4.8 Hz)) as those of **1** and **2** (Tables 1 and 2); hence, the dihedral angle between H-19 and H-20 in **4** and **5** is thought to be the same as those of **1** and **2**, respectively, i.e., **4** and **5** exhibited the 19*S* and 19*R* configurations, respectively. Thus, the absolute configuration of **4** (12*S*,19*S*,20*R*) and **5** (12*R*,19*R*,20*R*) is proposed. These stereostructural hypotheses will be positively supported by synthetic research or X-ray crystal structure analysis in the future.

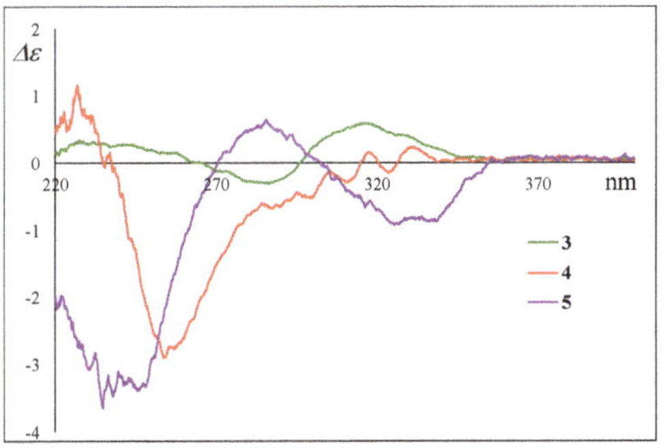

Figure 8. Experimental ECD spectra of **4** and **5**.

In this study, the cancer cell growth inhibitory property of the metabolites was examined using murine P388 leukemia, human HL-60 leukemia, and murine L1210 leukemia cell lines. Table 3 summarizes the results. **4** and **5** bearing a diene moiety (C-6 to C-8) exhibited significant cytotoxic activity against these cancer cells. In particular, the activity of **4** was equal to that of 5-fluorouracil. Contrary to our expectations, the difference in the stereochemistry was not related to the activity. Currently, investigation of related compounds isolated from this fungal metabolite is underway, as well as their structure-activity relationships.

Table 3. Cytotoxicity assay against P388 and HL-60 and L1210 cell lines.

Compounds	Cell line P388 IC_{50} (μM) [a]	Cell line HL-60 IC_{50} (μM) [a]	Cell line L1210 IC_{50} (μM) [a]
1	36.2	21.5	22.1
2	20.0	12.1	8.0
3	61.2	41.6	27.1
4	9.7	6.1	8.4
5	15.5	6.2	10.3
5-Fluorouracil [b]	7.2	4.5	1.1

[a] DMSO was used as vehicle. [b] Positive control.

3. Materials and Methods

3.1. General Experimental Procedures

NMR spectra were recorded on an Agilent-NMR-vnmrs (Agilent Technologies, Santa Clara, CA, USA) 600 with tetramethylsilane (TMS) as an internal reference. FABMS was recorded using a JEOL JMS-7000 mass spectrometer (JEOL, Tokyo, Japan). IR spectra was recorded on a JASCOFT/IR-680 Plus (Tokyo, Japan). Optical rotations were measured using a JASCO DIP-1000 digital polarimeter (Tokyo, Japan). Silica gel 60 (230–400 mesh, Nacalai Tesque, Inc., Kyoto, Japan) was used for column chromatography with medium pressure. ODS HPLC was run on a JASCO PU-1586 (Tokyo, Japan) equipped with a differential refractometer RI-1531 (Tokyo, Japan) and Cosmosil Packed Column 5C18-MSII (25 cm × 20 mm i.d., Nacalai Tesque, Inc., Kyoto, Japan). Analytical TLC was performed on precoated Merck aluminum sheets (DC-Alufolien Kieselgel 60 F254, 0.2 mm, Merck, Darmstadt, Germany) with the solvent system CH_2Cl_2-MeOH (19:1) (Nacalai Tesque, Inc., Kyoto, Japan), and compounds were viewed under a UV lamp (AS ONE Co., Ltd., Osaka, Japan) and sprayed with 10% H_2SO_4 (Nacalai Tesque, Inc., Kyoto, Japan) followed by heating.

3.2. Fungal Material

A strain of *Alternaria* sp. OUPS-117D-1 was initially isolated from the sea urchin *Anthocidaris crassispana*, collected in Osaka bay, Japan in May 2010. The fungal strain was identified by Techno Suruga Laboratory Co., Ltd., Shizuoka, Japan. The sea urchin, which wiped its surface with EtOH, was cracked by a scalpel and its inside was applied to the surface of nutrient agar layered in a Petri dish. Serial transfers of one of the resulting colonies provided a pure strain of *Alternaria* sp.

3.3. Culturing and Isolation of Metabolites

The fungal strain was cultured at 27 °C for six weeks in a liquid medium (70 L) containing 1% glucose, 1% malt extract and 0.05% pepton in artificial seawater adjusted to pH 7.5. The fungal strain filtrated culture broth was extracted thrice with MeOH (Nacalai Tesque, Inc., Kyoto, Japan). The combined extracts were evaporated in vacuo to afford a mixture of crude metabolites (52.8 g). The MeOH extract was chromatographed on a silica gel (Nacalai Tesque, Inc., Kyoto, Japan) column with a CH_2Cl_2-MeOH (Nacalai Tesque, Inc., Kyoto, Japan) gradient as the eluent. The MeOH-CH_2Cl_2 (5:95) eluate (22.6 g) was chromatographed again on a silica gel column with a hexane-EtOAc-MeOH (Nacalai Tesque, Inc., Kyoto, Japan) gradient as the eluent. The MeOH–EtOAc (2:98 and 5:95) eluate (F1 (1.9 g), F2 (1.3 g), respectively) were chromatographed on LH-20 (GE Healthcare Japan, Tokyo, Japan) using MeOH-CH_2Cl_2 (1:1) as the eluent. The fraction exhibiting cytotoxicity from F1 (105.1 mg) was purified by HPLC using MeOH-H_2O (80:20) as the eluent to afford **3** (4.6 mg), **4** (1.3 mg), and **5** (5.3 mg). The fraction exhibiting cytotoxicity from F2 (794.5 mg) was purified by HPLC using MeOH-H_2O (80:20) as the eluent to afford **1** (10.3 mg) and **2** (6.5 mg).

Altercrasin A (**1**). colorless oil; IR (film) ν_{max} 3345, 1730 1671 cm^{-1}; NMR data, see Table 1 and Table S0, and the previous report[4]; HRFABMS $[M + H]^+$ *m/z* 416.2436 (calcd for $C_{24}H_{34}NO_5$: 416.2437).

Altercrasin B (**2**). colorless oil; IR (film) ν_{max} 3368, 1729 1701 cm^{-1}; NMR data, see Table 1 and Table S1; HRFABMS $[M + H]^+$ *m/z* 416.2430 (calcd for $C_{24}H_{34}NO_5$: 416.2437).

Altercrasin C (**3**). colorless oil; IR (film) ν_{max} 3478, 1720 1710 cm^{-1}; NMR data, see Table 1 and Table S2; HRFABMS $[M + Na]^+$ *m/z* 392.1839 (calcd for $C_{22}H_{27}NO_4Na$: 392.1837).

Altercrasin D (**4**). colorless oil; IR (film) ν_{max} 3318, 2917, 1693 cm^{-1}; NMR data, see Table 2 and Table S3; HRFABMS $[M + H]^+$ *m/z* 398.2332 (calcd for $C_{24}H_{32}NO_4$: 398.2332).

Altercrasin E (**5**). colorless oil; IR (film) ν_{max} 3318, 2918 1701 cm^{-1}; NMR data, see Table 2 and Table S4; HRFABMS $[M + H]^+$ *m/z* 398.2332 (calcd for $C_{24}H_{32}NO_4$: 398.2332).

3.4. Assay for Cytotoxicity

Cytotoxic activities of **1–5** and 5-fluorouracil were examined with the 3-(4,5-dimethyl-2-thiazolyl)-2,5-diphenyl-2H-tetrazolium bromide (MTT) method. P388, HL-60, and L1210 cells were cultured in RPMI 1640 Medium (10% fetal calf serum) at 37 °C in 5% CO_2. The test materials were dissolved in dimethyl sulfoxide (DMSO) to give a concentration of 10 mM, and the solution was diluted with the Essential Medium to yield concentrations of 200, 20, and 2 μM, respectively. Each solution was combined with each cell suspension (1×10^{-5} cells/mL) in the medium, respectively. After incubating at 37 °C for 72 h in 5% CO_2, grown cells were labeled with 5 mg/mL MTT in phosphate-buffered saline (PBS), and the absorbance of formazan dissolved in 20% sodium dodecyl sulfate (SDS) in 0.1 N HCl was measured at 540 nm with a microplate reader (MTP-310, CORONA electric). Each absorbance values were expressed as percentage relative to that of the control cell suspension that was prepared without the test substance using the same procedure as that described above. All assays were performed three times, semilogarithmic plots were constructed from the averaged data, and the effective dose of the substance required to inhibit cell growth by 50% (IC_{50}) was determined.

4. Conclusions

In this study, four new decalin derivatives designated as altercrasins B–E (**2**–**5**) were isolated from a strain of *Alternaria* sp. OUPS-117D-1 originally derived from the sea urchin *A. crassispina*. Their chemical structures were confirmed by NMR spectral analysis, and their plausible stereochemistry was deduced by considering the NMR chemical shifts and spin–spin coupling constants, as well as the assignment of ECD Cotton effects. As a result of the assay for cytotoxicity, **4** and **5** bearing a diene moiety (C-6 to C-8) exhibited significant cytotoxic activity against these cancer cells, especially the HL-60 cell line. In especially, the activity of **4** was equal to that of 5-fluorouracil.

Supplementary Materials: The following are available online at http://www.mdpi.com/1660-3397/17/4/218/s1, Table S0: Spectral data including 2D NMR data for **1**, Table S1: Spectral data including 2D NMR data for **2**, Table S2: Spectral data including 2D NMR data for **3**, Table S3: Spectral data including 2D NMR data for **4**, Table S4: Spectral data including 2D NMR data for **5**, Figure S1: ^1H and ^{13}C NMR spectrum of **1** in acetone-d_6, Figure S2: ^1H-^1H COSY of **1**, Figure S3: NOESY of **1**, Figure S4: HMQC of **1**, Figure S5: HMBC of **1**, Figure S6: FABMS of **1**, Figure S7: ^1H and ^{13}C NMR spectrum of **2** in acetone-d_6, Figure S8: ^1H-^1H COSY of **2**, Figure S9: NOESY of **2**, Figure S10: HMQC of **2**, Figure S11: HMBC of **2**, Figure S12: FABMS of **2**, Figure S13: ^1H and ^{13}C NMR spectrum of **3** in acetone-d_6, Figure S14: ^1H-^1H COSY of **3**, Figure S15: NOESY of **3**, Figure S16: HMQC of **3**, Figure S17: HMBC of **3**, Figure S18: FABMS of **3**, Figure S19: ^1H and ^{13}C NMR spectrum of **4** in acetone-d_6, Figure S20: ^1H-^1H COSY of **4**, Figure S21: NOESY of **4**, Figure S22: HMQC of **4**, Figure S23: HMBC of **4**, Figure S24: FABMS of **4**, Figure S25: ^1H and ^{13}C NMR spectrum of **5** in acetone-d_6, Figure S26: ^1H-^1H COSY of **5**, Figure S27: NOESY of **5**, Figure S28: HMQC of **5**, Figure S29: HMBC of **5**, Figure S30: FABMS of **5**.

Author Contributions: Conceived and designed the experiments: T.Y., T.N. (Tatsuo Nehira), and T.K.; Performed the experiments: T.Y., A.S., and T.N. (Takumi Nishii); Analyzed the data: T.Y.; and Wrote the paper: T.Y.

Funding: This research received no external funding.

Acknowledgments: We thank Endo (Kanazawa University) for supply of the cancer cells. We are grateful to M. Fujitake and K. Minoura of this university for MS and NMR measurements, respectively.

Conflicts of Interest: The authors declare no conflict of interest.

References

1. Blunt, J.W.; Copp, B.R.; Keyzers, R.A.; Munro, M.H.G.; Prinsep, M.R. Marine natural products. *Nat. Prod. Rep.* **2017**, *34*, 235–294. [CrossRef] [PubMed]
2. Blunt, J.W.; Carroll, A.R.; Copp, B.R.; Davis, R.A.; Keyzers, R.A.; Prinsep, M.R. Marine natural products. *Nat. Prod. Rep.* **2018**, *35*, 8–53. [CrossRef] [PubMed]
3. Yamada, T.; Iritani, M.; Ohishi, H.; Tanaka, K.; Minoura, K.; Doi, M.; Numata, A. Pericosines, antitumour metabolites from the sea hare-derived fungus *Periconia byssoides*. Structures and biological activities. *Org. Biomol. Chem.* **2007**, *5*, 3979–3986. [CrossRef] [PubMed]
4. Yamada, T.; Kitada, H.; Kajimoto, T.; Numata, A.; Tanaka, R. The relationship between the CD Cotton effect and the absolute configuration of FD-838 and its seven stereoisomers. *J. Org. Chem.* **2010**, *75*, 4146–4153. [CrossRef] [PubMed]
5. Yamada, T.; Umebayashi, Y.; Kawashima, M.; Sugiura, Y.; Kikuchi, T.; Tanaka, R. Determination of the chemical structures of tandyukisins B–D, isolated from a marine sponge-derived fungus. *Mar. Drugs* **2015**, *13*, 3231–3240. [CrossRef] [PubMed]
6. Yamada, T.; Kikuchi, T.; Tanaka, R. Altercrasin A, a novel decalin derivative with spirotetramic acid, produced by a sea urchin-derived *Alternaria* sp. *Tetrahedron Lett.* **2015**, *56*, 1229–1232. [CrossRef]

7. Ueno, M.; Someno, T.; Sawa, R.; Iinuma, H.; Naganawa, H.; Ishizuka, M.; Takeuchi, T. Delaminomycins, novel nonpeptide extracellular matrix receptor antagonist and a new class of potent immunomodulator. II. Physico-chemical properties and structure elucidation of delaminomycin A. *J. Antibiotics.* **1993**, *46*, 979–984. [CrossRef]
8. Singh, S.B.; Zink, D.L.; Huber, J.; Genilloud, O.; Salazar, O.; Diez, M.T.; Basilio, A.; Vicente, F.; Byrne, K.M. Discovery of lucensimysin A and B from *Streptpmyces lucensis* MA7349 using an antisense strategy. *Org. Lett.* **2006**, *8*, 5449–5452. [CrossRef] [PubMed]
9. Singh, S.B.; Zink, D.L.; Herath, K.B.; Salazar, O.; Genilloud, O. Discovery and antibacterial activity of lucensimysin C from *Streptpmyces lucensis*. *Tetrahedron Lett.* **2008**, *49*, 2616–2619. [CrossRef]
10. Singh, S.B.; Zink, D.L.; Dorso, K.; Motyl, M.; Salazar, O.; Basilio, A.; Vicente, F.; Byrne, K.M.; Ha, S.; Genilloud, O. Isolation, structure, and antibacterial activities of lucensimysins D–G, discovered from *Streptpmyces lucensis* MA7349 using an antisense strategy. *J. Nat. Prod.* **2009**, *72*, 345–352. [CrossRef] [PubMed]
11. Jang, J.-H.; Asami, Y.; Jang, J.-P.; Kim, S.-O.; Moon, D.O.; Shin, K.-S.; Hashizume, D.; Muroi, M.; Saito, T.; Oh, H.; Kim, B.Y.; et al. Fusarisetin A, an acinar morphogenesis inhibitor from a soil fungus, *Fusarium* sp. FN080326. *J. Am. Chem. Soc.* **2011**, *133*, 6865–6867. [CrossRef] [PubMed]
12. Deng, J.; Zhu, B.; Lu, Z.; Yu, H.; Li, A. Total synthesis of (−)-fusarisetin A and reassignment of the absolute configuration of its natural counterpart. *J. Am. Chem. Soc.* **2012**, *134*, 920–923. [CrossRef] [PubMed]
13. Yin, J.; Wang, C.; Kong, L.; Cai, S.; Gao, S. Asymmetric synthesis and biosynthetic implications of (+)-fusarisetin A. *Angew. Chem. Int. Ed.* **2012**, *51*, 7786–7789. [CrossRef] [PubMed]
14. Pornpakakul, S.; Roengsumran, S.; Deechangvipart, S.; Petsom, A.; Muangsin, N.; Ngamrojnavanich, N.; Sriubolmas, N.; Chaichit, N.; Ohta, T. Diaporthichalasin, a novel CYP3A4 inhibitor from an endophytic *Diaporthe* sp. *Tetrahedron Lett.* **2007**, *48*, 651–655. [CrossRef]
15. Brown, S.G.; Jansma, M.J.; Hoye, T.R. Case study of empirical and computational chemical shift analyses: reassignment of the relative configuration of phomopsichalasin to that disporthichalasin. *J. Nat. Prod.* **2012**, *75*, 1326–1331. [CrossRef] [PubMed]

marine drugs

MDPI

Review

Natural Bioactive Thiazole-Based Peptides from Marine Resources: Structural and Pharmacological Aspects

Rajiv Dahiya [1,*,†], Sunita Dahiya [2,*,†], Neeraj Kumar Fuloria [3], Suresh Kumar [4], Rita Mourya [5], Suresh V. Chennupati [6], Satish Jankie [1], Hemendra Gautam [7], Sunil Singh [8], Sanjay Kumar Karan [9], Sandeep Maharaj [1], Shivkanya Fuloria [3], Jyoti Shrivastava [10], Alka Agarwal [11], Shamjeet Singh [1], Awadh Kishor [12], Gunjan Jadon [13] and Ajay Sharma [14]

1 School of Pharmacy, Faculty of Medical Sciences, The University of the West Indies, St. Augustine, Trinidad & Tobago; Satish.Jankie@sta.uwi.edu (S.J.); Sandeep.Maharaj@sta.uwi.edu (S.M.); Shamjeet.Singh@sta.uwi.edu (S.S.)

2 Department of Pharmaceutical Sciences, School of Pharmacy, University of Puerto Rico, Medical Sciences Campus, San Juan, PR 00936, USA

3 Department of Pharmaceutical Chemistry, Faculty of Pharmacy, AIMST University, Semeling, Bedong 08100, Kedah, Malaysia; neerajkumar@aimst.edu.my (N.K.F.); shivkanya_fuloria@aimst.edu.my (S.F.)

4 Institute of Pharmaceutical Sciences, Kurukshetra University, Kurukshetra 136119, Haryana, India; sureshmpharma@rediffmail.com

5 School of Pharmacy, College of Medicine and Health Sciences, University of Gondar, P.O. Box 196, Gondar 6200, Ethiopia; ritz_pharma@yahoo.co.in

6 Department of Pharmacy, College of Medical and Health Sciences, Wollega University, P.O. Box 395, Nekemte, Ethiopia; sureshchennupati@rediffmail.com

7 Arya College of Pharmacy, Dr. A.P.J. Abdul Kalam Technical University, Nawabganj, Bareilly 243407, Uttar Pardesh, India; drhemendragautam@gmail.com

8 Department of Pharmaceutical Chemistry, Ideal Institute of Pharmacy, Wada, Palghar 421303, Maharashtra, India; rssunil29@gmail.com

9 Department of Pharmaceutical Chemistry, Seemanta Institute of Pharmaceutical Sciences, Jharpokharia, Mayurbhanj 757086, Orissa, India; sanjay_karan21@rediffmail.com

10 Department of Pharmaceutical Chemistry, The Oxford College of Pharmacy, Hongasandra, Bangalore 560068, Karnataka, India; jyotishrivastavapharmacy@gmail.com

11 Department of Pharmaceutical Chemistry, U.S. Ostwal Institute of Pharmacy, Mangalwad, Chittorgarh 313603, Rajasthan, India; agarwalalka2014@gmail.com

12 Department of Pharmaceutical Biotechnology, Shrinathji Institute of Pharmacy, Nathdwara 313301, Rajsamand, Rajasthan, India; awadh.k1771@gmail.com

13 Department of Pharmaceutical Chemistry, Shrinathji Institute of Pharmacy, Nathdwara 313301, Rajsamand, Rajasthan, India; jadon_gunjan@yahoo.in

14 Department of Pharmacognosy and Phytochemistry, School of Pharmaceutical Sciences, Delhi Pharmaceutical Sciences and Research University, New Delhi 110017, India; ajaysharmapharma1979@gmail.com

* Correspondence: rajiv.dahiya@sta.uwi.edu (R.D.); sunita.dahiya@upr.edu (S.D.); Tel.: +1-868-493-5655 (R.D.); +1-787-758-2525 (ext. 5413) (S.D.)

† These authors contributed equally to this work.

Received: 25 May 2020; Accepted: 19 June 2020; Published: 24 June 2020

Abstract: Peptides are distinctive biomacromolecules that demonstrate potential cytotoxicity and diversified bioactivities against a variety of microorganisms including bacteria, mycobacteria, and fungi via their unique mechanisms of action. Among broad-ranging pharmacologically active peptides, natural marine-originated thiazole-based oligopeptides possess peculiar structural features along with a wide spectrum of exceptional and potent bioproperties. Because of their complex nature and size divergence, thiazole-based peptides (TBPs) bestow a pivotal chemical platform in drug discovery processes to generate competent scaffolds for regulating allosteric binding sites and peptide–peptide interactions. The present study dissertates on the natural reservoirs and exclusive structural components of marine-originated TBPs, with a special focus on their most pertinent pharmacological profiles, which may impart vital resources for the development of novel peptide-based therapeutic agents.

Keywords: azole-based peptide; marine sponge; peptide synthesis; cytotoxicity; cyanobacteria; thiazole; bioactivity

---

1. Introduction

Heterocycles are known to govern a lot of processes of vital significance inside our body, including transmission of nerve impulses, hereditary information, and metabolism. A variety of the naturally occurring congeners, including reserpine, morphine, papaverine, and quinine, are heterocycles in origin, and many of the synthetic bioactives viz. methotrexate and isoniazid contain heterocyclic pharmacophores [1]. Among heterocycles, thiazoles have received special attention as promising scaffolds in the area of medicinal chemistry because this azole has been found alone or incorporated into the diversity of therapeutic active agents such as sulfathiazole, combendazole, niridazole, fanetinol, bleomycin, and ritonavir, which are associated with antibiotic, fungicidal, schistozomicidal, anti-inflammatory, anticancer, and anti-HIV properties [2,3]. Peptides are bioactive compounds of natural origin available in all living organisms and are known for their vital contribution in a wide array of biological activity. Due to their therapeutic abilities, peptides have received growing interest in recent years. In the human body, peptides perform a lot of essential functions including the engagement of peptide hormones like insulin, glucagon-like peptide-1 (GLP-1), and glucagon and in blood glucose regulation and are used to treat novel targets for certain disease conditions, including Alzheimer's disease, diabetes mellitus type 2, and obesity [4–7].

As unique structural features make azole-containing heterocyclic peptides (especially thiazoles) attractive lead compounds for drug development as well as nice tools for advance research, efforts should be made by scientists to develop biologically active thiazole-based peptide derivatives (TBPs). TBPs are obtained from diverse resources, primarily from cyanobacteria, sponges, and tunicates. A thiazole ring can be part of a cyclic structure or connected in a linear chain of peptides either alone or with other heterocycles like oxazole (e.g., thiopeptide antibiotics), imidazole, and indole (in the forms of histidine and tryptophan), thiazoline, oxazoline, etc. Cyclic peptides have an advantage over their linear counterparts as cyclization offers a reduction in conformational freedom, resulting in higher receptor-binding affinities. Understanding the structure–activity relationship (SAR), different modes of action, and routes of synthesis as tools are of vital significance for the study of complex molecules like heterocyclic bioactive peptides, which have a broad spectrum of pharmacological activities associated with them. Further, the sudden increase in the number of peptide drug products is another good reason to study this particular category of compounds on a priority basis. Keeping in view the vital significance of TBPs, the current article focuses on different bioactive marine-derived thiazole-based polypeptides with complex structures and their potent resources, synthetic methodologies, stereochemical aspects, structural activity relationships, diverse modes of action, and bioproperties.

1.1. Resources

Various natural sources of TBPs and other heterocyclic rings containing cyclopolypeptides comprise cyanobacteria [8–40], ascidians [41–62], marine sponges [63–70], and sea slugs [71–73]. Moreover, actinomycetes, sea hare, red alga, and higher plants [74–80] were found to be other potential resources of TBPs.

1.2. Linear vs. Cyclic Peptides

In linear peptides with amino acid units between 10 to 20, secondary structures like α-helices and β-strands begin to form, which impose constraints that reduce the free energy of linear peptides. Compared to linear peptides, cyclopeptides are typically considered to have even greater potential as therapeutic agents due to their increased chemical and enzymatic stability, receptor selectivity, and improved pharmacodynamic properties. Although peptide cyclization generally induces structural constraints, the site of cyclization within the sequence can affect the binding affinity of cyclic peptides. Cyclization is a well-known technique to increase the potency and in vivo half-life of peptide molecules by locking their conformation. Hence, both the biological activity and the stability of peptides can be improved by cyclization. The reduction in conformational freedom brought about by cyclization often results in higher receptor-binding affinities. Overall, cyclization of peptides is a vital tool for structure–activity studies and drug development because ring formation limits the flexibility of the peptide chain and allows for the induction or stabilization of active conformations. Moreover, cyclic peptides are less sensitive to enzymatic degradation [81].

The cyclization process often increases the stability of peptides, can prolong their bioeffect, and can create peptides with the ability to penetrate tumors in order to enhance the potency of anticancer drugs [82,83]. Cyclization is envisioned to enhance the selective binding, uptake, potency, and stability of linear precursors. The prolonged activity may even be the result of additional resistance to enzymatic degradation by exoproteases. Cyclic peptides are of considerable interest as potential protein ligands and might be more cell permeable than their linear counterparts due to their reduced conformational flexibility.

Further, cyclic nature of peptides was found to be crucial to their bioactivity in the case of depsipeptides. For example, corticiamide A is a member of a family of structurally related cyclic depsipeptides with tryptophan moiety that include the discodermins, halicylindramides, polydiscamide A, and microspinosamide A. However, corticiamide A is the only member of the family to contain a *p*-Br-Phe at residue 11 and an *N*-MeAsn. Microspinosamide A and polydiscamide A contained the unusual β-Me-Ile at residue 6, whereas the same amino acid is found at residue 5 in corticiamide A. All these peptides were known to be cytotoxic in the low μM range and to inhibit the growth of bacteria and fungi in addition to inhibition of the cytopathic effect of HIV-1 in mosaic human T cell leukemia cells-Syncitial Sensitive (CEM-SS) by microspinosamide A. Interestingly, the cyclic nature of these peptides was important for their bioactivity, with linear versions exhibiting a loss of activity of at least 1 order of magnitude [84,85].

2. Chemistry

2.1. Structural Features of Thiazole (Tzl)-Containing Cyclooligopeptides

Aestuaramides, banyascyclamides, ulongamides (**1–3**), guineamides (**4**,**5**), microcyclamides MZ602 and MZ568, trichamide, tawicyclamides (**6**,**7**), obyanamide (**8**), cyclodidemnamide and cyclodidemnamide B, lyngbyabellins, oriamide (**9**), scleritodermin A (**10**), haligramide A (**11**), waiakeamide (**12**), haligramide B (**13**), mollamide C (**15**), jamaicensamide A (**16**), myotamides, didmolamides, dolastatin 3, homodolastatin 3, sanguinamides, cyclotheonellazoles, aeruginazole A, aeruginazole DA1497, aeruginazole DA1304, and aeruginazole DA1274 are examples of heterocyclic thiazole-based polypeptides having diverse unusual structural features from marine organisms.

Cyanobactin cyclopolypeptide aestuaramide A contained valylthiazole (Val-Tzl) and prolylthiazole (Pro-Tzl) residues in addition to proline, valine, and methionine units and a reverse *O*-Tyr isoprene moiety (Ptyr). Aestuaramide B was found to be an unprenylated analogue of aestuaramide A, whereas aestuaramide C was found to be a forward C-prenylated derivative. Aestuaramide D–F and aestuaramide J–L were found to be the sulfoxide derivatives of aestuaramides A–C and aestuaramides G–I, respectively. Similarily, aestuaramides G–L were reverse O-prenylated, unprenylated, or forward C-prenylated congeners, with or without Met oxidation, but contained alanylthiazole (Ala-Tzl) instead of a Val-Tzl unit of aestuaramides A–F. Cyclic peptides such as aestuaramides may be exceptionally widespread metabolites in natural ecosystems [10].

Banyascyclamides B and C are modified cyclopolypeptides, closely related in structure, and composed of two thiazole-alanine units. The cyclohexapeptide banyascyclamide C exhibited close structural similarity with banyascyclamide A but differed in having L-phenylalanyl-L-threonine moiety instead of L-Phe-mOzl residue of banyascyclamide A. Similarily, banyascyclamide B differed from banyascyclamide C in having L-leucyl-L-threonine moiety instead of L-phenylalanyl-L-threonine residue [11].

The cyanobacterium-derived ulongamide A (**1**) and other ulongamides B–F are alanine-derived thiazole carboxylic acid (L-Ala-Tzl-ca) containing cyclodepsipeptides which possessed a novel β-amino acid residue, 3-amino-2-methylhexanoic acid (Amha). Further, there was the presence of 2-hydroxyisovaleric acid (Hiva) in ulongamide D (**2**) and 2-hydroxy-3-methylpentanoic acid (Hmpa) in ulongamide E and ulongamide F (**3**), which had replaced the L-lactic acid moiety present in ulongamides A–C. Ulongamides A–E displayed weak in vitro cytotoxicity against ubiquitous KERATIN-forming tumor cell subline (KB) and LoVo cells [13] (Figure 1).

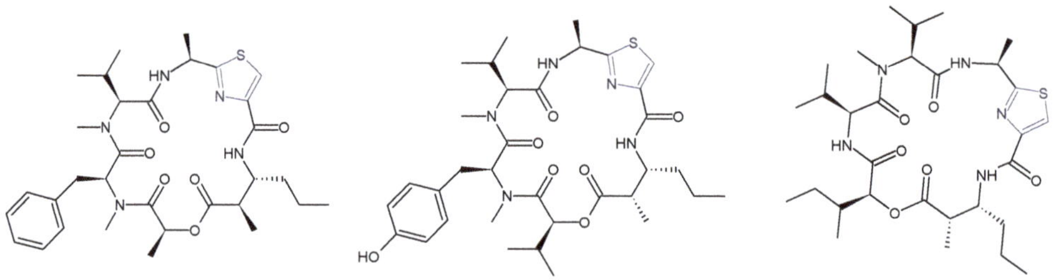

1 **2** **3**

Figure 1. Structures of ulongamide A (**1**), ulongamide D (**2**), and ulongamide F (**3**) with alanylthiazole (Ala-Tzl) and 3-amino-2-methylhexanoic acid (Amha) moieties.

The cyanobacterium-derived guineamide A (**4**) contained the common L-alanine-disubstituted-thiazole unit, unique β-amino acid 2-methyl-3-aminopentanoic acid (Mapa), lactic acid (L-Lac), *N*-methylated amino acids viz. *N*-methylphenylalanine (L-*N*-MePhe), and *N*-methylvaline (L-*N*-MeVal), but guineamide B (**5**) deviated from guineamide A (**4**) in having 2-hydroxyisovaleric acid (L-Hiv) and 2-methyl-3-aminobutanoic acid (Maba) units instead of L-Lac and Mapa units. The absolute stereochemistry of the 2-methyl-3-aminopentanoic acid (Mapa) unit in guineamide A (**4**) was found to be 2*S*,3*R*. From a biosynthetic perspective, the guineamides were found to be interesting molecules because of the presence of unusual α-amino and β-hydroxy acid residues. Further, guineamide B (**5**) exhibited moderate cytotoxic activity against a mouse neuroblastoma cell line [14] (Figure 2).

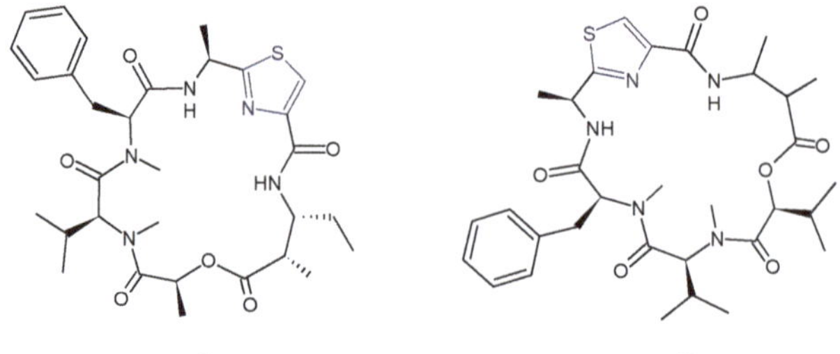

4 **5**

Figure 2. Structures of guineamide A (**4**) and guineamide B (**5**) with Ala-Tzl and L-*N*-Methylated amino acid units.

Microcyclamides MZ602 and MZ568 contained isoleucylthiazole moiety in common but differed in having phenylalanine and glycine amino acids in the former and valine and alanine in the latter. Trichamide possessed serylthiazole and leucylthiazole moieties in addition to histidine amino acid [18].

The cyanobacterium-derived lyngbyabellin A is a significantly cytotoxic dichlorinated peptolide with unusual structural features, including a dichlorinated α-hydroxy acid and two functionalized thiazole carboxylic acid units. This depsipeptide was found to be a potent disrupter of the cellular microfilament network [27]. Lyngbyabellin B is related cyclic depsipeptide in which one thiazole unit was replaced by a thiazoline ring, with the placement of the ring between the glycine residue and the α,β-dihydroxyisovaleric acid rather than adjacent to the valine-derived unit, and the isoleucine-derived unit in lyngbyabellin A was replaced by a valine-derived moiety in lyngbyabellin B. Lyngbyabellin B displayed potent toxicity toward brine shrimp and the fungus *Candida albicans* and was found to be slightly less cytotoxic in vitro than lyngbyabellin A against KB and LoVo cells, respectively [86]. The structures of lyngbyabellin E and H showed the presence of two 2,4-disubstituted thiazole rings and differed7 in having the α,β-dihydroxyisovaleric acid (dhiv) unit in lyngbyabellin E replaced by the 2-hydroxyisovaleric acid (hiva) unit in lyngbyabellin H. Intriguingly, lyngbyabellin E and H appeared to be more active against the H460 human lung tumor cell lines. From the bioactivity results, it appeared that lung tumor cell toxicity is enhanced in the cyclic representatives with an elaborated side chain [28].

In addition to two thiazole rings and a chlorinated 2-methyloctanoate residue, lyngbyabellin N contained an unusual dimethylated valine terminus and a leucine statine residue. The planar structure of lyngbyabellin N was closely related to that of lyngbyabellin H except for the replacement of the polyketide portion with an *N,N*-dimethylvaline (DiMeVal) residue [29]. The cytotoxic lyngbyabellin J contained the *gem*-dichloro moiety as part of a 7,7- dichloro-3-acyloxy-2-methyloctanoate residue in addition to the α,β-dihydroxy-β-methylpentanoic acid (Dhmpa, C_{19-24}) unit and two disubstituted thiazole rings [30].

Tawicyclamides A and B (**6**,**7**) represent a novel category of cyclooligopeptides, bearing alternative sequences of two thiazoles and one thiazoline amino acid but lacking the oxazoline ring, which is characteristic of ascidian-derived heptapeptides lissoclinamides and the octapeptides patellamides/ulithiacyclamides. Moreover, the presence of a *cis*-valine-proline amide bond facilitates an unusual three-dimensional conformation to ascidian-derived tawicyclamides A and B (**6**,**7**). Tawicyclamide B (**7**) differs from tawicyclamide A (**6**) in having a leucine moiety in place of the phenylalanine residue of tawicyclamide A [41] (Figure 3).

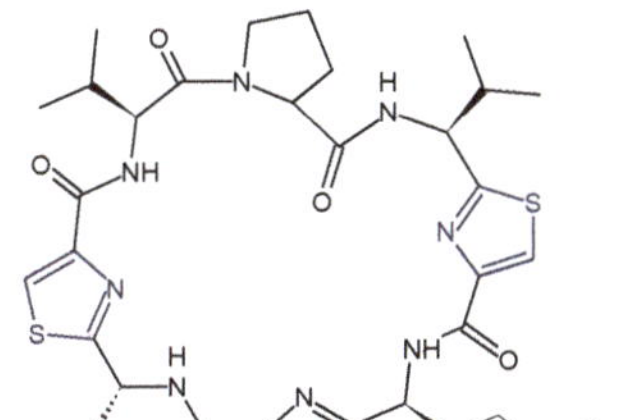

6

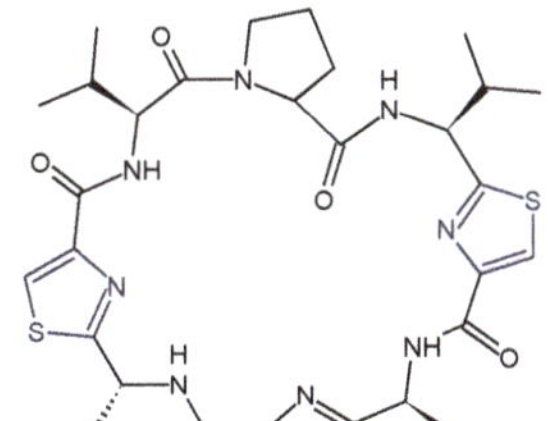

7

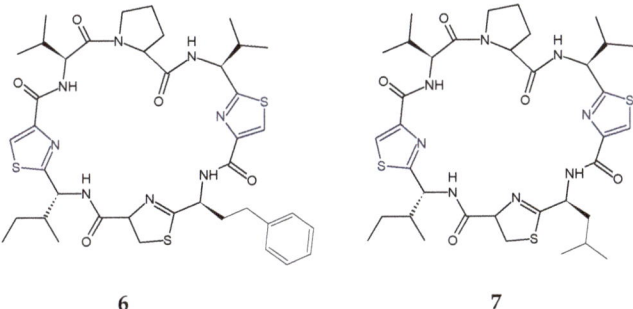

Figure 3. Structures of tawicyclamide A (**6**) and tawicyclamide B (**7**) with valylthiazole (Val-Tzl) and L-isoleucyl-thiazole (Ile-Tzl) moieties.

In the structure of depsipeptide–obyanamide (**8**), the alanylthiazole (Ala-Tzl) unit and 3-aminopentanoic acid (Apa) were present [12,42] whereas the sponge-derived cytotoxic cyclic peptide, oriamide (**9**), was found to contain a new 4-propenoyl-2-tyrosylthiazole amino acid (PTT) moiety. Further, a novel conjugated thiazole moiety viz. 2-(1-amino-2-*p*-hydroxyphenylethane)-4-

(4-carboxy-2,4-di-methyl-2*Z*,4*E*-propadiene)-thiazole (ACT) was found to be part of the structure of tubulin inhibitory sponge-derived cyclopolypeptide scleritodermin A (**10**), along with *O*-methyl-*N*-sulfoserine and keto-*allo*-isoleucine units [64] (Figure 4).

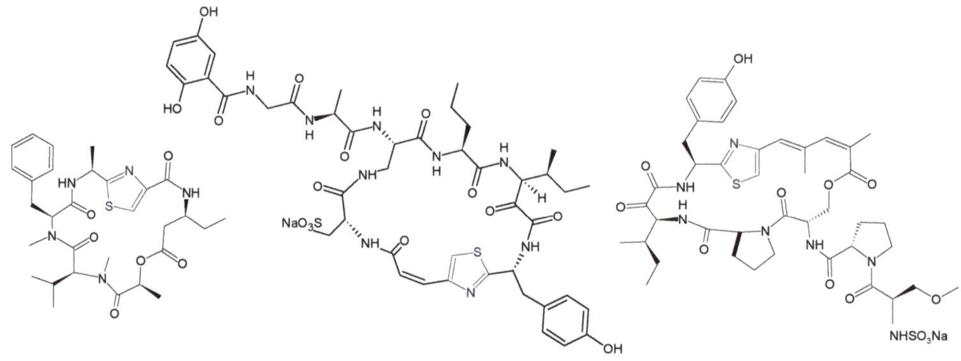

8 **9** **10**

Figure 4. Structures of obyanamide (**8**) with Ala-Tzl moiety, oriamide (**9**) with 4-propenoyl-2-tyrosylthiazole amino acid (PTT) moiety, and scleritodermin A (**10**) with 2-(1-amino-2-*p*-hydroxyphenylethane)-4-(4-carboxy-2,4-di-methyl-2*Z*,4*E*-propadiene)-thiazole (ACT) moiety.

In the structure of the bisthiazole-containing macrocyclic peptide, cyclodidemnamide B, two thiazole moieties viz. prolylthiazole (L-Pro-Tzl) and leucylthiazole (D-Leu-Tzl) were found to be present. The ascidian-derived cyclodidemnamide was found to be similar to reverse prenyl substituted cytotoxic cycloheptapeptide mollamide only in possessing the same dihyrothiazole-proline dipeptide unit (C_{20}–C_{27}), but it also contained leucylthiazole and phenylalanyl-methyl oxazoline moieties [43,62].

The sponge-derived cytotoxic hexapeptides haligramide A and B (**11**,**13**) were found to contain the phenylalanylthiazole (Phe-Tzl) moiety in addition to three proline units. Haligramide A (**11**) was the bismethionine analogue of waiakeamide (**12**), bearing Phe-Tzl moiety. Haligramide B (**13**) contained both methionine and methionine sulfoxide residues in comparison to haligramide A (**11**) which contained only methionine residues and waiakeamide (**12**), another sponge-derived cyclohexapeptide that contained methionine sulfoxide residues only [63,66] (Figure 5).

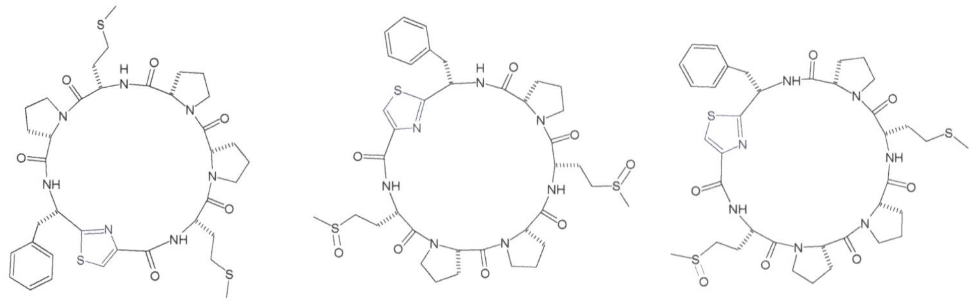

11 **12** **13**

Figure 5. Structures of haligramide A (**11**), waiakeamide (**12**), and haligramide B (**13**) with phenylalanylthiazole (Phe-Tzl) moieties.

A unique amino acid, 2-bromo-5-hydroxytryptophan (BhTrp), and an unusual ureido linkage were found to be present in the composition of sponge-derived peptide konbamide with calmodulin antagonistic activity [87]. Further, the cytotoxic depsipeptide polydiscamide A contained a novel amino acid 3-methylisoleucine in addition to heterocyclic tryptophan moiety [65,88].

The notaspidean mollusk-derived cytotoxic cyclic hexapeptide keenamide A (**14**) contained a leuylthiazoline (Leu-Tzn) unit together with serylisoprene residue in its structure and differed from mollamide C (**15**), a tunicate-derived cyclohexapeptide, in having thiazoline moiety instead of thiazole [72]. Trunkamide A contained a thiazoline heterocycle and two residues of Ser and Thr with the hydroxy function modified as reverse prenyl (rPr). The structure of jamaicensamide A (**16**), a sponge-derived peptide having β-amino-α-keto and thiazole-homologated η-amino acid residues, was found to contain 2-aminobutanoic acid (Aba), 5-hydroxytryptophan (HTrp), and a terminal 2-hydroxy-3-methylpentanamide (Hmp) unit [44,89] (Figure 6).

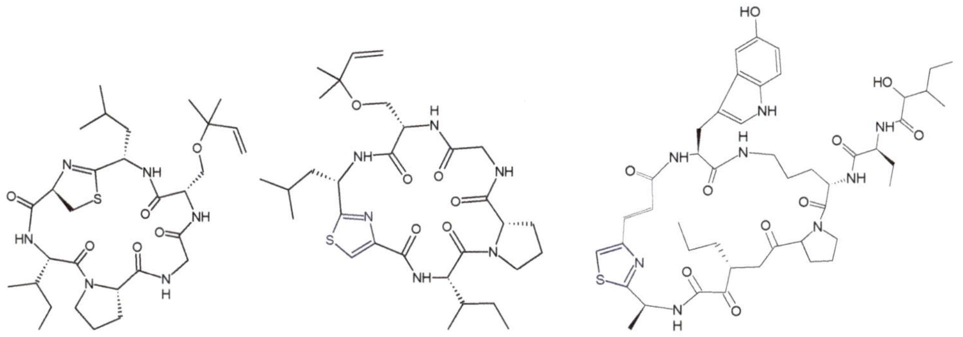

14 **15** **16**

Figure 6. Structures of keenamide A (**14**) with leuylthiazoline (Leu-Tzn) moiety, mollamide C (**15**) with Leu-Tzl moiety, and jamaicensamide A (**16**) with Ala-Tzl and 2-hydroxy-3-methylpentanamide (Hmp) residues.

Myotamides A and B are ascidian-derived cycloheptapeptides that contained three unusual amino acids containing heteroatoms including one thiazole (Tzl) and two thiazoline (Tzn) rings in addition to valine, proline, isoleucine, and methionine. Mayotamide A embodied the same Val-Pro-Tzn sequence as was found in ascidian-derived cyclic heptapeptide cyclodidenmamide and also contained an additional thiazoline (Tzn) ring. Myotamide A differed from myotamide B in having isoleucine moiety, which was replaced by valine moiety in the latter. Both cyclopolypeptides exhibited cytotoxicity against tumor cell lines [45].

Didmolamide B is a thiazole-containing ascidian-derived cyclopolypeptide that contained two L-alanylthiazole residues, and L-phenylalanine and L-threonine moieties. The threonine residue of didmolamide B was modified to a methyloxazoline (mOzn) heterocycle in the case of didmolamide A. Didmolamide B was found to exhibit mild cytotoxicity against several cultured tumor cell lines [48].

Dolastatin 3 is a cyanobacterium- as well as sea hare-derived cyclopolypeptide that contained two L-glutaminyl-thiazole (L-Gln-Tzl) and glycyl-thiazole (Gly-Tzl) units in addition to L-valine, L-leucine, and L-proline residues. The cyanobacterium-derived homodolastatin 3 differed from dolastatin 3 by the addition of a methylene group, i.e., an L-isoleucine residue in place of the L-valine residue of dolastatin 3. The cyclopentapeptide dolastatin 3 was found to exhibit HIV-1 integrase inhibitory activity as well as P388 lymphocytic leukemia (PS) cell growth inhibitory activity. Kororamide is another cyanobacterium-derived polypeptide having two L-tyrosinyl-thiazole (L-Tyr-Tzl) and leucyl-thiazoline (Leu-Tzn) units in addition to L-leucine, L-isoleucine, L-serine, L-proline, and L-asparagine residues [9,90].

The sponge-derived cyclotheonellazoles A–C are unusual cyclopolypeptides containing nonproteinogenic acids, the most unique being 4-propenoyl-2-tyrosylthiazole (PTT), 3-amino-4-methyl-2-oxohexanoic acid (Amoha), and diaminopropionic acid (Dpr), along with two or three proteinogenic amino acids like glycine and alanine. Cyclotheonellazoles B and C shared the same basic structure with cyclotheonellazole A, in which leucine (in cyclotheonellazole B) and homoalanine (in cyclotheonellazole C) replaced the 2-aminopentanoic acid residue of cyclotheonellazole A. Cyclotheonellazoles were found to be nanomolar inhibitors of chymotrypsin and sub-nanomolar inhibitors of elastase [68].

The nudibranch-derived sanguinamide A is a modified heptapeptide containing a 2-substituted thiazole-4-carboxamide moiety. Structural analysis of this peptide indicated the presence of two residues, L-proline and L-isoleucine, present in alternative continuous sequences in addition to amino acid moieties phenylalanine and alanine with an L-configuration. In this cycloheptapeptide, azole-modified amino acid was found to be L-isoleucyl-thiazole (L-Ile-Tzl). In comparison to sanguinamide A, the cyclic octapeptide sanguinamide B was found to contain additional heteroaromatic oxazole and thiazole rings [73].

The cyanobacterium-derived polythiazole peptide aeruginazole DA1497 contained leuylthiazole (Leu-Tzl), alanylthiazole (Ala-Tzl), phenylalanylthiazole (Phe-Tzl), and valylthiazole (Val-Tzl) residues and exhibited bioproperties against Gram-positive bacterium *Staphylococcus aureus*. However, in related cyclopolypeptides, aeruginazole DA1304 and aeruginazole DA1274 moieties like asparaginylthiazole (Asn-Tzl), Leu-Tzl and isoleucylthiazole (Ile-Tzl) were found to be present. L-Asn-Tzl moiety was also observed in the polythiazole containing cyanobacterium-derived polypeptide aeruginazole A in addition to D-Leu-Tzl and L-Val-Tzl residues. This cyclododecapeptide was found to potently inhibit the Gram-positive bacterium *Bacillus subtilis* [8,91].

2.2. Structural Features of Tzl-Containing Linear Peptides

In addition to cyclopolypeptides, heterocyclic thiazole ring-based linear peptides are also obtained from marine organisms. Micromide (**17**), apramides (**18**,**19**), dolastatin 10 (**20**), symplostatin 1 (**21**), dolastatin 18 (**22**), lyngbyapeptins A and C (**23**,**24**), and lyngbyabellin F (**25**) and I (**26**) are the best examples of linear peptides containing thiazole rings.

Micromide (**17**) is a highly *N*-methylated linear peptide containing structural features common to many cyanobacterial metabolites, including a D-amino acid, a modified cysteine unit in the form of a thiazole ring and *N*-methylated amino acids. The structrural components of this peptide included moieties like 3-methoxyhexanoic acid, *N*-Me-Gly-thiazole, and other *N*-methylated amino acids viz. *N*-Me-Phe, *N*-Me-Ile, *N*-Me-Val, etc. Micromide (**17**) was found to exhibit cytotoxicity against KB cells [92]. On the other hand, the cyanobacterium-derived apramides A–G are linear lipopeptides containing a thiazole-containing modified amino acid unit. Structural analysis of apramide A (**18**) suggested the presence of a 2-methyl-7-octynoic acid moiety (Moya) and six amino acid residues (*N*-Me-Ala, Pro, *N*,*O*-diMe-Tyr, and 3 units of *N*-Me-Val) and a C-terminally modified amino acid unit (*N*-Me-Gly-thz). Structures of apramide B and apramide C (**19**) differed from apramide A (**18**) in having the presence of a 7-octynoic acid unit (Oya) and 2-methyl-7-octenoic acid moiety (Moea) in lieu of the Moya moiety of apramide A (**18**). Apramides D–F differed from apramide A (**18**), B, and C (**19**), only by bearing a Pro-Tzl unit instead of the *N*-Me-Gly-Tzl residue, which had caused a drastic impact on the conformational behavior. The lipopeptide apramide A (**18**) was found to enhance elastase activity [93] (Figure 7).

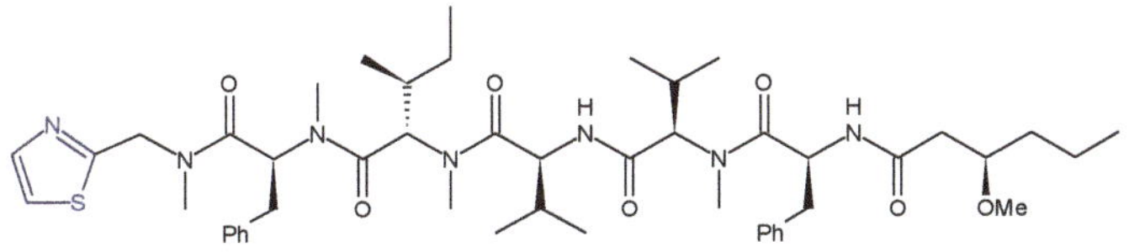

17

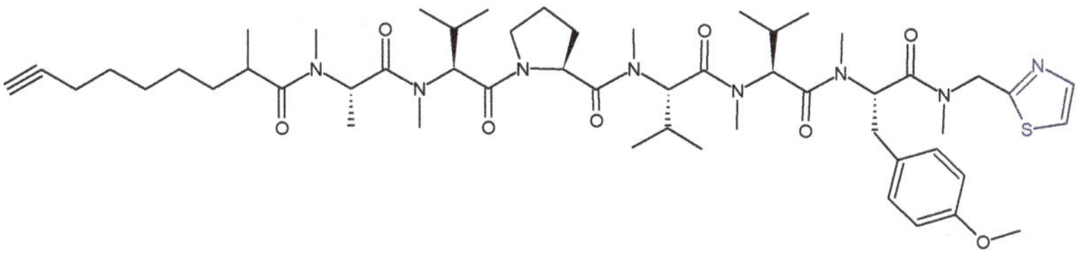

18

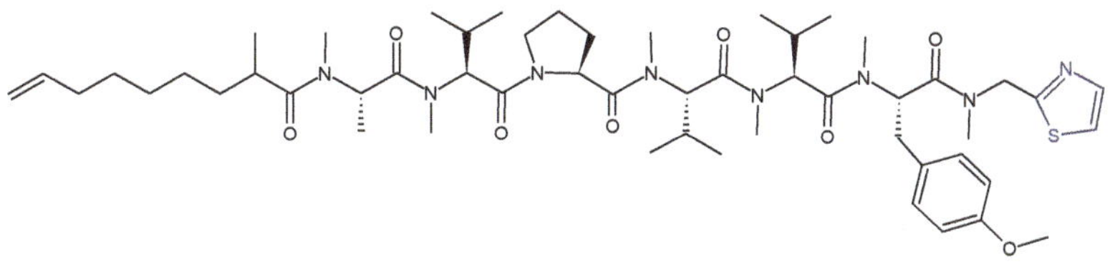

19

Figure 7. Structures of micromide (**17**), apramide A (**18**), and apramide C (**19**) with terminal *N*-Me-Gly-Tzl residues.

The dolastatins are sea hare- and marine cyanobacterium-derived compounds that exhibit cytotoxic properties. Dolastatin 10 (**20**) is a linear thiazole-containing heterocyclic peptide bearing *N*,*N*-dimethylvaline, (3*R*,4*S*,5*S*)-dolaisoleucine, (2*R*,3*R*,4*S*)-dolaproine, and (*S*)-dolaphenine [94]. Like dolastatin 10 (**20**), cyanobacterium-derived symplostatin 1 (**21**) is a potent microtubule inhibitor. Symplostatin 1 (**21**) differed from dolastatin 10 (**20**) by the replacement of the *iso*-propyl group by a *sec*-butyl group on the first *N*-dimethylated amino acid. Symplostatin 1 (**21**) is a very potent cytotoxin but not as potent as dolastatin 10 (**20**), whereas synthetic analogues lacking the *N*,*N*-dimethylamino acid residue were reported to be markedly less cytotoxic. The structure of symplostatin 1 (**21**) differed from dolastatin 10 (**20**) by only one additional CH_2 unit in the *N*-terminal residue. The absolute configuration of the stereocenter at C-26 in symplostatin 1 (**21**) was found to be 26*S*. The biological evaluation of symplostatin 1 (**21**) revealed that it is highly active against certain tumors and comparable in its activity with isodolastatin H. Both dolastain 10 (**20**) as well as its methyl analog, symplostatin 1 (**21**) were found to be potent microtubule depolymerizers [95,96].

Dolastatin 18 (**22**) is another cancer cell growth inhibitory linear peptide bearing thiazole moiety from the sea hare, the structure of which is derived from two α-amino acids (Leu and MePhe), a dolaphenine (Doe) unit, and the new carboxylic acid 2,2-dimethyl-3-oxohexanoic acid (dolahexanoic acid, Dhex). Dolastatin 18 (**22**) was found to significantly inhibit growth of human cancer cell lines [97] (Figure 8).

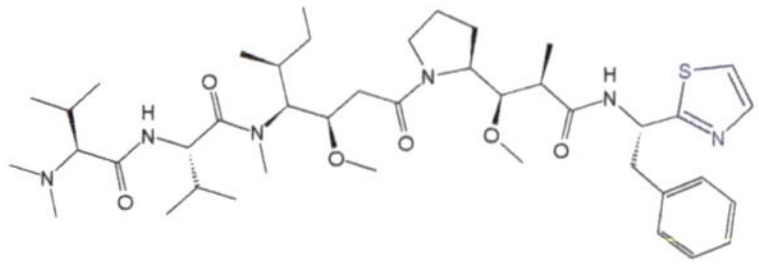

20

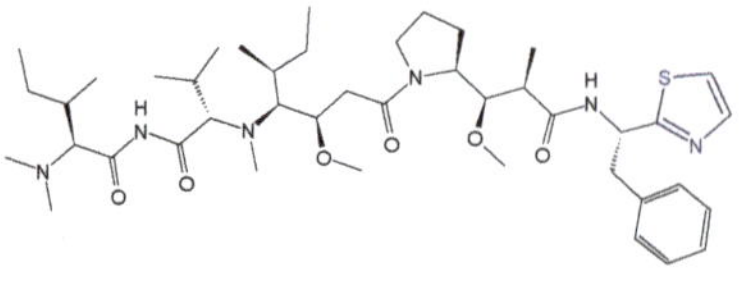

21

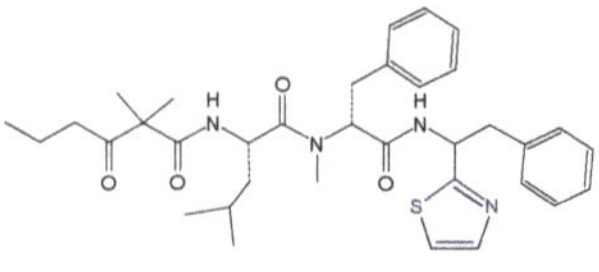

22

Figure 8. Structures of dolastatin 10 (**20**), symplostatin 1 (**21**), and dolastatin 18 (**22**) with terminal Phe-Tzl residues.

Lyngbyapeptins are thiazole-containing lipopeptides with a rare 3-methoxy-2-butenoyl moiety with a high level of *N*-methylation. The cyanobacterium-derived lyngbyapeptin A (**23**) is a linear modified peptide with a 2-substituted thiazole ring. In comparison to lyngbyapeptin A (**23**), lyngbyapeptin B and C possess the same/similar characteristic C- and N-terminal modification and differed by containing other amino acid units in between. Structural analysis of lyngbyapeptin B indicated the presence of two *N*,*O*-dimethyltyrosine residues, an *N*-methylvaline unit, a thiazole-containing modified alanine (Ala-thz) unit, and a 3-methoxy-2-butenoic acid (Mba) moiety with the absolute stereochemistry *S* for the methylated amino acids. The structure of lyngbyapeptin C (**24**) differed from that of lyngbyapeptin B in having the presence of an *N*-terminal unit and 3-methoxy-2-pentenoic acid (Mpa) residue. The structure of lyngbyapeptin D (**27**) differed from that of lyngbyapeptin A (**23**) in having *N*-Me-Val residue instead of *N*-Me-Ile in addition to *N*-Me-Leu, a thiazole-containing modified proline (Pro-thz) unit and *N*,*O*-dimethyltyrosine (*N*,*O*-diMe-Tyr) [98,99]. Lyngbyabellin F (**25**) and I (**26**) are linear dichlorinated lipopeptides that showed the presence of two 2,4-disubstituted thiazole rings. Lyngbyabellin I (**26**) and F (**25**) were found to be cytotoxic to human lung tumor and neuro-2a mouse neuroblastoma cells [100] (Figure 9).

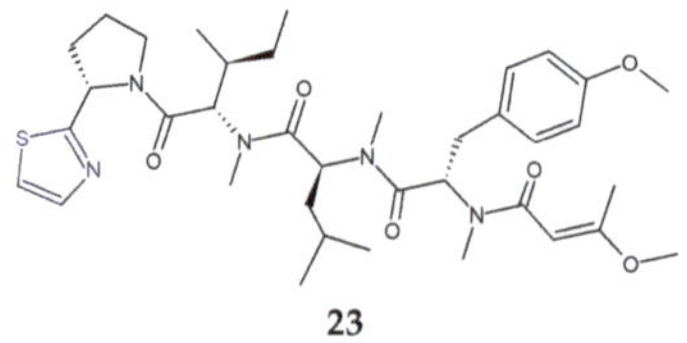

23

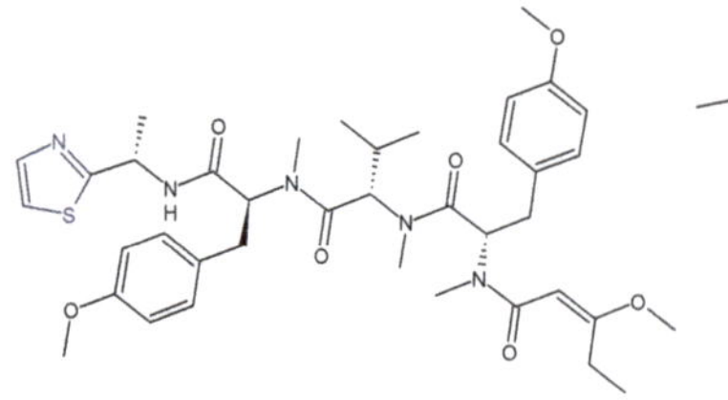

24

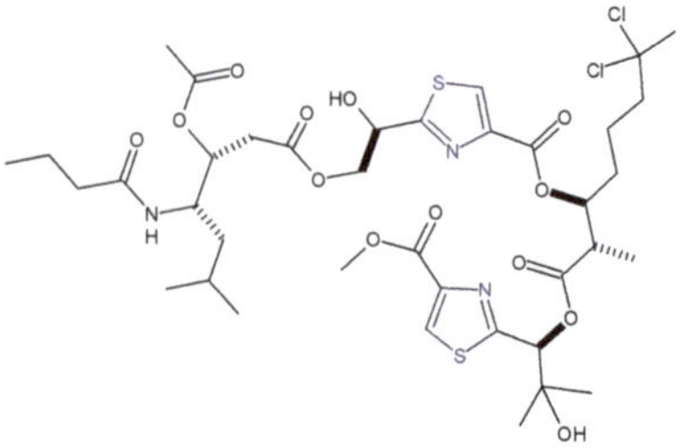

25

Figure 9. *Cont.*

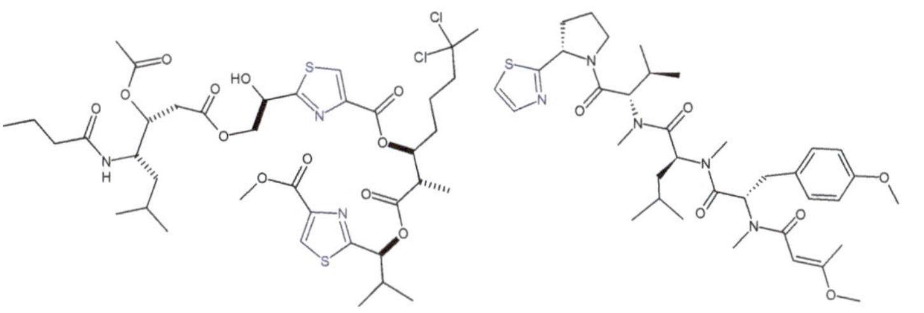

26 **27**

Figure 9. Structures of lyngbyapeptin A (**23**) with Pro-Tzl moiety, lyngbyapeptin C (**24**) withAla-Tzl moiety, lyngbyabellin F (**25**) with α,β-dihydroxyisovaleric acid (DHIV)-Tzl residue, lyngbyabellin I (**26**) with Val-Tzl moiety, and lyngbyapeptin D (**27**) with Pro-Tzl moiety.

2.3. *Structural Features of Thiazole (Tzl)- and Oxazole (Ozl)-Containing Cyclopeptides*

In addition to cyclic peptides with thiazole/thiazoline rings, mixed heterocyclic ring-based cyclopeptides are also derived from marine resources. Comoramide A, didmolamides A–C (**28–30**), vemturamides (**31,32**), dolastatins E and I (**34,35**), microcyclamide (**36**), bistratamides (**37–41**), raocyclamides (**42,43**), tenuecyclamides, patellamides, and lissoclinamides are bioactive cyclooligopeptides containing thiazole and oxazole rings.

Comoramides are cyanobactins that contained prenylated amino acids. The ascidian-derived cyclopeptide comoramide A was isolated with threonine heterocyclized in position 5 and prenylated in position 3 and was found to contain six amino acids in its structure, including two amino acids that existed as a 5-methyloxazoline (mOzn) heterocycle and as a thiazoline ring (Tzn). The additional amino acid moieties present were L-alanine, L-phenylalanine, and L-isoleucine. Like patellin, trunkamide A, mollamide, and hexamollamide, comoramide A was found to be a unique type of peptide that contained threonine residue for which the side chain is modified as dimethylallyl ether. This cyclohexapeptide exhibited structural similarilty with another ascidian-derived cycloheptapeptide mollamide in two amino acids viz. Ile-Tzn and Phe-Thr. Comoramide A was found to be cytotoxic against the A549, HT29, and MEL-28 tumor cell lines [45].

Didmolamides A and B (**28,29**) are ascidian-derived cyclohexapeptides that contained two L-alanylthiazole residues and one L-phenylalanine moiety in common but didmolamide A (**28**) contained 5-methyloxazoline (mOzn) heterocycle in addition, which is replaced by L-threonine moiety in didmolamide B (**29**). Morover, didmolamide C (**30**) differs from didmolamides A and B (**28,29**) in the oxidation state of the heterocyclic rings, having two thiazoline rings (instead of thiazoles) in didmolamide C (**30**). Additionally, didmolamide C (**30**) was found to contain a methyloxazole ring instead of a methyloxazoline ring of didmolamide A (**28**). Didmolamide A (**28**) displayed mild cytotoxicity against the A549, HT29, and MEL28 tumor cell lines [48,101] (Figure 10).

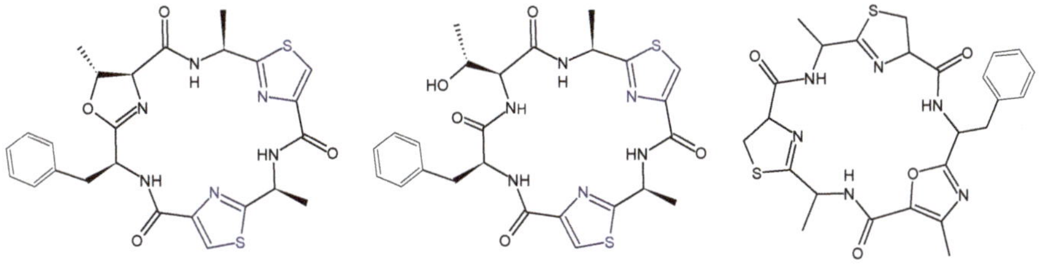

28 **29** **30**

Figure 10. Structures of didmolamide A (**28**) with Ala-Tzl moieties, didmolamide B (**29**) with Ala-Tzl moieties, and didmolamide C (**30**) with Ala-Tzn moieties.

Venturamides (**31**,**32**) are cyanobacterium-derived thiazole- and methyloxazole-containing cyclohexapeptides that exhibited antimalarial and cytotoxic activities. Structural analysis of venturamide B (**32**) indicated the presence of D-alanine, D-valine, and D-*allo*-threonine in addition to three heteroaromatic moieties. The polypeptide venturamide B (**32**) was identified as cyclo-D-*allo*-Thr-Tzl-D-Val-Tzl-D-Ala-mOzl. The cyclic hexapeptide venturamide B (**32**) differed from venturamide A (**31**) in having a D-threonine unit in place of the D-alanine adjacent to the thiazole ring. There was a close similarity between the structures of venturamide A (**31**) and blue-green alga-derived cyclopeptide dendroamide A (**33**): however, D-valine and D-alanine are exchanged with each other, adjacent to two thizaole heterocycles at C-12 and C-20. Venturamides (**31**,**32**) showed strong in vitro activity against *Plasmodium falciparum*, with only mild cytotoxicity to mammalian Vero cells. Also, mild activity against *Trypanasoma cruzi*, *Leishmania donovani*, and MCF-7 cancer cells was also reported for venturamides [34] (Figure 11).

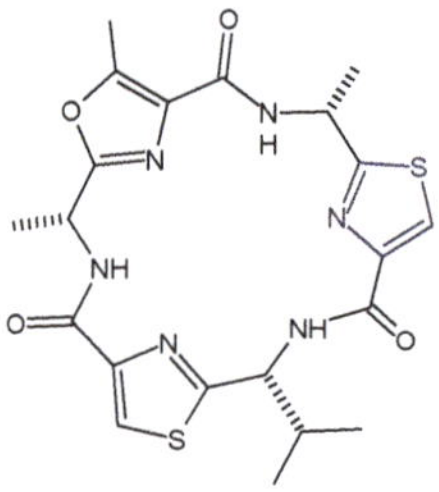

31

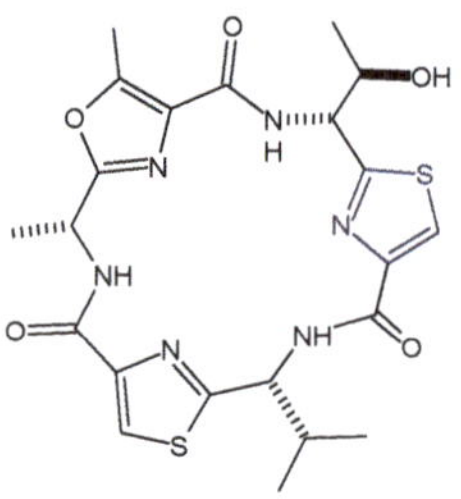

32

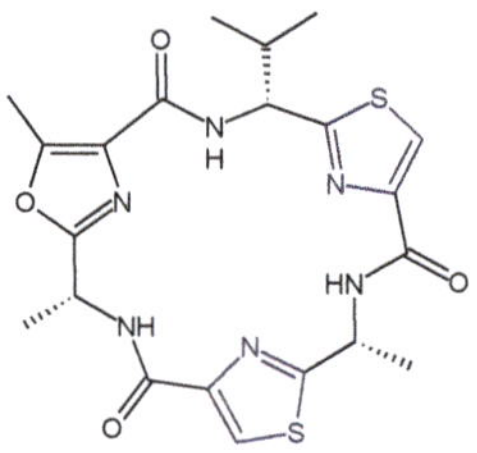

33

Figure 11. Structures of venturamide A (**31**) with Ala-Tzl and Val-Tzl residues, venturamide B (**32**) with Thr-Tzl and Val-Tzl residues, and dendroamide A (**33**) with Val-Tzl and Ala-Tzl residues.

The sea hare-derived cyclopolypeptides dolastatins E and I (**34**,**35**) were found to contain three kinds of five-membered heterocycles viz. oxazole/methyloxazole (Ozl/mOzl), thiazole (Tzl), and thiazoline/oxazoline (Tzn/Ozn), in addition to one residue each of D-alanine and L-alanine and one residue of D-isoleucine in dolastatin E (**34**) while one residue each of L-alanine, L-valine, and L-isoleucine in the case of dolastatin I (**35**). Although both of these cyclic hexapeptides displayed cytotoxicity against HeLa S_3 cells, in comparison, dolastatin I (**35**) was found to be more cytotoxic than dolastatin E [75,76]. On the other hand, in addition to two thiazole (Tzl) and one methyloxazole (mOzl) rings, the cyanobacterium-derived cyclopeptide microcyclamide (**36**) contained two usual amino acids, L-isoleucine and L-alanine, and one *N*-methylhistidine residue. Overall, the hexapeptidic structure was composed of three units viz. thiazole-methylhistidinyl, thiazole-isoleucinyl, and methyloxazole-alanyl units. This cyclic hexapeptide displayed a moderate cytotoxic activity against P388 murine leukemia cells [35] (Figure 12).

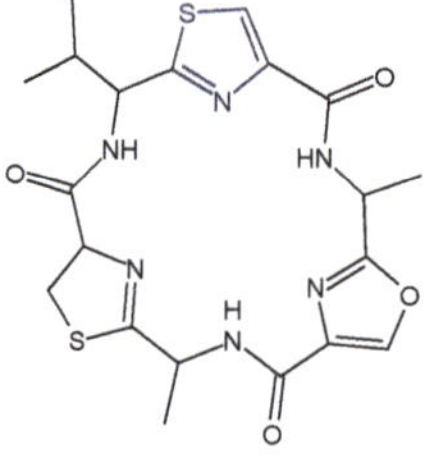

34

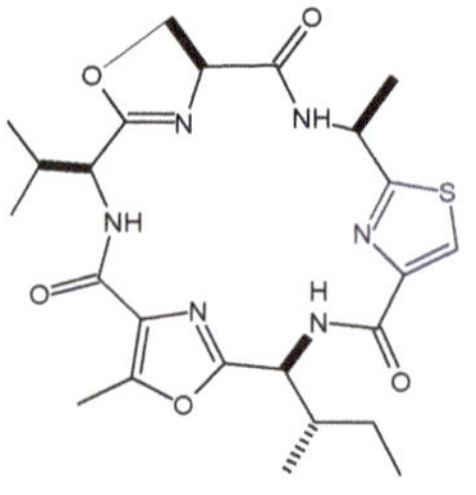

35

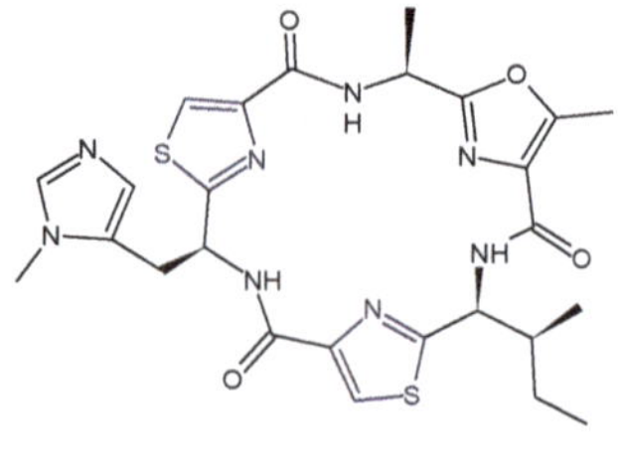

36

Figure 12. Structures of dolastatin E (**34**) with Ile-Tzl moiety, dolastatin I (**35**) with Ala-Tzl moiety, and microcyclamide (**36**) with Ile-Tzl and *N*-Me-His-Tzl residues.

The ascidian-derived bistratamide A and B contained heteroaromatic rings viz. methyloxazoline (mOzn) and thiazoline (Tzn) rings in common in addition to one residue each of alanine, phenylalanine, and L-valine. However, bistratamide A differed from bistratamide B only in the conversion of one thiazoline ring to a thiazole, i.e., these hexapeptides differed only by the the presence or absence of one double bond. Both these cyclohexapeptides displayed activity toward human cell lines viz. MRC5CV1 fibroblasts and T24 bladder carcinoma cells. Bistratamides C and D (**37**,**38**) possessed one thiazole ring in common in addition to two L-valine residues. However, bistratamide C (**37**) differed from bistratamide D (**38**) in having an L-alanine moiety instead of additional L-valine. Moreover, the other two heteroaromatic rings in bistratamide D (**38**) were methyloxazoline and oxazole, whereas in bistratamide C (**37**), oxazole and thiazole rings were present. Bistratamides E and F were found to contain three residues of L-valine in addition to thiazole and methyloxazoline rings. Bistratamide F differed from bistratamide E in having an additional oxazoline ring instead of a second thiazole ring in bistratamide E. Similarily, bistratamides G and H (**39**,**40**) were found to contain three residues of L-valine in addition to thiazole and methyloxazole rings. Bistratamide G (**39**) differed from bistratamide H (**40**) in having an additional oxazole ring instead of a second thiazole ring in bistratamide H (**40**). Further, bistratamide I (**41**) contained three residues of L-valine in addition to one thiazole and one oxazole ring. The ascidian-derived bistratamides M and N (**46**,**47**) are oxazole-thiazole-containing cyclic hexapeptides that displayed moderate cytotoxicity against four human tumor cell lines including NSLC A-549 human lung carcinoma cells, MDA-MB-231 human breast adenocarcinoma cells, HT-29 human colorectal carcinoma cells, and PSN1 human pancreatic carcinoma cells. Moreover, bistratamides G-I (**39**–**41**) and J showed weak to moderate activity against the HCT-116 human colon tumor cell line [50,59–61] (Figure 13).

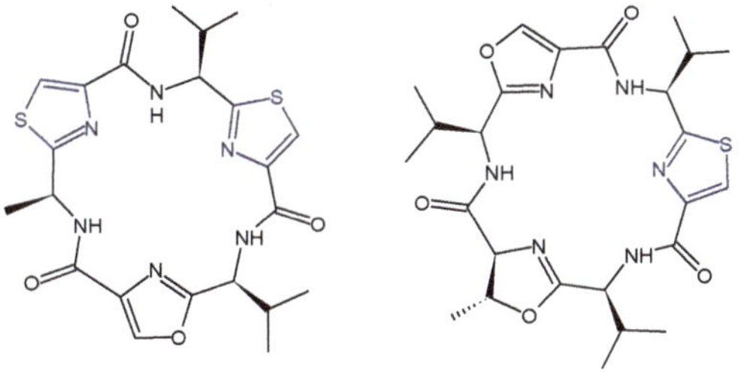

37 **38**

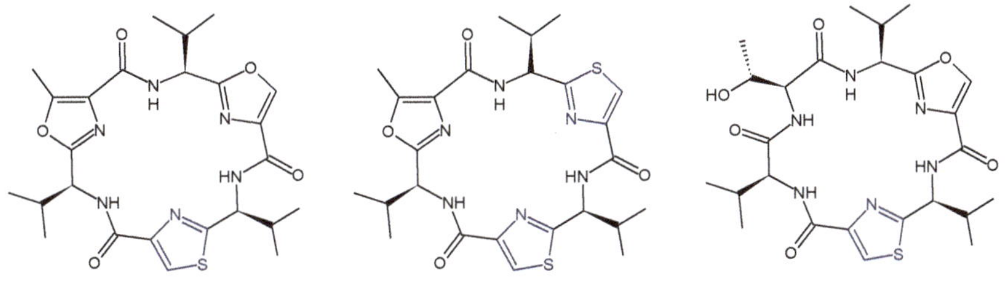

39 **40** **41**

Figure 13. Structures of bistratamide C (**37**) with Val-Tzl and Ala-Tzl residues, bistratamide D (**38**) with Val-Tzl moiety, bistratamide G (**39**) with Val-Tzl moiety, bistratamide H (**40**) with two Val-Tzl residues, and bistratamide I (**41**) with Val-Tzl moiety.

Raocyclamides (**42**,**43**) are cyclooligopeptides in which the ring system contains amide links only, and they contain three heteroaromatic rings symmetrically arranged in a peptide chain with different connected aliphatic amino acids providing structural diversity. Raocyclamides A and B (**42**,**43**) are cyanobacterium-derived oxazole- and thiazole-containing cyclic hexapeptides with cytotoxic properties. Raocyclamide A (**42**) contained three standard amino acid residues viz. D-isoleucine, L-alanine, and D-phenylalanine and three modified amino acids viz. thiazole, oxazole, and oxazoline. In comparison, raocyclamide B (**43**) contained four standard amino acid residues viz. D-isoleucine, L-alanine, D-phenylalanine, and D-serine and two modified amino acids viz. thiazole and oxazole. Raocyclamide A (**42**) differed from raocyclamide B (**43**) in having an additional heterocyclic ring "oxazoline" with a D-configuration instead of a D-serine residue. Raocyclamide A (**42**) was found to be moderately cytotoxic against sea urchin embryos [32] (Figure 14).

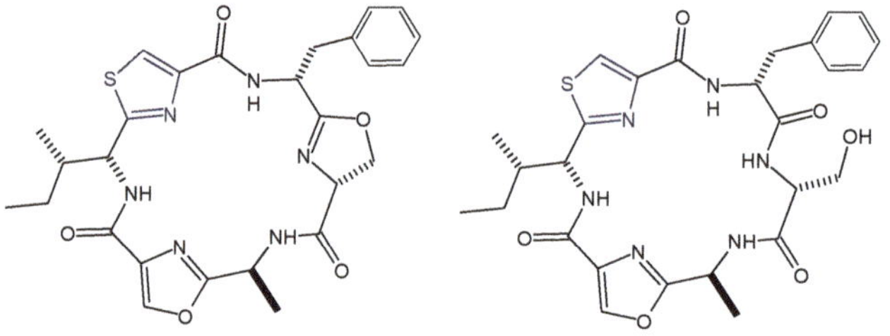

42 **43**

Figure 14. Structures of raocyclamide A (**42**) and raocyclamide B (**43**) with D-Ile-Tzl residues.

The ascidian-derived lissoclinamides 1–10 and cyanobacterium-derived tenuecyclamide A and B are other cyclopolypeptides containing thiazole, thiazoline, methyloxazole, and methyloxazoline rings which displayed cytotoxicity against SV40 transformed fibroblasts and transitional bladder carcinoma cells as well as inhibited the division of sea urchin embryos [102–105].

Various heterocyclic marine-derived thiazole-based cyclopolypeptides including those having thiazoline (Tzn), oxazole (Ozl), oxazoline (Ozn), 5-methyloxazole (mOzl), 5-methyloxazoline (mOzn), 5-hydroxytryptophan (Htrp), N-methylimidazole (mImz), histidine (His), tryptophan (Trp), 2-bromo-5-hydroxytryptophan (Bhtrp), and N-methyltryptophan (Metrp) rings in addition to thiazole, together with their molecular formulas and composition, are tabulated in Table 1.

Table 1. Heterocyclic thiazole-based cyclopolypeptides from marine resources.

Year	Cyclic Peptide	Molecular Formula	Composition	Heterocyclic Ring (s) *
1980	Ulicyclamide [53]	$C_{33}H_{39}N_7O_5S_2$	cyclooligopeptide	Tzl, mOzn
1980	Ulithiacyclamide [53]	$C_{32}H_{42}N_8O_6S_4$	bicyclic peptide	Tzl, mOzn
1982	Patellamide A [39]	$C_{35}H_{50}N_8O_6S_2$	cyclooctapeptide	Tzl, Ozn, mOzn
1982	Patellamide B [39]	$C_{38}H_{48}N_8O_6S_2$	cyclooctapeptide	Tzl, mOzn
1982	Patellamide C [39]	$C_{37}H_{46}N_8O_6S_2$	cyclooctapeptide	Tzl, mOzn
1983	Ascidiacyclamide [106]	$C_{36}H_{52}N_8O_6S_2$	cyclopolypeptide	Tzl, mOzn
1989	Lissoclinamide 4 [56]	$C_{38}H_{43}N_7O_5S_2$	cycloheptapeptide	Tzl, Tzn, mOzn
1989	Lissoclinamide 5 [56]	$C_{38}H_{41}N_7O_5S_2$	cycloheptapeptide	Tzl, mOzn
1989	Ulithiacyclamide B [57]	$C_{35}H_{40}N_8O_6S_4$	bicycle peptide	Tzl, mOzn
1989	Patellamide D [80]	$C_{38}H_{48}N_8O_6S_2$	cyclooctapeptide	Tzl, mOzn
1990	Lissoclinamide 8 [55]	$C_{38}H_{43}N_7O_5S_2$	cycloheptapeptide	Tzl, Tzn, mOzn
1990	Lissoclinamide 7 [55]	$C_{38}H_{45}N_7O_5S_2$	cycloheptapeptide	Tzn, mOzn
1992	Tawicyclamide A [41]	$C_{39}H_{51}N_8O_5S_3$	cyclooctapeptide	Tzl, Tzn
1992	Tawicyclamide B [41]	$C_{36}H_{53}N_8O_5S_3$	cyclooctapeptide	Tzl, Tzn
1992	Patellamide E [58]	$C_{39}H_{50}N_8O_6S_2$	cyclooctapeptide	Tzl, mOzn
1992	Bistratamide C [59]	$C_{22}H_{26}N_6O_4S_2$	cyclohexapeptide	Tzl, Ozl

Table 1. *Cont.*

Year	Cyclic Peptide	Molecular Formula	Composition	Heterocyclic Ring (s) *
1992	Bistratamide D [59]	$C_{25}H_{34}N_6O_5S$	cyclohexapeptide	Tzl, Ozl, mOzn
1995	Keramamide J [67]	$C_{33}H_{58}N_{10}O_{11}S$	cyclopolypeptide	Tzl, Trp
1995	Keramamide G [67]	$C_{43}H_{56}N_{10}O_{11}S$	cyclopolypeptide	Tzl, Htrp
1995	Keramamide H [67]	$C_{43}H_{57}N_{10}O_{12}BrS$	cyclopolypeptide	Tzl, Bhtrp
1995	Cyclodidemnamide [62]	$C_{34}H_{43}N_7O_5S_2$	cycloheptapeptide	Tzl, Tzn, Ozn
1995	Dolastatin E [76]	$C_{21}H_{26}N_6O_4S_2$	cyclohexapeptide	Tzl, Tzn, Ozl
1995	Lissoclinamide 3 [54]	$C_{33}H_{41}N_7O_5S_2$	cycloheptapeptide	Tzl, mOzn
1995	Patellamide F [54]	$C_{37}H_{46}N_8O_6S_2$	cyclooctapeptide	Tzl, Ozn, mOzn
1995	Nostocyclamide [107]	$C_{27}H_{32}N_6O_6S$	cyclohexapeptide	Tzl, mOzl
1996	Waiakeamide [66,108]	$C_{37}H_{49}N_7O_8S_3$	cyclohexapeptide	Tzl
1996	Raocyclamide B [32]	$C_{27}H_{32}N_6O_6S$	cyclohexapeptide	Tzl, Ozl
1996	Raocyclamide A [32]	$C_{27}H_{30}N_6O_5S$	cyclohexapeptide	Tzl, Ozl, Ozn
1996	Dendramide A [40]	$C_{21}H_{24}N_6O_4S_2$	cyclohexapeptide	Tzl, mOzl
1996	Dendramide B [40]	$C_{21}H_{24}N_6O_4S_3$	cyclohexapeptide	Tzl, mOzl
1996	Dendramide C [40]	$C_{21}H_{24}N_6O_5S_3$	cyclohexapeptide	Tzl, mOzl
1997	Oriamide [65]	$C_{44}H_{54}N_{15}O_9S_2Na$	cyclopolypeptide	Tzl
1997	Dolastatin I [75]	$C_{24}H_{32}N_6O_5S$	cyclohexapeptide	Tzl, mOzl, Ozn
1998	Ulithiacyclamide E [51]	$C_{35}H_{44}N_8O_8S_4$	bicyclic peptide	Tzl
1998	Comoramide B [45]	$C_{34}H_{50}N_6O_7S$	cyclohexapeptide	Tzn
1998	Mayotamide A [45]	$C_{30}H_{43}N_7O_4S_4$	cycloheptapeptide	Tzl, Tzn
1998	Mayotamide B [45]	$C_{29}H_{41}N_7O_4S_4$	cycloheptapeptide	Tzl, Tzn
1998	Keramamide K [109]	$C_{44}H_{60}N_{10}O_{11}S$	cyclopolypeptide	Tzl, Metrp
1998	Ulithiacyclamide F [51]	$C_{35}H_{42}N_8O_7S_4$	bicycle peptide	Tzl, mOzn
1998	Ulithiacyclamide G [51]	$C_{35}H_{42}N_8O_7S_4$	bicycle peptide	Tzl, mOzn
1998	Comoramide A [45]	$C_{34}H_{48}N_6O_6S$	cyclohexapeptide	Tzn, mOzn
1998	Patellamide G [51]	$C_{38}H_{50}N_8O_7S_2$	cyclooctapeptide	Tzl, mOzn
1998	Tenuecyclamide A [105]	$C_{19}H_{20}N_6O_4S_2$	cyclohexapeptide	Tzl, mOzl
1998	Tenuecyclamide C [105]	$C_{20}H_{22}N_6O_4S_3$	cyclohexapeptide	Tzl, mOzl
1998	Tenuecyclamide D [105]	$C_{20}H_{22}N_6O_5S_3$	cyclohexapeptide	Tzl, mOzl
2000	Haligramide A [63]	$C_{37}H_{49}N_7O_6S$	cyclohexapeptide	Tzl
2000	Haligramide B [63]	$C_{37}H_{49}N_7O_7S$	cyclohexapeptide	Tzl
2000	Dolastatin 3 [9]	$C_{25}H_{36}N_6O_5S_2$	cyclopentapeptide	Tzl
2000	Homodolastatin 3 [9]	$C_{30}H_{42}N_8O_6S_2$	cyclopentapeptide	Tzl
2000	Lyngbyabellin A [27]	$C_{29}H_{40}N_4O_7S_2Cl_2$	cyclodepsipeptide	Tzl
2000	Lyngbyabellin B [86]	$C_{28}H_{40}N_4O_7S_2Cl_2$	cyclodepsipeptide	Tzl, Tzn
2000	Kororamide [9]	$C_{45}H_{64}N_{10}O_{10}S_2$	cyclononapeptide	Tzl, Tzn
2000	Lissoclinamide 9 [52]	$C_{35}H_{45}N_7O_5S_2$	cycloheptapeptide	Tzl, Tzn, mOzn
2000	Ceratospongamide [77]	$C_{41}H_{49}N_7O_6S$	cycloheptapeptide	Tzl, mOzn
2000	Microcyclamide [35]	$C_{26}H_{30}N_8O_4S_2$	cyclohexapeptide	Tzl, mOzl, mImz
2001	Nostocyclamide M [36]	$C_{20}H_{22}N_6O_4S_3$	cyclohexapeptide	Tzl, mOzl
2002	Cyclodidemnamide B [42]	$C_{32}H_{47}N_7O_6S_2$	cycloheptapeptide	Tzl
2002	Obyanamide [12]	$C_{30}H_{41}N_5O_6S$	cyclodepsipeptide	Tzl
2002	Ulongamide A [13]	$C_{32}H_{45}N_5O_6S$	cyclodepsipeptide	Tzl
2002	Ulongamide D [13]	$C_{34}H_{49}N_5O_7S$	cyclodepsipeptide	Tzl
2002	Ulongamide E [13]	$C_{35}H_{51}N_5O_7S$	cyclodepsipeptide	Tzl
2002	Ulongamide B [13]	$C_{32}H_{45}N_5O_7S$	cyclodepsipeptide	Tzl

Table 1. *Cont.*

Year	Cyclic Peptide	Molecular Formula	Composition	Heterocyclic Ring (s) *
2002	Ulongamide C [13]	$C_{36}H_{45}N_5O_7S$	cyclodepsipeptide	Tzl
2002	Ulongamide F [13]	$C_{30}H_{49}N_5O_6S$	cyclodepsipeptide	Tzl
2002	Banyascyclamide B [11]	$C_{22}H_{30}N_6O_5S_2$	cyclohexapeptide	Tzl
2002	Banyascyclamide C [11]	$C_{25}H_{28}N_6O_5S_2$	cyclohexapeptide	Tzl
2002	Banyascyclamide A [11]	$C_{25}H_{26}N_6O_4S_2$	cyclohexapeptide	Tzl, mOzn
2002	Leucamide A [70]	$C_{29}H_{37}N_7O_6S$	cycloheptapeptide	Tzl, Ozl, mOzl
2003	Guineamide A [14]	$C_{31}H_{44}N_5O_6S$	cyclodepsipeptide	Tzl
2003	Guineamide B [14]	$C_{32}H_{45}N_5O_6S$	cyclodepsipeptide	Tzl
2003	Didmolamide A [48]	$C_{25}H_{26}N_6O_4S_2$	cyclohexapeptide	Tzl
2003	Didmolamide B [48]	$C_{25}H_{28}N_6O_5S_2$	cyclohexapeptide	Tzl
2003	Bistratamide J [50]	$C_{25}H_{36}N_6O_5S_2$	cyclohexapeptide	Tzl
2003	Bistratamide I [50]	$C_{25}H_{36}N_6O_5S_2$	cyclohexapeptide	Tzl, Ozl
2003	Bistratamide H [50]	$C_{25}H_{32}N_6O_4S_2$	cyclohexapeptide	Tzl, mOzl
2003	Bistratamide E [50]	$C_{25}H_{34}N_6O_4S_2$	cyclohexapeptide	Tzl, mOzn
2003	Bistratamide G [50]	$C_{25}H_{32}N_6O_5S$	cyclohexapeptide	Tzl, Ozl, mOzl
2003	Bistratamide F [50]	$C_{26}H_{36}N_6O_5S$	cyclohexapeptide	Tzl, Ozn, mOzn
2003	Myriastramide C [69]	$C_{42}H_{53}N_9O_7S$	cyclooctapeptide	Tzl, Ozl, Trp
2003	Bistratamide B [60]	$C_{27}H_{32}N_6O_4S_2$	cyclohexapeptide	Tzl, Tzn, mOzn
2004	Scleritodermin A [64]	$C_{42}H_{54}N_7O_{10}SNa$	cyclopolypeptide	Tzl
2005	Lyngbyabellin E [28]	$C_{37}H_{51}N_3O_{12}S_2Cl_2$	cyclodepsipeptide	Tzl
2005	Lyngbyabellin H [28]	$C_{37}H_{51}N_3O_{11}S_2Cl_2$	cyclodepsipeptide	Tzl
2005	Mechercharmycin A [79]	$C_{35}H_{32}N_8O_7S$	cyclooligopeptide	Tzl, Ozl
2006	Trichamide [17]	$C_{44}H_{66}N_{16}O_{12}S_2$	cyclopolypeptide	Tzl, His
2007	Urukthapelstatin A [78]	$C_{34}H_{30}N_8O_6S_2$	cyclooligopeptide	Tzl, Ozl
2007	Venturamide A [34]	$C_{21}H_{24}N_6O_4S_2$	cyclohexapeptide	Tzl, mOzl
2007	Venturamide B [34]	$C_{22}H_{26}N_6O_5S_2$	cyclohexapeptide	Tzl, mOzl
2008	Mollamide C [46]	$C_{30}H_{46}N_6O_6S$	cyclohexapeptide	Tzl
2008	Aerucyclamide B [37]	$C_{24}H_{33}N_6O_4S_2$	cyclohexapeptide	Tzl, mOzn
2008	Aerucyclamide A [37]	$C_{24}H_{34}N_6O_4S_2$	cyclohexapeptide	Tzl, Tzn, mOzn
2008	Aerucyclamide D [38]	$C_{26}H_{31}N_6O_4S_3$	cyclohexapeptide	Tzl, Tzn, mOzn
2008	Aerucyclamide C [38]	$C_{24}H_{32}N_6O_5S$	cyclohexapeptide	Tzl, Ozl, mOzn
2009	Sanguinamide A [73]	$C_{37}H_{52}N_7O_6S$	cycloheptapeptide	Tzl
2009	Sanguinamide B [73]	$C_{33}H_{43}N_8O_6S_2$	cyclooctapeptide	Tzl, Ozl
2010	Microcyclamide MZ602 [18]	$C_{28}H_{38}N_6O_7S$	cyclohexapeptide	Tzl
2010	Microcyclamide MZ568 [18]	$C_{25}H_{40}N_6O_7S$	cyclohexapeptide	Tzl
2010	Aeruginazole A [91]	$C_{53}H_{66}N_{13}O_{11}S_3$	cyclododecapeptide	Tzl
2010	Lyngbyabellin J [30]	$C_{37}H_{51}N_3O_{12}S_2Cl_2$	cyclodepsipeptide	Tzl
2010	27-deoxylyngbyabellin A [30]	$C_{29}H_{40}N_4O_6S_2Cl_2$	cyclodepsipeptide	Tzl
2012	Aeruginazole DA1497 [8]	$C_{68}H_{91}N_{17}NaO_{14}S_4$	cyclopolypeptide	Tzl
2012	Aeruginazole DA1304 [8]	$C_{61}H_{72}N_{14}NaO_{13}S_3$	cyclopolypeptide	Tzl
2012	Aeruginazole DA1274 [8]	$C_{60}H_{70}N_{14}NaO_{12}S_3$	cyclopolypeptide	Tzl
2012	Lyngbyabellin N [29]	$C_{40}H_{58}N_4O_{11}S_2Cl_2$	cyclodepsipeptide	Tzl
2012	Largazole [16]	$C_{29}H_{38}N_4O_5S_3$	cyclodepsipeptide	Tzl, Tzn
2012	Marthiapeptide A [74]	$C_{30}H_{31}N_7O_3S_4$	cyclooligopeptide	Tzl, Tzn
2012	Calyxamide A [110]	$C_{45}H_{61}N_{11}O_{12}S$	cyclooligopeptide	Tzl, Htrp

Table 1. *Cont.*

Year	Cyclic Peptide	Molecular Formula	Composition	Heterocyclic Ring (s) *
2012	Calyxamide B [110]	$C_{45}H_{61}N_{11}O_{12}S$	cyclooligopeptide	Tzl, Htrp
2013	Aestuaramide A [10]	$C_{40}H_{51}N_7O_6S_3$	cyclopolypeptide	Tzl
2013	Aestuaramide B [10]	$C_{35}H_{43}N_7O_6S_3$	cyclopolypeptide	Tzl
2013	Aestuaramide C [10]	$C_{40}H_{51}N_7O_6S_3$	cyclopolypeptide	Tzl
2014	Balgacyclamide A [33]	$C_{25}H_{37}N_6O_5S$	cyclooligopeptide	Tzl, mOzn
2014	Balgacyclamide B [33]	$C_{25}H_{39}N_6O_6S$	cyclooligopeptide	Tzl, mOzn
2014	Balgacyclamide C [33]	$C_{28}H_{37}N_6O_6S$	cyclooligopeptide	Tzl, mOzn
2016	Jamaicensamide A [89]	$C_{45}H_{61}N_9O_{10}S$	cyclooligopeptide	Tzl, Htrp
2017	Cyclotheonellazole A [68]	$C_{44}H_{54}N_9O_{14}S_2Na_2$	cyclopolypeptide	Tzl
2017	Cyclotheonellazole B [68]	$C_{45}H_{57}N_9O_{14}S_2Na$	cyclopolypeptide	Tzl
2017	Cyclotheonellazole C [68]	$C_{43}H_{52}N_9O_{14}S_2Na_2$	cyclopolypeptide	Tzl
2017	Bistratamide M, N [61]	$C_{21}H_{24}N_6O_4S_2$	cyclohexapeptide	Tzl, Ozl

* Tzl: Thiazole, Tzn: Thiazoline, Ozl: Oxazole, Ozn: Oxazoline, mOzl: 5-methyloxazole, mOzn: 5-methyloxazoline, Htrp: 5-hydroxytryptophan, mImz: N-methylimidazole, His: histidine, Trp: tryptophan, Bhtrp: 2-bromo-5-hydroxytryptophan, Metrp: N-methyltryptophan.

2.4. Structural Features of Thiopeptide Antibiotics

Thiopeptides are a novel family of antibiotics which are associated with a lot of pharmacological properties including immunosuppressive, antineoplastic, antimalarial, and potent antimicrobial activity against Gram-positive bacteria. Due to their interesting structures and bioprofile against bacteria, thiopeptides have attracted the attention of researchers and scientists as a new class of emerging antibiotics. The most important characteristic feature of the thiopeptides is the central nitrogen-containing six-membered ring with diverse oxidation states. On the basis of different oxidation states of the central ring of thiopeptides, they can belong to the "a series" with a totally reduced central piperidine, the "b series" with a 1,2-dehydropiperidine ring, and the "c series" with a piperidine ring fused with imidazoline. All members of series a, b, and c have a macrocycle which contains a quinaldic acid moiety. The d series shows a trisubstituted pyridine ring, and the e series is known for the hydroxyl group in the central tetrasubstituted pyridine ring. The e series also presents a macrocycle formed by a modified 3,4-dimethylindolic acid moiety. The central ring in thiopeptides serves as a scaffold to at least one macrocycle and a tail, containing different thiazoles and oxazoles which are developed by dehydration/dehydrosulfanylation of amino acid like serine, cysteine, etc. TP-1161, YM-266183, YM-266184, kocurin, baringolin, geninthiocin, Ala-geninthiocin, and Val-geninthiocin are examples of thiopeptides from marine resources [111].

TP-1161 belongs to the "d series" of thiopeptide antibiotics, produced by a marine sediment-derived *Nocardiopsis* sp. Structural features of this thiopeptide include the three 2,4-disubstituted thiazoles and one 2,4-disubstituted oxazole moiety in addition to the presence of a trisubstitued pyridine (Pyr) functional unit and an unusual aminoacetone moiety. TP-1161 displayed good activity against a panel of Gram-positive bacteria including *Staphylococcus aureus*, *Staphylococcus haemolyticus*, *Staphylococcus epidermidis*, *Enterococcus faecium*, and *Enterococcus faecalis* [112].

YM-266183 and YM-266184 are novel thiopeptide antibiotics produced by *Bacillus cereus* isolated from a marine sponge and structurally related to a known family of antibiotics that include thiocillins and micrococcins. Structural analysis of these thiopeptides indicated the presence of several unusual amino acids with heteroaromatic moieties, including the six thiazole rings, a 2,3,6-trisubstituted pyridine residue to which three of thiazole units are attached, a 2-amino-2-butanoic acid unit with an aminoacetone residue, a (Z)-2-amino-2-butenoic acid unit attached to a threonine residue, and a 3-hydroxyvaline moiety. There was a close similarity in structures of YM-266183 and YM-266184 except for the presence of a methoxy group (C55) in YM-266184 instead of the hydroxy group of

YM-266183. These new antibacterial substances were found to exhibit activity against drug-resistant bacteria [113].

Kocurin is a new anti-methicillin-resistant *Staphylococcus aureus* (MRSA) bioactive compound, belonging to the thiazolyl peptide family of antibiotics, obtained from sponge-derived *Kocuria* and *Micrococcus* spp. Structural analysis of this thiopeptide indicated the presence of several heteroaromatic moieties, including one thiazoline and four thiazole rings, one methyloxazole ring and a 2,3,6-trisubstituted pyridine residue to which two of thiazole units and one methyloxazole unit are attached, aromatic amino acids like phenylalanine and tyrosine, and two proline units. Kocurin was found to be closely related to two known thiazolyl peptide antibiotics with similar modes of action: GE37468A and GE2270. The antimicrobial activity profile of kocurin indicated the extreme potency against Gram-positive bacteria with minimum inhibitory concentration (MIC) values of 0.25–0.5 µg/mL against methicillin-resistant *Staphylococcus aureus* (MRSA) [114].

Baringolin is a novel thiopeptide of the d series, containing a central 2,3,6-trisubstituted pyridine, derived from fermentation of the marine-derived bacterium *Kucuria* sp. The macrocycle in baringolin contained three thiazoles—a methyloxazole and pyridine ring, a thiazoline ring with an α-chiral center, and a pyrrolidine motif derived from a proline residue—in addition to three natural amino acids viz. tyrosine, phenylalanine, and asparagine. The long peptidic tail was found to be a pentapeptide containing three methylidenes resulting from dehydration of serine that is attached to the pyridine through a fourth thiazole. This thiopeptide displayed important antibacterial activity against *Staphylococcus aureus*, *Micrococcus luteus*, *Propionibacterium acnes*, and *Bacillus subtilis* at nanomolar concentrations [115].

Ala-geninthiocin, geninthiocin, and Val-geninthiocin are new broad-spectrum thiopeptide antibiotics produced from the cultured marine *Streptomyces* sp. Structural analysis of all three thiopeptides indicated the presence of heteroaromatic moieties, including one thiazole and two oxazole rings, one methyloxazole ring, and a 2,3,6-trisubstituted pyridine residue to which two of thiazole units are attached at the 2 and 3 positions, including proteinogenic amino acid viz. L-threonine. The peptide structure of Ala-geninthiocin is largely similar to geninthiocin, the only difference being the presence of an L-Alanine residue instead of dealanine at the C-terminal amide. Further, Val-geninthiocin contained L-valine moiety instead of L-hydroxyvaline of geninthiocin. Ala-geninthiocin was found to exhibit good activity against Gram-positive bacteria including *Staphylococcus aureus*, *Bacillus subtilis*, *Mycobacterium smegmatis*, and *Micrococcus luteus* as well as cytotoxicity against A549 human lung carcinoma cells. When compared to geninthiocin, Ala-geninthiocin displayed better cytotoxicity but antibiotic activity against Gram-positive bacteria was comparatively low. Val-geninthiocin was found to possess more antifungal activity against *Mucor hiemalis* and cytotoxicity against A549 human lung carcinoma cells and L929 murine fibrosarcoma in comparison to geninthiocin. Further, Ala-geninthiocin and Val-geninthiocin displayed weak to moderate antifungal activity against *Candida albicans*, whereas geninthiocin was inactive. Ala-geninthiocin and geninthiocin displayed moderate antibiotic activity against Gram-negative bacteria *Chromobacterium violaceum*, whereas val-geninthiocin was inactive [116].

2.5. Structural Features of Bridged Heterocyclic Peptide Bicycles

Bicyclic peptides form one of the promising platforms for drug development owing to their biocompatibility and chemical diversity to proteins. Bioactive bicyclic peptides exist as disulfide-bridged peptide bicycles (e.g., ulithiacyclamide A, B, E, F, and G), histidino-tyrosine bridged peptide bicycles (e.g., aciculitins A–C), histidino-alanine bridged peptide bicycles (e.g., Theonellamides A, B, C, F, and G and Theogrenamide) and are derived from marine sponges/tunicates, plants, and mushrooms.

Ulithiacyclamide A is a strong cytotoxic disulfide-bridged peptide bicycle characterized by a symmetrical dimeric structure consisting of oxazoline and thiazole rings in addition to a transannular disulfide isolated from marine tunicate/ascidian *Lissoclinum patella*. The structure of ulithiacyclamide B closely resembled the structure of ulithiacyclamide with the exception of the replacement of one of the two D-leucine units with D-phenylalanine residue, resulting in an asymmetrical dimeric structure. Because the configuration of both leucine and phenylalanine was D, both thiazole amino acids possessed *R* configurations in ulithiacyclamide. The structures of ulithiacyclamides E, F, and G are related in structure to ulithiacyclamide B but with either both (in the case of ulithiacyclamide E) or just one of the two (in the cases of ulithiacyclamides F and G) oxazoline rings existing as their hydrolyzed L-threonine counterpart. Ulithiacyclamides F and G were found to be isomers and contained one oxazoline including one "free" threonine unit and were anhydro forms of ulithiacyclamide E. Ulithiacyclamide and ulithiacyclamide B exhibited cytotoxicity against the KB cell line with IC_{50} values of 35 and 17 ng/mL, respectively [51,53,56,57,117].

Aciculitins A–C are cytotoxic and antifungal glycopeptidolipids from the lithistid sponge *Aciculites orientalis*. They consist of a bicyclic peptide structure that contains a histidine-tyrosine bridge, with an unusual combination of tyrosine and histidine residues joined through the 3′-position of tyrosine and the 5′-position of histidine [118]. Theonegramide is a peculiar antifungal peptide that presents an intra-cycle histidine-alanine bridge in which the imidazole ring is substituted by a D-arabinose moiety. The alanine portion of histidinoalanine was found to have the (*R*)-configuration while the histidine portion with the (*S*)-configuration [119]. Theonellamides (TNMs) are members of a distinctive family of sterol-binding bioactive bicyclic dodecapeptides, with theonellamide F being a novel antifungal bicyclic dodecapeptide with an unprecedented histidinoalanine bridge composed of unusual amino acid residues like τ-L-histidino-D-alanine, (2*S*,4*R*)-2-amino-4-hydroxyadipic acid (Ahad), and (3*S*,4*S*,5*E*,7*E*)-3-amino-4-hydroxy-6-methyl-8- (*p*-bromophenyl)-5,7-octadienoic acid (Aboa). Theonellamide F was found to be a useful agent for investigating membrane structures in cells and inhibited growth of various pathogenic fungi including *Candida* sp., *Trichophyton* sp., and *Aspergillus* sp. [120,121].

Moroidin is a unique bicyclic peptide bearing residues like histidine, tryptophan, arginine, and β-leucine, isolated from the seeds of the Chinese herb *Celosia argentea* (Amaranthaceae), that remarkably inhibited the polymerization of tubulin [122]. Celogentins are unique cyclopolypeptides containing a bicyclic ring system; an unusual C–N bond formed by Trp and His residues; and an unusual amino acid, β-substituted Leu, isolated from the seeds of *Celosia argentea*. Celogentins A–C inhibited the polymerization of tubulin, and celogentin C was found to be 4 times more potent than moroidin in the inhibitory activity [123]. Phalloidin is a rigid bicyclic peptide containing an unusual cysteine-tryptophan linkage, isolated from the death cap mushroom *Amanita phalloides*. This cycloheptapeptide is commonly used in imaging applications to selectively label F-actin in fixed cells, permeabilized cells, and cell-free experiments [124]. α-Amanitin is a highly toxic hydrophobic bicyclic octapeptide found in a genus of mushrooms known as Amanita, including *Amanita phalloides*, *Amanita verna*, and *Amanita virosa*. The cytotoxicity found in amanitin is the result of inhibition of RNA polymerases, in particular RNA polymerase II, which precludes mRNA synthesis [124].

2.6. Structural Features of Other Heterocyclic Peptides from Marine Resources

Azonazine is a unique anti-inflammatory peptide with a macrocyclic heterocyclic core of the benzofuro indole ring system with diketopiperazine residue and possesses structural similarity with diazonamide A. The absolute configuration of this marine sediment-derived fungus-originated complex peptide was established as 2*R*,10*R*,11*S*,19*R*. The first total synthesis of hexacyclic dipeptide ent-(−)-azonazine was accomplished using a hypervalent iodine-mediated biomimetic oxidative cyclization to construct the highly strained core [125].

The pyridine ring (in the form of 3-hydroxypicolinic acid, 3HyPic) also forms part of cyclopeptide structures such as fijimycins and etamycin. Fijimycins A–C are cyclic depsipeptides from a marine-derived *Streptomyces* sp. which possessed in vitro antibacterial activity against three methicillin-resistant *Staphylococcus aureus* (MRSA) strains. The depsipeptide fijimycin A was found to contain eight subunits including α-phenylsarcosine (L-PhSar), *N*,β-dimethylleucine (L-DiMeLeu), sarcosine (Sar), 4-hydroxyproline (D-Hyp), and 3-hydroxypicolinic acid (3HyPic). Fijimycin A was defined as a stereoisomer of etamycin A containing D-α-phenylsarcosine. While comparing the structure of fijimycin B with fijimycin A, there was disappearance of α-phenylsarcosine (PhSar) and the existence of an *N*-methylleucine (L-*N*MeLeu) residue. Comparison of structures of fijimycins C and A suggested that the alanine (Ala) moiety in fijimycin A was replaced by a serine (Ser) unit. Etamycin A, also called virifogrisein I, was isolated from cultures of a terrestrial *Streptomyces* species which exhibited considerable activity against Gram-positive bacteria as well as *Mycobacterium tuberculosis*.

Fijimycins A and C and etamycin A exhibited strong antibiotic activities against the three MRSA strains (ATCC33591, Sanger 252, UAMS1182). However, fijimycin B showed weak inhibition against both ATCC33591 and UAMS1182, which indicated that the α-phenylsarcosine unit might be vital for significant antibacterial activity. The similar antimicrobial activities of the stereoisomers fijimycin A and etamycin A suggested that substituting D- for L-α-phenylsarcosine had little effect on the anti-MRSA activities [126].

Jaspamide P is a sponge-derived modified jaspamide derivative possessing antimicrofilament activity and characterised by a modification of the *N*-methylabrine (*N*-methyl-2-bromotrypthophan) residue. Structural analysis of this cyclopeptide indicated the presence of a 4-methoxy-1,3-benzoxazine-2-one heteroaromatic system. Jaspamide P was found to exhibit cytotoxic activity against HT-29 and MCF-7 tumour cell lines. Modifications of the methylabrine residue, claimed as essential for the observed biological activity, appeared to have little influence on the observed antiproliferative effect [127].

Wainunuamide is an unusual histidine containing cycloheptapeptide, containing three proline units. There were adjacent *cis* and *trans* proline residues in the structure of wainunuamide. Similar patterns were also found in cyclooligopeptide phakellistatin 8 and were found to be powerful β-turn inducers. The stereochemistry of all residues including histidine, phenylalanine, and leucine was found to be L. Wainunuamide exhibited weak cytotoxic activity in A2780 ovarian tumor and K562 leukemia cancer cells [128].

Ohmyungsamycins A and B are marine bacterium-derived cytotoxic and antimicrobial cyclic depsipeptides composed of 12 amino acid residues, including unusual amino acids such as *N*-methyl-4-methoxy-L-tryptophan, *β*-hydroxy-L-phenylalanine, and *N*,*N*-dimethylvaline. Ohmyungsamycins A and B showed significant inhibitory activities against diverse cancer cells as well as antibacterial effects against both Gram-positive and Gram-negative bacteria. Sungsanpin is a serine-rich lasso peptide containing 15 amino acid units from a deep-sea streptomycete in which eight amino acids form a cyclic peptide and the remaining seven amino acids including L-tryptophan unit form a tail that loops through the ring. It is the first example of a lasso peptide from a marine-derived microorganism and displays inhibitory activity with the human lung cancer cell line A549 in a cell invasion assay [129].

Desotamide and destolamide B are L-tryptophan containing bioactive peptides from marine microbe *Streptomyces scopuliridis* SCSIO ZJ46. These cyclohexapeptides displayed good antibacterial activities against *Streptococcus pnuemoniae*, *Staphylococcus aureus*, and *methicillin-resistant Staphylococcus epidermidis* (MRSE). In a complementary fashion, the antibacterial activities of destolamides revealed the "Tryptophan" moiety to be essential, thereby highlighting a critical structural element to this advancing antibacterial scaffold [130].

3. Stereochemical Aspects

Stereochemistry includes the study of the relative arrangement of atoms or groups in a molecule in three-dimensional space and its understanding is crucial for the study of complex molecules like heterocyclic peptides, which are of paramount biological significance.

cis,*cis*- and *trans*,*trans*-ceratospongamides (**44**,**45**) are new bioactive thiazole-containing cyclic heptapeptides from the marine red alga *Ceratodictyon spongiosum* and symbiotic sponge *Sigmadocia symbiotica*. The structures of ceratospongamides (**44**,**45**) contained two L-phenylalanine residues, one (L-isoleucine)-L-methyloxazoline residue, one L-proline residue, and one (L-proline)thiazole residue and were found to be proline amide conformers. The change in conformation of a cyclooligopeptide ceratospongamide from "*trans*" to "*cis*" resulted in complete loss of bioactivity, e.g., *trans, trans*-isomer of ceratospongamide (**45**) was found to be a potent inhibitor of the expression of a key enzyme in the inflammatory cascade, secreted phospholipase A_2 ($sPLA_2$), with an ED_{50} of 32 nM in a cell-based model for anti-inflammation, whereas *cis,cis*-isomer (**44**) was inactive [77] (Figure 15).

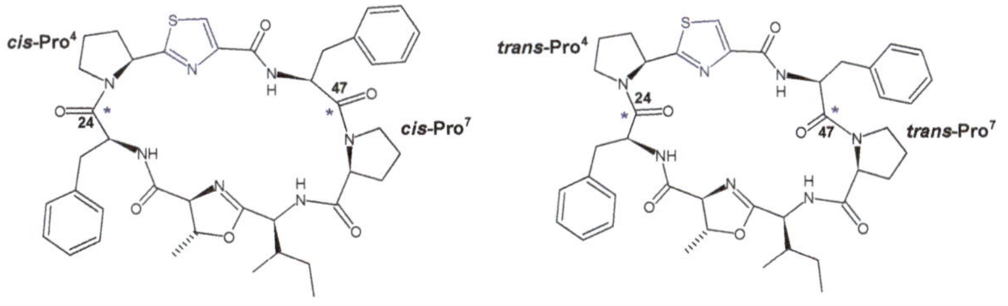

44 **45**

Figure 15. Structures of *cis,cis*-ceratospongamide (**44**) and *trans,trans*-ceratospongamide (**45**) with Pro-Tzl residues (*change in stereochemistry at C-24 and C-47 carbonyls).

Ulithiacyclamides are thiazole-containing cyclopolypeptides, isolated from the ascidian *Lissoclinum patella*. Bicyclic isomeric ulithiacyclamides F and G contained one oxazoline and one "free" threonine and were found to be anhydro forms of ulithiacyclamide E. Ulithiacyclamides F and G exhibited anti-multiple drug resistant (MDR) activity against vinblastine-resistant CCRF-CEM human leukemic lymphoblasts [51].

Lissoclinamides 4, 5, 7, and 8 are all cyclic heptapeptides derived from sea squirt *Lissoclinum patella* that have the same sequence of amino acids around the ring and differ from one another only in their stereochemistry or the number of thiazole and thiazoline rings. For lissoclinamide 8, the valine residue was at position 31, the same sequence that occurs in lissoclinamide 4. Therefore, the only difference between lissoclinamides 4 and 8 resided in the stereochemistry of one or two of the amino acids. The D configuration was assigned to "Phe-Tzl" and the L-configuration was assigned to "Val-Tzn" moiety in lissoclinamide 4. However, both lissoclinamides 4 and 8 contained similar residues like L-Pro-mOzn and L-Phe. Further, there was similarity in the structural components of lissoclinamides 2 and 3; the only difference was in the stereochemistry around Ala-Tzl moiety, D in the case of the former and L in the latter [55,56].

Lyngbyabellins are thiazole-containing halogenated peptolides derived from cyanobacteria, possessing cytotoxic properties. The configurations at C-15 and C-16 in lyngbyabellin A were found to be 15*S* and 16*S*. Further, C-26 and C-3 in the peptolide has the *S* configuration. The stereochemical assignments of lyngbyabellins E and H were found to be 2*S*, 3*S*, 14*R*, 20*S*, 26*R*, and 27*S*. The stereoconfigurations assigned to lyngbyabellin N was 2*S*, 3*S*, 14*R*, and 20*S*. The absolute configuration of the *N,N*-dimethylvaline (DiMeVal) residue in lyngbyabellin N was found to be L, whereas the absolute configurations of the leucine statine were determined to be 3*R* and 4*S*. The absolute configurations of lyngbyabellin J were found to be 2*S*, 3*S*, 14*R*, 20*R*, 21*S*, 27*R*, and 28*S*. An overall cyclic constitution was not required for potent cytotoxic properties in lyngbyabellins as acyclic peptides like lyngbyabellins F and I also exhibited significant cytotoxic properties [27–30].

The cyclopolypeptides bistratamides M and N (**46**,**47**) were found to be isomers of each other and differed in the configuration of alanine residue attached to the thiazole ring. The configuration was L in bistratamide M (**46**) and was found to be D in bistratamide N (**47**). Bistratamide M (**46**) was found to be slightly more cytotoxic against lung, breast, and pancreatic carcinoma cells in comparison to bistratamide N (**47**). Similarly, bistratamides K and L (**50**,**51**) are isomers, differing in the configuration of alanine residue attached to the thiazole ring. The configuration was D in bistratamide K (**50**) and was found to be L in bistratamide L (**51**). Further, bistratamide G (**39**) was found to be *O*-isostere of bistratamide H (**40**) and bistratamide J was found to be *S*-isostere of bistratamide I (**41**). The compounds containing two thiazole rings were found to be more active than those containing a thiazole ring and an oxazole ring [50,61]. Moreover, the gross structure of cytotoxic cyclopeptide keramamide G (**49**) was found to be almost the same as that of keramamide F (**48**), the only change being the different stereochemistry at C-13 of the α-keto-β-amino acid (Figure 16).

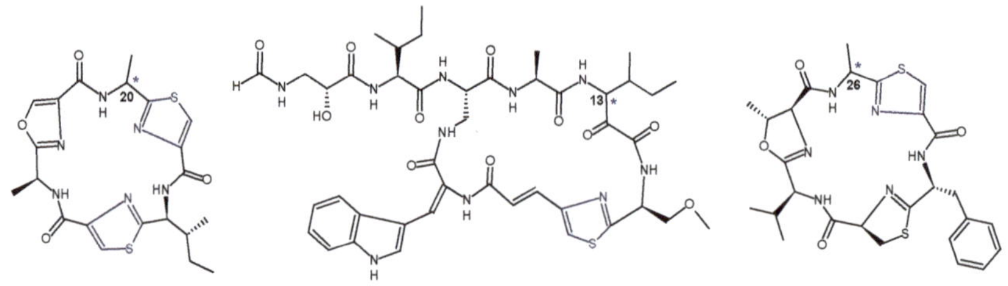

46: *20L **47:** *20D **48:** *13R **49:** *13S **50:** 26D **51:** *26L

Figure 16. Structures of bistratamide M (**46**) with configuration L at C-20, bistratamide N (**47**) with configuration D at C-20, keramamide F (**48**) with stereochemistry *R* at C-13, keramamide G (**49**) with stereochemistry *S* at C-13, bistratamide K (**50**) with configuration D at C-26, and bistratamide L (**51**) with configuration L at C-26.

Grassypeptolides D and E are diasteromeric cyclic peptides from a red sea *Leptolyngbya* cyanobacterium. These cyclodepsipeptides were found to contain two aromatic residues, phenyllactic acid (Pla), *N*-methylphenylalanine (*N*-Me-Phe); *β*-amino acid residue 2-methyl-3-aminobutyric acid (Maba); and 2-aminobutyric acid (Aba) residue. Further, structural analysis indicated the presence of a 2-methylthiazoline carboxylic acid derived from *N*-methylphenylalanine (*N*-Me-Phe-4-Me-thn-ca) and an Aba-thn-ca unit. Grassypeptolides D and E showed significant cytotoxicity to HeLa (IC_{50}: 335 and 192 nM) and mouse neuro-2a blastoma cells (IC_{50}: 599 and 407 nM). These depsipeptides were found to be threonine/N-methylleucine diastereomers and possesssed different configurations for both L-Thr and *N*-Me-L-Leu in grassypeptolide E (**53**) relative to grassypeptolide D (**52**). Grassypeptolide D (7*R*,11*R*; D-*allo*-Thr and *N*-Me-D-Leu) (**52**) was found to be approximately 1.5-fold less cytotoxic to HeLa cervical carcinoma and neuro-2a mouse blastoma cells than grassypeptolide E (7*S*,11*S*; L-Thr and *N*-Me-L-Leu) (**53**). Moreover, grassypeptolides A and C were found to be the *N*-methylphenylalanine epimers with stereochemistry (7*R*,11*R*,25*R*,29*R*) and (7*R*,11*R*,25*R*,29*S*), respectively. Grassypeptolide C showed 16–23-fold greater potency than grassypeptolide A against colorectal adenocarcinoma HT29 and cervical carcinoma HeLa cells [25] (Figure 17).

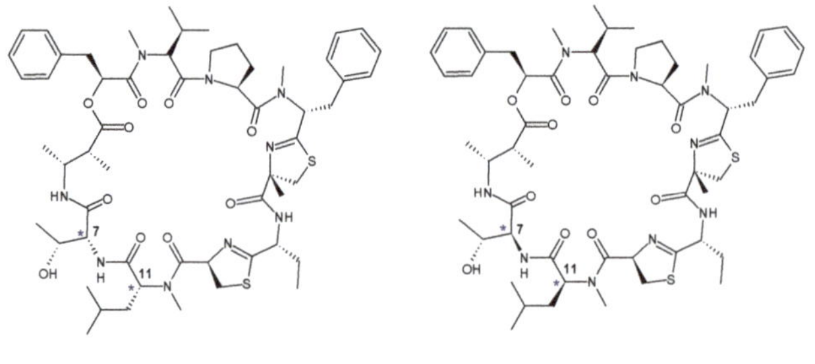

52: *7*R*,11*R* **53:** *7*S*,11*S*

Figure 17. Structures of grassypeptolide D (**52**) with stereochemistry *R* at C-7 and C-11 of D-*allo*-Thr and *N*-Me-D-Leu residues and grassypeptolide E (**53**) with stereochemistry *S* at C-7 and C-11 of L-Thr and *N*-Me-L-Leu residues.

Nostocyclamide M (**54**) and tenuecyclamide C (**55**) were found to be diasteromers. Nostocyclamide M (**54**) has the same constitution as tenuecyclamide C (**55**) but differs in the configuration of methionine in the structure. Adjacent to one of thiazole ring, D-methionine was present in cyclic hexapeptide nostocyclamide M (**54**) wheresas there was L-methionine in cyclic hexapeptide tenuecyclamide C (**55**). Nostocyclamide M (**54**) displayed allelopathic activity like nostocyclamide but was inactive against grazers unlike the latter [36] (Figure 18).

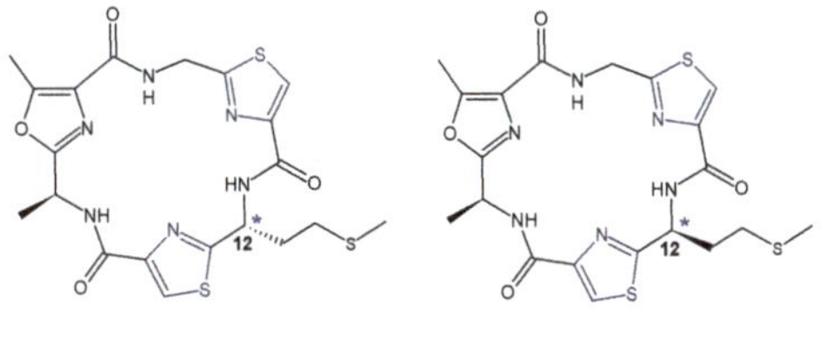

54: *12*D* **55:** *12*L*

Figure 18. Structures of nostocyclamide M (**54**) with Gly-Tzl and Met-Tzl residues, having methionine configuration D at C-12, and tenuecyclamide C (**55**) with Gly-Tzl and Met-Tzl residues, having methionine configuration L at C-12.

Ulongamides (**1–3**) are thiazole-containing cytotoxic cyclic depsipeptides with a novel β-amino acid, 3-amino-2-methylhexanoic acid (Amha), stereochemistry which differentiates ulongamides A–C from ulongamides D–F. The former has the Amha residue in 2*R*,3*R* configuration, while the latter contains an Amha unit in 2*S*,3*R* configuration. The 2-hydroxy-3-methylpentanoic acid (Hmpa) residue was found to be part of ulongamide E and F (**3**) structures, and the configuration of the residue was 2*S*,3*S*. Furthermore, stereochemistry of the 2-hdroxyisovaleric acid (Hiva) unit present in ulongamide D (**2**) was found to be *S* [13].

Calyxamides A and B (**56,57**) are cyclic peptides containing 5-hydroxytryptophan (Htrp), isolated from the marine sponge *Discodermia calyx*. These peptides contained residues like 2,3-diaminopropionic acid (Dpr) in addition to (*O*-methylseryl)thiazole moiety. Calyxamides A and B (**56,57**) possessed the same planar structure but are isomeric at the 3-position of the 3-amino-2-keto-4-methylhexanoic acid (AKMH) residue like keramamides F and G (13*S* and 13*R*). Structures of calyxamides differ in stereochemistry on isoleucine moiety adjacent to (*O*-methylseryl)thiazole moiety. Calyxamide B (**57**) was found to be the diastereomer of calyxamide A (**56**) and displayed more cytotoxicity against P388 murine leukemia cells, with an IC_{50} value of 0.9 μM, in comparison to calyxamide A (IC_{50}: 3.9 μM) (**56**) [110] (Figure 19).

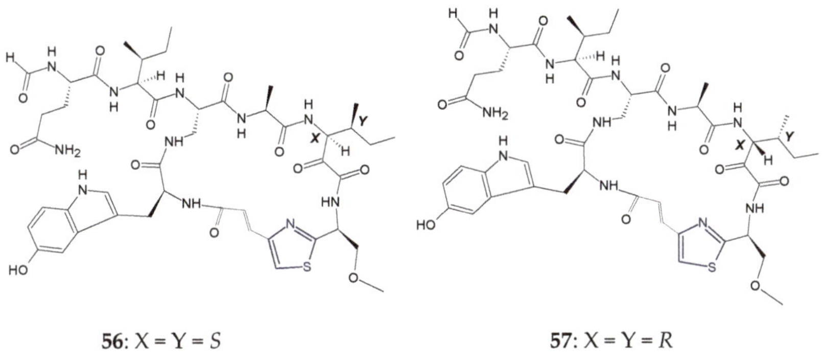

56: X = Y = *S* **57:** X = Y = *R*

Figure 19. Structures of calyxamide A (**56**) with *O*-Me-Ser-Tzl moiety, having stereochemistry *S* at the 3-position of 3-amino-2-keto-4-methylhexanoic acid (AKMH) residue, and Calyxamide B (**57**) with *O*-Me-Ser-Tzl moiety, having stereochemistry *R* at the 3-position of AKMH residue.

Aciculitamides A and B are bicyclic *E* and *Z* isomeric peptides obtained from the lithistid sponge *Aciculites orientalis* and result from oxidation of the imidazole ring of aciculitins A–C, bicycles containing an unusual histidino-tyrosine bridge. Aciculitamide A did not show any cytotoxicity against HCT-116 and/or antifungal activity [118].

Sclerotides A and B are cyclopolypeptides from marine-derived fungus, *Aspergillus sclerotiorum* PT06-1. These cyclic hexapeptides contained amino acid residues like L-threonine, L-alanine, phenylalanine, serine, anthranilic acid (AA), and dehydrotryptophan (Δ-Trp). Sclerotides A and B were found to be *Z* and *E* isomers and differed in stereochemistry of dehydrotryptophan. Sclerotide B showed more antifungal activity against *Candida albicans* with MIC values of 3.5 μM in comparison to sclerotide A (MIC: 7 μM). In addition, sclerotide B exhibited weak cytotoxic activity against the HL-60 cell line (IC_{50}: 56.1 μM) and selective antibacterial activity against *Pseudomonas aeruginosa* (MIC: 35.3 μM) [131].

4. Synthesis of Heterocyclic Peptides

Despite of lot of challenges associated with synthesizing complex peptide molecules [132–135], syntheses of diverse aromatic/heteroaromatic peptides were accomplished by several research groups employing diverse techniques of peptide synthesis including solid-phase peptide synthesis (SPPS), liquid-phase peptide synthesis (LPPS), and a mixed solid-phase/solution synthesis strategy, irrespective of whether these congeners belong to linear analogues [136–151] or are cyclic in nature [152–169]. Literature is enriched with reports involving synthesis of various heterocyclic cyclopolypeptides bearing thiazole/thiazoline/tryptophan/histidine moieties viz. cyclodidemnamide B [42], dolastatin 3 [90], aeruginazole A [170], didmolamide B (**29**) [171], dolastatin 10 (**20**) [172], scleritodermin A (**10**) [173], obyanamide (**8**) [174,175], marthiapeptide A [176], diandrine C [177], diandrine A [178], sarcodactylamide [179], segetalin C [180], segetalin E [181], annomuricatin B [182], and gypsin D [183].

The first total synthesis of thiazole and methyloxazoline-containing cyclohexapeptides didmolamides A and B was accomplished by the solid phase assembly of thiazole-containing amino acids and Fmoc-protected α-amino acids. The synthesis of thiazole-containing didmolamide B (**29**) was also achieved using solution phase peptide synthesis. The crucial thiazole amino acid was synthesized by MnO_2 oxidation of a thiazoline prepared from an Ala-Cys dipeptide using bis(triphenyl)oxodiphosphonium trifluoromethanesulfonate. The final macrolactamization was accomplished efficiently by benzotriazole-1-yl-oxy-tris-pyrrolidino-phosphonium hexafluorophosphate (PyBOP) and 4-dimethylaminopyridine (DMAP) [171].

A practical approach to asymmetric synthesis of dolastatin 10 (**20**) was found to involve SmI2-induced cross-coupling and asymmetric addition of chiral N-sulfinyl imine [172].

The synthesis of the C1–N15 fragment of the marine natural product scleritodermin A (**10**) was accomplished through a short and stereocontrolled sequence. The highlights of this route included synthesis of a novel conjugated thiazole moiety 2-(1-amino-2-*p*-hydroxyphenylethane)-4-(4-carboxy-2,4-dimethyl-2Z,4E-propadiene)-thiazole (ACT) fragment and the formation of the α-keto amide linkage by the use of a highly activated α,β-ketonitrile [173]. The total synthesis of a cytotoxic *N*-methylated thiazole-containing cyclic depsipeptide obyanamide (**8**) was accomplished that included the preparation of two protected fragments before macrocyclization, starting from material (S)-2-aminobutyric acid. The synthesis has led to a reassignment of the C-3 configuration in β-amino acid residue. As a result, the configuration at C-3 position has been amended as *R* [174,175].

The cytotoxic polythiazole-containing cyclopeptide marthiapeptide A having a linked trithiazole–thiazoline system was synthesized via two routes. The initial strategy involved a macrocyclization of the linear precursor via a peptide-coupling reaction between the amine on the alanine residue and the carboxylic acid end of isoleucine. However, the cyclization was not successful, which was attributed to the closing point being too close to the rigid heterocyclic thiazole moiety. The second strategy involved closing between the thiazoline and peptide in which successful cyclization can be attributed to the flexibility of the thiazoline, which allows a connection between the molecule's head and tail [176].

5. Structural Activity Relationships

Structural activity relationships (SAR) are prime keys to diverse aspects of drug discovery, ranging from primary screening to extensive lead optimization. SAR can be used to predict bioactivity from the molecular structure. This powerful technology is used in drug discovery to guide the acquisition or synthesis of desirable new compounds as well as to further characterize existing molecules. The principle of structure–activity relationship indicated that there is a relationship between molecular structures and their biological activity and solely depends on the recognition of which structural characteristics correlate with chemical and biological reactivity.

The lissoclinamides, heterocyclic peptides isolated from sea squirt Lissoclinum patella, are derived from a cyclic heptapeptide in which a threonine has been cyclised to an oxazoline and two cysteines have been cyclised to give a thiazole or thiazoline. While comparing natural and synthetic lissoclinamides, it was found that the replacement of thiazoline rings with oxazolines decreased activity to a greater extent than replacement of oxazoline rings with thiazolines [184]. This study further showed that it was not the individual components of the macrocycle that conferred high activity, but rather, the overall conformation of this molecule was responsible for the bioactivity. While comparing structures of lissoclinamides 4 and 5, it was observed that these compounds differ only in the oxidation state of a single thiazole unit but that this difference makes lissoclinamide 5 two orders of magnitude less cytotoxic than lissoclinamide 4 against bladder carcinoma (T24) cells [55].

In raocyclamides (**42**,**43**), the presence of oxazoline moiety was found to be essential for cytotoxicity against sea urchin embryos. The cyanobacterium-derived cyclopolypeptides raocyclamide A and B (**42**,**43**) possessed thiazole and oxazoline rings in their composition, but raocyclamide A (**42**) contained an additional oxazoline moiety in its structure. This structural change results in a lot of variation in the biological response. While comparing the bioeffects of these cyclopolypeptides, it was found that raocyclamide A (**42**) inhibited the division of embryos of *Paracentrotus lividus* with an effective dose for 100% inhibition (ED_{100}) of 30 μg/mL, whereas raocyclamide B (**43**) was inactive even at the concentrations of 250 μg/mL [32].

Replacement of D-valine moiety with D-methionine adjacent to one of the thiazole rings in the structure of macrocyclic thiazole and methyloxazole-containing allelochemical nostocyclamide resulted in cyanobacterial cyclopeptide nostocyclamide M (**54**) with inactivity toward grazers, but this structural modification does not affect the allelopathic activity against anabaena 7120 [36].

The reduction of isoleucylthiazole (Ile-Tzl) residue of a thiazole- and methyloxazoline-containing cyclooligopeptide of cyanobacterial origin, aerucyclamide B, to an isoleucylthiazoline (Ile-Tzn) residue resulted in a close analogue aerucyclamide A. From this one structural modification, the antiplasmodial activity was found to decrease by 1 order of magnitude. Further, the cyclohexapeptide aerucyclamide C underwent hydrolysis reaction using trifluoroacetic acid to form ring-opened products microcyclamide 7806A and microcyclamide 7806B. This change in structure from rigid, disk-like cyclamides to methyloxazoline (mOzn) ring-opened hydrolysis products resulted in loss of antimicrobial and cytotoxic activities [38]. In comparison, aerucyclamide B was the most active antiplasmodial compound among aerucyclamides against chloroquine-resistant strain K1 of *P. falciparum*, with selectivity against a rat myoblast cell line, whereas against parasite T. brucei rhodesiense, the most active compound was aerucyclamide C.

The cyclic structure of oxazole-rich, thiazole-containing polypeptide mechercharmycin A was found to be essential for its strong antitumor activity against human lung cancer and leukemia cells. The cyclic ring opening of mechercharmycin A resulted in linear peptide mechercharmycin B which did not displayed any inhibitory activity toward any of the cell lines [79].

The ascidian-derived cytotoxic cyclic hexapeptides, bistratamides A and B, differed from each other only by the presence or absence of one double bond. The conversion of one thiazoline in bistratamide A to a thiazole in bistratamide B, i.e., oxidation of thiazoline to thiazole, resulted in a less toxic compound. For example, comparing bioactivities of bistratamides A and B, the former has an IC_{50} value of about 50 μg/mL and latter has an IC_{50} value greater than 100 μg/mL against human cell lines including fibroblasts and bladder carcinoma cells [60].

Replacement of the alanine unit adjacent to the thiazole ring by a threonine unit in cyanobacterium-derived modified cyclohexapeptide venturamide A (**31**) resulted in a related cyclic hexapeptide venturamide B (**32**). This structural change reflected an increase in antimalarial activity against *Plasmodium falciparum* and cytotoxic activity toward mammalian Vero cells. However, with this modification, a decrease in bioactivity against *Trypanasoma cruzi* and MCF-7 cancer cells was observed [34].

The lyngbyabellin family of thiazole-containing peptolides are known to exhibit moderate to potent cytotoxicity against a number of different cancer cell types through the promotion of actin polymerization. In the HCT116 colon cancer cell line assay, reproducible IC_{50} values (40.9 ± 3.3 nM) were obtained for lyngbyabellin N, confirming the potent cytotoxic effect of this new member of the lyngbyabellin class and suggesting that the side chain of lyngbyabellin N was an essential structural feature for this potent activity. However, this trend was not entirely consistent within this structure class as other lyngbyabellin analogs lacking the side chain were found to exhibit bioactivity against HT29 and HeLa cells [29]. When compared to lyngbyabellin A, lyngbyabellin J displayed slightly less bioactivity against HT29 colorectal adenocarcinoma and HeLa cervical carcinoma cells. The cytoskeletal actin-disrupting lyngbyabellin 27-deoxylyngbyabellin A was found to be more potent than lyngbyabellin A against HT29 and HeLa carcinoma cell lines (IC_{50} values: 27-deoxylyngbyabellin A, 0.012 and 0.0073 μM; lyngbyabellin A, 0.047 and 0.022 μM), indicating the importance of hydroxylation at the C-27 position. However, lyngbyabellin A, its 27-deoxy analog, and lyngbyabellin J exhibited more cytotoxic activity against the two cell lines when compared to peptolide lyngbyabellin B (IC_{50} values: 1.1 and 0.71 μM). The configuration of the hydroxy acid-derived unit esterified to the 7,7-dichloro-3-acyloxy-2-methyloctanoic acid residue (here, Dhmpa) was not found to have a profound effect on the activity. Furthermore, close analysis of bioactivity data indicated that the cytotoxicity of cyclic and acyclic lyngbyabellins appeared to be similar [30].

The antithrombin cyclopolypeptides and cyclotheonellazoles had structural features similar to another *Theonella* sponge-derived peptide oriamide (**9**) in having nonproteinogenic amino acids like 4-propenoyl-2-tyrosylthiazole and 3-amino-4-methyl-2-oxohexanoic acid and showed potent inhibitory activity against the serine protease enzymes chymotrypsin and elastase. Cyclotheonellazole complexes with elastase/chymotrypsin exhibit a tetrahedral transition state involving the keto group of Amoha and Ser195 of elastase, while the side chain of Amoha fits in the enzyme S1 pocket. Cyclotheonellazole A, which contains a 2-aminopentanoic acid residue, was found to be the most potent inhibitor. This was probably due to a better compatibility with the enzyme S2 subsite. Cyclotheonellazoles B and C contained the amino acids leucine and homoalanine, and it appeared that the length and the branching of the aliphatic chain influenced the bioactivity. Further, these cyclopeptides were inactive against the malaria parasite plasmodium falciparum at IC_{50} values of greater than 20 μg/mL [68].

Ulongamides (**1–3**) are cyanobacterium-derived β-amino acid- and thiazole-containing cyclic peptides with weak cytotoxic properties. In cyclodepsipeptide ulongamide F (**3**), the lack of an aromatic amino acid or the N-methyl group adjacent to the hydroxyl acid (N-methylphenylalanine/N-methyl tyrosine in ulongapeptides A–E and L-valine in ulongapeptide F) was found to be detrimental to bioactivity. This was evident from the observation that ulongamide F (**3**) was inactive at <10 μM against KB and LoVo cells in comparison to ulongapeptides A (**1**) and D (**2**), which displayed cytotoxicity against both cell lines [13].

6. Biological Activity

Although thiazole-containing cyclopolypeptides of marine origin are associated with a number of bioactivities including antitubercular, antibacterial, antifungal, and inhibitory activity against serine protease enzymes chymotrypsin and elastase; anti-HIV activity; antiproliferative activity; antimalarial activity; and inhibitory activity against the transcription factor activator protein-1, the majority of them were found to exhibit anticancer activity. Various pharmacological activity-associated marine-derived Tzl-containing cyclopolypeptides along with susceptible cell line/organism with minimum inhibitory concentration are tabulated in Table 2.

Table 2. Heterocyclic Tzl-based peptides (TBPs) with diverse pharmacological activities.

TBPs	Resource	Bioactivity	
		Susceptibilty	**MIC[a] Value**
Haligramide A [63]	marine sponge *Haliclona nigra*	Cytotoxicity against A-549 (lung), HCT-15 (colon), SF-539 (CNS[b]), and SNB-19 (CNS) human tumor cell lines	5.17–15.62 μg/mL
Haligramide B [63]	marine sponge *Haliclona nigra*	Cytotoxicity against A-549 (lung), HCT-15 (colon), SF-539 (CNS), and SNB-19 (CNS) human tumor cells	3.89–8.82 μg/mL
Scleritodermin A [64]	marine sponge *Scleritoderma nodosum*	Cytotoxicity against colon HCT116, ovarian A2780, and breast SKBR3 cell lines	0.67–1.9 μM
Obyanamide [12]	marine cyanobacterium *Lyngbya confervoides*	Cytotoxicity against KB[c] and LoVo cells	0.58 and 3.14 μg/mL
Waiakeamide [66]	marine sponge *Ircinia dendroides*	Anti-TB activity against *Mycobacterium tuberculosis*	7.8 μg/mL
Ulongamide A [13]	marine cyanobacterium *Lyngbya* sp.	Cytotoxicity against KB and LoVo cells	1 and 5 μM
Guineamide B [14]	marine cyanobacterium *Lyngbya majuscula*	Cytotoxicity against mouse neuroblastoma cell line	15 μM
Calyxamide A [110]	marine sponge *Discodermia calyx*	Cytotoxicity against P388 murine leukemia cells	3.9 and 0.9 μM
Bistratamide J [50]	marine ascidian *Lissoclinum bistratum*	Cytotoxic activity against the human colon tumor (HCT-116) cell line	1.0 μg/mL
Didmolamide A and B [48]	marine tunicate *Didemnum molle*	Cytotoxicity against several cultured tumor cell lines (A549, HT29, and MEL28)	10–20 μg/mL
Aeruginazole A [91]	freshwater cyanobacterium *Microcystis* sp.	Antibacterial activity againt *B. subtilis* and *S. albus* Cytotoxicity against MOLT-4 human leukemia cell line and peripheral blood lymphocytes	2.2 and 8.7 μM 41 and 22.5 μM
Cyclotheonellazole A, B and C [68]	marine sponge *Theonella* aff. *swinhoei*	Inhibitory activity against serine protease enzyme chymotrypsin Inhibitory activity against serine protease enzyme elastase	0.62, 2.8, and 2.3 nM 0.034, 0.10, and 0.099 nM
Microcyclamide MZ602 [18]	cyanobacterium *Microcystis* sp.	Inhibition activity of chymotrypsin	75 μM
Dolastatin 3 [9]	marine cyanobacterium *Lyngbya majuscula*	Inhibition of HIV-1 integrase (for the terminal-cleavage and strand-transfer reactions)	5 mM and 4.1 mM
Lyngbyabellin A [27]	marine cyanobacterium *Lyngbya majuscula*	Cytotoxicity against KB cells (human nasopharyngeal carcinoma cell line) and LoVo cells (human colon adenocarcinoma cell line) Cytotoxicity against HT29 colorectal adenocarcinoma and HeLa cervical carcinoma cells Cytoskeletal-disrupting effects in A-10 cells	0.03 and 0.50 μg/mL 1.1 and 0.71 μM 0.01–5.0 μg/mL
Lyngbyabellin B [86]	marine cyanobacterium *Lyngbya majuscula*	Toxicity to brine shrimp (*Artemia salina*) Antifungal activity against *Candida albicans* (ATCC 14053) in a disk diffusion assay Cytotoxicity against HT29 colorectal adenocarcinoma and HeLa cervical carcinoma cells	3.0 ppm 100 μg/disk 1.1 and 0.71 μM
Lyngbyabellin E [28]	marine cyanobacterium *Lyngbya majuscula*	Cytotoxicity against NCI-H460 human lung tumor and neuro-2a mouse neuroblastoma cells Cytoskeletal-disrupting effects in A-10 cells	0.4 and 1.2 μM 0.01–6.0 μM

Table 2. *Cont.*

TBPs	Resource	Bioactivity	
		Susceptibilty	MIC[a] Value
Lyngbyabellin H [28]	marine cyanobacterium *Lyngbya majuscula*	Cytotoxicity against NCI-H460 human lung tumor and neuro-2a mouse neuroblastoma cells	0.2 and 1.4 μM
Lyngbyabellin N [29]	marine cyanobacterium *Moorea bouilloni*	Cytotoxic activity against HCT116 colon cancer cell line	40.9 nM
27-Deoxy-lyngbyabellin A [30]	marine cyanobacterium *Lyngbya bouillonii*	Cytotoxicity against HT29 colorectal adenocarcinoma and HeLa cervical carcinoma cells	0.012 and 0.0073 μM
Lyngbyabellin J [30]	marine cyanobacterium *Lyngbya bouillonii*	Cytotoxicity against HT29 colorectal adenocarcinoma and HeLa cervical carcinoma cells	0.054 and 0.041 μM
Raocyclamide A [32]	filamentous cyanobacterium *Oscillatoria raoi*	Cytotoxicity against embryos of sea urchin *Paracentrotus lividus*	30 μg/mL (ED_{100})[d]
Tenuecyclamide A, C and D [105]	cultured cyanobacterium *Nostoc spongiaeforme* var. *tenue*	Cytotoxicity against embryos of sea urchin *Paracentrotus lividus*	10.8, 9.0, and 19.1 μM (ED_{100})
Dolastatin I [75]	sea hare *Dolabella auricularia*	Cytotoxicity against HeLa S_3 cells	12 μg/mL
Marthiapeptide A [74]	marine actinomycete *Marinactinospora thermotolerans* SCSIO 00652	Antibacterial activities against *Micrococcus luteus, Staphylococcus aureus, Bacillus subtilis,* and *Bacillus thuringiensis* Cytotoxicity against SF-268 (human glioblastoma) cell line, MCF-7 (human breast adenocarcinoma) cell line, NCI-H460 (human lung carcinoma) cell line, and HepG2 (human hepatocarcinoma) cancer cell line	2.0, 8.0, 4.0, and 2.0 μg/mL 0.38, 0.43, 0.47, and 0.52 μM
Keramamide G, H and J [67]	marine sponge *Theonella* sp.	Cytotoxicity against L1210 murine leukemia cells and KB human epidermoid carcinoma cells	10 μg/mL
Keramamide K [109]	marine sponge *Theonella* sp.	Cytotoxicity against L1210 murine leukemia cells and KB human epidermoid carcinoma cells	0.72 and 0.42 μg/mL
Lissoclinamide 8 [55]	sea squirt *Lissoclinum patella*	Cytotoxicity against T24 (bladder carcinoma cells), MRC5CV1 (fibroblasts), and lymphocytes	6, 1, and 8 μg/mL
Mechercharmycin A [79]	marine bacterium *Thermoactinomyces* sp. YM3-251	Cytotoxic activity against A549 (human lung cancer) cells and Jurkat cells (human leukemia)	4.0×10^{-8} M and 4.6×10^{-8} M
Leucamide A [70]	marine sponge *Leucetta microraphis*	Cytotoxicity against HM02, HepG2, and Huh7 tumor cell lines	5.2, 5.9, and 5.1 μg/mL
Bistratamide H [50]	marine ascidian *Lissoclinum bistratum*	Cytotoxic activity against the human colon tumor (HCT-116) cell line	1.7 μg/mL
Patellamide E [58]	marine ascidian *Lissoclinum patella*	Cytotoxicity against human colon tumor cells in vitro	125 μg/mL
Microcyclamide [35]	cultured cyanobacterium *Microcystis aeruginosa*	Cytotoxicity against P388 murine leukemia cells	1.2 μg/mL
Dolastatin E [76]	sea hare *Dolabella auricularia*	Cytotoxicity against HeLa-S_3 cells	22–40 μg/mL
Aerucyclamide A [38]	freshwater cyanobacterium *Microcystis aeruginosa* PCC 7806	Antiparasite activity against *Plasmodium falciparum* K1 and *Trypanosoma brucei rhodesiense* STIB 900	5.0 and 56.3 μM
Aerucyclamide B [38]	freshwater cyanobacterium *Microcystis aeruginosa* PCC 7806	Antiparasite activity against *Plasmodium falciparum* K1 and *Trypanosoma brucei rhodesiense* STIB 900	0.7 and 15.9 μM
Aerucyclamide C [38]	freshwater cyanobacterium *Microcystis aeruginosa* PCC 7806	Antiparasite activity against *Plasmodium falciparum* K1 and *Trypanosoma brucei rhodesiense* STIB 900	2.3 and 9.2 μM
Aerucyclamide D [38]	freshwater cyanobacterium *Microcystis aeruginosa* PCC 7806	Antiparasite activity against *Plasmodium falciparum* K1 and *Trypanosoma brucei rhodesiense* STIB 900	6.3 and 50.1 μM

Table 2. *Cont.*

TBPs	Resource	Bioactivity	
		Susceptibilty	MIC[a] Value
Aerucyclamide A, B and C [37,38]	freshwater cyanobacterium *Microcystis aeruginosa* PCC 7806	Grazer toxicity against the freshwater crustacean *Thamnocephalus platyurus*	30.5, 33.8, and 70.5 μM
Aerucyclamide B and C [38]	freshwater cyanobacterium *Microcystis aeruginosa* PCC 7806	Cytotoxic activity against Rat Myoblast L6 cells	120 and 106 μM
Urukthapelstatin A [78]	marine-derived bacterium *Mechercharimyces asporophorigenens* YM11-542	Cytotoxicity against A549 human lung cancer cells	12 nM
Mechercharmycin A [79]	marine-derived bacterium *Thermoactinomyces* sp.	Cytotoxicity against A549 human lung cancer cells and Jurkat cells	4.0×10^{-8} M and 4.6×10^{-8} M
Ulithiacyclamide [56,117]	marine tunicate *Lissoclinum patella*	Cytotoxic activity against L1210, MRC5CV1, T24, and CEM cell lines (continuous exposure)	0.35, 0.04, 0.10, and 0.01 μg/mL
Ulicyclamide [117]	marine tunicate *Lissoclinum patella*	Cytotoxic activity against L1210 murine leukemia cells	7.2 μg/mL
Patellamide A [117]	marine tunicate *Lissoclinum patella*	Cytotoxic activity against L1210 murine leukemia and human ALL cell line (CEM)	3.9 and 0.028 μg/mL
Patellamide B, C [117]	marine tunicate *Lissoclinum patella*	Cytotoxic activity against L1210 murine leukemia cells	2.0 and 3.2 μg/mL
Venturamide A [34]	marine cyanobacterium *Oscillatoria* sp.	Antiparasitic activity against *Plasmodium falciparum, Trypanasoma cruzi* Cytotoxicity against mammalian Vero cells and MCF-7 cancer cells	8.2 and 14.6 μM 86 and 13.1 μM
Venturamide B [34]	marine cyanobacterium *Oscillatoria* sp.	Antiparasitic activity against *Plasmodium falciparum, Trypanasoma cruzi* Cytotoxicity against mammalian Vero cells	5.2 and 15.8 μM 56 μM
Bistratamides A and B [60]	aplousobranch ascidian *Lissoclinum bistratum*	Cytotoxicity against MRC5CV1 fibroblasts and T24 bladder carcinoma cells	50 and 100 μg/mL
Bistratamide M [61]	marine ascidian *Lissoclinum bistratum*	Cytotoxicity against breast, colon, lung, and pancreas cell lines	18, 16, 9.1, and 9.8 μM
Balgacyclamide A [33]	freshwater cyanobacterium *Microcystis aeruginosa* EAWAG 251	Antimalarial activity against *Plasmodium falciparum* K1	9 and 59 μM
Balgacyclamide B [33]	freshwater cyanobacterium *Microcystis aeruginosa* EAWAG 251	Antiparasitic activity against *Trypanosoma brucei rhodesiense* STIB 900	8.2 and 51 μM

[a] MIC—minimum inhibitory concentration, [b] CNS—central nervous system, [c] KB—ubiquitous KERATIN-forming tumor cell subline, [d] ED_{100}—effective dose for 100% inhibition.

7. Mechanism of Action

Heterocyclic thiazole-based peptides act by a variety of mechanisms including inhibiting microtubule assembly/mitosis, arresting nuclear division, inducing tumor cell apoptosis, causing microtubule depolymerization, inhibiting the protein secretory pathway through preventing cotranslational translocation, inducing G1 cell cycle arrest and an apoptotic cascade, inhibiting the phosphorylation of ERK and Akt, disrupting the cellular actin microfilament network, overproducing 1,3-β-D-glucan, activating the caspase-3 protein expression and decrease in B-cell lymphoma 2 (Bcl-2) levels, inhibiting nuclear factor kappa-light-chain-enhancer of activated B cells (NF-κB) luciferase and nitrite production, etc.

Dolastatin 10 (**20**) is a pentapeptide with potential antineoplastic activity, derived from marine mollusk Dolabella auricularia. Its mechanism of action involves the inhibition of tubulin polymerization, tubulin-dependent guanosine triphosphate hydrolysis, and nucleotide exchange, and it is a potent noncompetitive inhibitor of vincristine binding to tubulin. Binding to tubulin, dolastatin 10 (**20**) inhibits microtubule assembly, resulting in the formation of tubulin aggregates and inhibition of mitosis. This thiazole-containing linear peptide also induces tumor cell apoptosis through a mechanism involving bcl-2, an oncoprotein that is overexpressed in some cancers. Microtubule inhibitors from several chemical classes can block the growth and development of malarial parasites, reflecting the importance of microtubules in various essential parasite functions. Dolastatin 10 (**20**) was a more potent inhibitor of *P. falciparum* than any other microtubule inhibitor like dolastatin 15. Dolastatin 10 (**20**) caused arrested nuclear division and apparent disassembly of mitotic microtubular structures in the parasite, indicating that compounds binding in the "Vinca domain" of tubulin can be highly potent antimalarial agents [185].

Symplostatin 1 (**21**), an analog of dolastatin 10 (**20**), is a potent antimitotic with antiproliferative effects that act by causing microtubule depolymerization, formation of abnormal mitotic spindles that lead to mitotic arrest, and initiation of apoptosis involving the phosphorylation of the anti-apoptotic protein Bcl-2. Symplostatin 1 (**21**) inhibited the polymerization of tubulin in vitro, consistent with its mechanism of action in cells and suggesting that tubulin may be its intracellular target. Additionally, symplostatin 1 (**21**) was found to inhibit the proliferation and migration of endothelial cells, suggesting that it may have antiangiogenic activity [186].

Largazole is a cyclic peptide with thiazole/thiazoline residues, including a number of unusual structural features, including a 3-hydroxy-7-mercaptohept-4-enoic acid unit and a 16-membered macrocyclic cyclodepsipeptide skeleton. Largazole showed potent and highly selective inhibitory activities against class I HDACs (histone deacetylases) and displayed superior anticancer properties. Largazole was found to strongly stimulate histone hyperacetylation in the tumor, showed efficacy in inhibiting tumor growth and induced apoptosis in the tumor. This effect is likely mediated by modulation of levels of cell cycle regulators, by antagonism of the AKT pathway through IRS-1 downregulation, and by reduction of epidermal growth factor receptor levels [187].

Lyngbyabellins are hectochlorin-related peptides with thiazole moieties that are associated with actin polymerization activity. These lipopeptides were found to induce perceptible thickening of the cytoskeletal elements with a relatable increase in binucleated cells. Lyngbyabellin A was found to disrupt the cellular actin microfilament network in A10 and, accordingly, disrupted cytokinesis in colon carcinoma cells, causing the formation of apoptotic bodies. Lyngbyabellin E exhibited actin polymerization ability and was found to completely block the cellular microfilaments, forming binucleated cells [188].

Scleritodermin A (**10**) is a cytotoxic cyclic peptide with an unusual N-sulfated side chain and a novel conjugated thiazole moiety as well as an α-ketoamide group. Scleritodermin A (**10**) has significant in vitro cytotoxicity against a panel of human tumor cells lines, and this depsipeptide acts through inhibition of tubulin polymerization and the resulting disruption of microtubules, which is the target of a number of clinically useful natural product anticancer drugs [64].

Theonellamides are sponge-derived antifungal and cytotoxic bicyclic dodecapeptides with a histidine-alanine bridge. Specific binding of these peptides to 3β-hydroxysterols resulted in overproduction of 1,3-β-D-glucan and membrane damage in yeasts. The inclusion of cholesterol or ergosterol in phosphatidylcholine membranes significantly enhanced the membrane affinity of theonellamide A because of its direct interaction with 3β-hydroxyl groups of sterols. Membrane action of theonellamide A proceeds via binding to the membrane surface through direct interaction with sterols and modification of the local membrane curvature in a concentration-dependent manner, resulting in dramatic membrane morphological changes and membrane disruption. Theonellamides represents a new class of sterol-binding molecules that induce membrane damage and activate Rho1-mediated 1,3-beta-D-glucan synthesis [189].

Phalloidin is a tryptophan containing bicyclic phallotoxin, which functions by binding and stabilizing filamentous actin (F-actin) and effectively prevents the depolymerization of actin fibers. Due to its tight and selective binding to F-actin, derivatives of phalloidin-containing fluorescent tags are used widely in microscopy to visualize F-actin in biomedical research. Though phallotoxins are highly toxic to liver cells, they add little to the toxicity of ingested death cap, as they are not absorbed through the gut [190].

Jaspamide (Jasplakinolide) is a cytotoxic cyclodepsipeptide with bromotryptophan moiety that induces apoptosis in human leukemia cell lines and brain tumor Jurkat T cels by activation of caspase-3 protein expression and decrease in Bcl-2 levels. Apoptosis induced by Jaspamide was associated with caspase-3 activation, decreased Bcl-2 protein expression, and increased Bax levels, suggesting that jaspamide induced a caspase-independent cell death pathway for cytosolic and membrane changes in apoptosis cells and a caspase-dependent cell death pathway for poly (ADP-ribose) polymerase (PARP) protein degradation [191].

Azonazine is a unique peptide with a macrocyclic heterocyclic core of the benzofuro indole ring system with diketopiperazine residue. This hexacyclic dipeptide displayed anti-inflammatory activity and was found to act by inhibiting NF-κB luciferase and nitrite production [192].

8. Issues Associated with Marine Peptides in Drug Development

Marine peptides are fascinating therapeutic candidates due to their diverse bioactivities. They demonstrate significant chemical and biological diversity for drug development including minimized drug–drug interaction, less tissue accumulation, and low toxicity. Approximately 40% of existing small molecules and 70% of new candidates under development pipelines suffer from the low solubility problem, which is a major reason for their suboptimal drug delivery as well as failures in their development process. Approaches such as cyclodextrin complexation and solid dispersions have been employed to address this challenge and recommend the better formulation over their existing dosage forms [193–198]. Likewise, peptides, being biomacromolecules, also exhibit various challenges such as limited water solubility, stability aspects, as well as structural and synthesis complexities, limiting their full exploitation in drug development [199,200]. Table 3 portrays various issues associated with peptide drug development. Amidst the major challenges, difficulty in optimization of the required peptide length to achieve pharmacologically useful levels for receptor activation accounts for the hindered drug development of marine-based peptides. The optimization depends on variables including the size, accessibility, and fit of ligand-binding surfaces, ligand stability, and receptor residency time. Further, the high proteolytic instability of peptide-based therapeutics can be conquered by alteration of the side chains and amide bonds, which in turn makes the peptide resistant to proteolytic degradation [201]. The challenges of low bioavailability and short half-life can be overpowered by three approaches: (i) modification of the peptide backbone through the introduction of D-amino acids or unnatural amino acids, (ii) alteration of the peptide bonds with reduced amide bonds or β-amino acids, and (iii) attachment of a fatty acid. Approaches (i) and (ii) drive the peptide backbone through introducing cyclization, reduced flexibility, and enzyme digestion. Approach (iii) could lead to more specific binding to the target leading to enhanced half-life and bioavailability with fewer side effects [202]. Intracellular delivery of peptides has been a subject of interest due to their membrane-binding ability to exert action on the cell surface. Also, involving the protein transduction domain allows intracellular peptide delivery. Although the liposomal and nanoparticle drug delivery takes advantage of fusing the peptides for intracellular drug delivery, they also face the problem of low encapsulation efficiency [202]. During the process development of peptide synthesis, it is difficult to identify the critical process parameters to achieve expected purity and yield. In addition, the peptide synthesis process also depends on the specifications or requirements and targeted volumes. However, the establishment of acceptable standards and proven ranges may be lacking, which in turn accelerates their manufacturing costs during drug development.

Table 3. Issues associated with marine peptide drug development.

Sr. No.	Associated Issue
1.	Low bioavailability and short half-life due to instability of peptides in the body
2.	Formulation challenges and synthesis challenges including aggregation and solubility problems
3.	Difficulty optimizing peptide length to pharmacologically useful levels for receptor activation
4.	Expensive synthesis and manufacturing cost
5.	Difficulty in delivering expected purities and yields

9. Peptide Market and Clinical Trials

As a class of drugs, peptides are increasingly important in medicine. The Food and Drug Administration (FDA) has seen a rapid increase in the number of new drug applications submitted for peptide drug products. The availability of generic versions of these products will be critical to increasing public access to these important medications. However, ensuring the quality and equivalence between generic and brand-name peptide drug products raises a number of challenges, and those challenges differ according to the type of peptide drug. For peptide drug products with a specifically defined sequence of amino acids, the challenge has been with impurities that may be inadvertently introduced during the production process that may affect a proposed generic drug's safety profile. Peptide-related impurities can be especially difficult to detect, analyze, and control because they usually have similar sequences to the drug itself. As per the current calculations, the market for peptide and protein drugs is estimated around 10% of the entire pharmaceutical market and will make up an even larger proportion of the market in the future. Since the early 1980s, more than 200 therapeutic proteins and peptides are approved for clinical use by the US-FDA [203].

Promising preclinical data led to clinical evaluation of a thiazole-containing linear pentapeptide, dolastatin 10 (**20**), isolated from sea hare as well as cyanobacterium. The potent antimitotic compound, dolastatin 10 (**20**), was evaluated in many phase I and phase II clinical trials for solid tumor, including a multi-institutional phase II clinical trial for soft tissue sarcoma treatment [204]. Dolastatin 10 (**20**) was withdrawn from clinical trials due to adverse effects such as peripheral neurophathy in cancer patients. Dolastatin 10 (**20**) was not found to be successful in human clinical trials, but it acted as a valuable source for a number of related compounds with clinical significance like ILX651, LU103793, and soblidotin [205,206]. Chemical modification efforts to reduce toxicity resulted in the synthesis of TZT-1027 (soblidotin or auristatin PE), a microtubule-disrupting compound, which entered a phase II clinical trial in patients with advanced or metastatic soft tissue sarcomas and lung cancer. Soblidotin has not progressed further beyond phase II clinical trials due to the associated hematological toxicities [207].

Although due to poor water solubility dolastatin 15 could not enter clinical trials, the investigations on this linear depsipeptide encouraged the development of its synthetic analogs like synthadotin and cematodin which have entered clinical trials. Preclinical studies confirmed the antitumor potential of the orally active microtubule inhibitor synthadotin against padiatric sarcomas. This depsipeptide has completed three phase II trials for the treatment of hormone refractory prostate cancer and metastatic melanoma that indicated toward the favorable toxicity profiles of synthadotin [208]. Another synthetic analog of dolastatin 15, cemadotin, underwent many phase I and phase II clinical trials against metastatic breast cancer and malignant melanoma. However, clinical trials were discontinued because of inconsiderable cytotoxicity caused by cemadotin in phase II trials and to acute myocardial infarction and neutropenia in phase I clinical trials [209].

Further modifications of soblidotin/auristatin E led to the development of monomethyl auristatin E (MMAE) and monomethyl auristatin F (MMAF), each of which included a secondary amine at their N-terminus. MMAE and MMAF have been used as warheads to link monoclonal antibodies and are presently in many clinical trials for the treatment of cancer, and eventually various antibody-drug conjugates received FDA approval [210,211].

10. Conclusions and Future Prospects

In present times, there is an increased frequency of resistance for conventional drugs. This fact necessitates the focus of drug research to be shifted toward a new era where bioactive compounds are developed with novel mechanisms of action. TBPs with unique structural features claim their candidature to overcome the existing issues. Various bioactive heteroaromatic peptides have been isolated from different organisms ranging from marine sponges, mollusks, and tunicates to terrestrial cyanobacteria and other microbes including fungi and bacteria. On this basis, various mimetics of bioactive peptides have been synthesized using solid and solution phase techniques of peptide synthesis. Despite enormous potential, utilization of these bioactive peptides is limited due to their stability and bioavailability issues. This review portrays recent updates and future perspectives of TBPs to attract the attention of researchers and scientists leading the efforts toward their clinical translation from the bench to the bedside.

Author Contributions: R.D., S.D., N.K.F., J.S. and R.M. conceived and designed the structure of the review. R.D., S.D., S.V.C., A.S., H.G. and A.A. conducted literature research and drafted the entire manuscript. S.D., S.M., S.S., S.F. and S.J. edited the manuscript. R.D., S.D., S.K., G.J., A.K., N.K.F., S.F., S.J. and S.K.K. supervised and contributed to the key parts of the text associated with it. All authors have read and agreed to the published version of the manuscript.

Funding: This work was partially funded by the Campus Research and Publication Fund Committee of The University of the West Indies, St. Augustine, Trinidad & Tobago.

Acknowledgments: The authors wish to thank chief librarians of Faculty of Medical Sciences, The University of the West Indies, St. Augustine, Trinidad & Tobago, WI and University of Puerto Rico, San Juan, PR, USA for providing literature support.

Conflicts of Interest: The authors declare no conflict of interest.

References

1. Gomtsyan, A. Heterocycles in drugs and drug discovery. *Chem. Heterocyl. Compd.* **2012**, *48*, 7–10. [CrossRef]
2. Kumawat, M.K. Thiazole containing heterocycles with antimalarial activity. *Curr. Drug Discov. Technol.* **2018**, *15*, 196–200. [CrossRef] [PubMed]
3. Pathak, D.; Dahiya, R.; Pathak, K.; Dahiya, S. New generation antipsychotics: A review. *Indian. J. Pharm. Educ. Res.* **2006**, *40*, 77–83.
4. Fang, W.Y.; Dahiya, R.; Qin, H.L.; Mourya, R.; Maharaj, S. Natural proline-rich cyclopolypeptides from marine organisms: Chemistry, synthetic methodologies and biological status. *Mar. Drugs* **2016**, *14*, 194. [CrossRef]
5. Dahiya, R.; Pathak, D. Cyclic peptides: New hope for antifungal therapy. *Egypt. Pharm. J.* **2006**, *5*, 189–199.
6. Tiwari, J.; Gupta, G.; Dahiya, R.; Pabreja, K.; Kumar Sharma, R.; Mishra, A.; Dua, K. Recent update on biological activities and pharmacological actions of liraglutide. *Excli J.* **2017**, *16*, 742–747.
7. Singh, Y.; Gupta, G.; Shrivastava, B.; Dahiya, R.; Tiwari, J.; Ashwathanarayana, M.; Sharma, R.K.; Agrawal, M.; Mishra, A.; Dua, K. Calcitonin gene-related peptide (CGRP): A novel target for Alzheimer's disease. *CNS Neurosci. Ther.* **2017**, *23*, 457–461. [CrossRef]
8. Adiv, S.; Ahronov-Nadborny, R.; Carmeli, S. New aeruginazoles, a group of thiazole-containing cyclic peptides from Microcystis aeruginosa blooms. *Tetrahedron* **2012**, *68*, 1376–1383. [CrossRef]
9. Mitchell, S.S.; Faulkner, D.J.; Rubins, K.; Bushman, F.D. Dolastatin 3 and two novel cyclic peptides from a Palauan collection of Lyngbya majuscula. *J. Nat. Prod.* **2000**, *63*, 279–282. [CrossRef]
10. McIntosh, J.A.; Lin, Z.; Tianero, M.D.; Schmidt, E.W. Aestuaramides, a natural library of cyanobactin cyclic peptides resulting from isoprene-derived Claisen rearrangements. *ACS Chem. Biol.* **2013**, *8*, 877–883. [CrossRef]
11. Ploutno, A.; Carmeli, S. Modified peptides from a water bloom of the cyanobacterium *Nostoc* sp. *Tetrahedron* **2002**, *58*, 9949–9957. [CrossRef]
12. Williams, P.G.; Yoshida, W.Y.; Moore, R.E.; Paul, V.J. Isolation and structure determination of obyanamide, a novel cytotoxic cyclic depsipeptide from the marine cyanobacterium Lyngbya confervoides. *J. Nat. Prod.* **2002**, *65*, 29–31. [CrossRef] [PubMed]

13. Luesch, H.; Williams, P.G.; Yoshida, W.Y.; Moore, R.E.; Paul, V.J. Ulongamides A-F, new beta-amino acid-containing cyclodepsipeptides from Palauan collections of the marine cyanobacterium *Lyngbya* sp. *J. Nat. Prod.* **2002**, *65*, 996–1000. [CrossRef] [PubMed]
14. Tan, L.T.; Sitachitta, N.; Gerwick, W.H. The guineamides, novel cyclic depsipeptides from a Papua New Guinea collection of the marine cyanobacterium Lyngbya majuscula. *J. Nat. Prod.* **2003**, *66*, 764–771. [CrossRef] [PubMed]
15. Luesch, H.; Yoshida, W.Y.; Moore, R.E.; Paul, V.J. New apratoxins of marine cyanobacterial origin from Guam and Palau. *Bioorg. Med. Chem.* **2002**, *10*, 1973–1978. [CrossRef]
16. Hong, J.; Luesch, H. Largazole: From discovery to broad-spectrum therapy. *Nat. Prod. Rep.* **2012**, *29*, 449–456. [CrossRef] [PubMed]
17. Sudek, S.; Haygood, M.G.; Youssef, D.T.A.; Schmidt, E.W. Structure of Trichamide, a cyclic peptide from the bloom-forming cyanobacterium Trichodesmium erythraeum, predicted from the genome sequence. *Appl. Environ. Microbiol.* **2006**, *72*, 4382–4387. [CrossRef]
18. Zafrir-Ilan, E.; Carmeli, S. Two new microcyclamides from a water bloom of the cyanobacterium *Microcystis* sp. *Tetrahedron Lett.* **2010**, *51*, 6602–6604. [CrossRef]
19. Luesch, H.; Yoshida, W.Y.; Moore, R.E.; Paul, V.J.; Corbett, T.H. Total structure determination of apratoxin A, a potent novel cytotoxin from the marine cyanobacterium Lyngbya majuscula. *J. Am. Chem. Soc.* **2001**, *123*, 5418–5423. [CrossRef]
20. Gutiérrez, M.; Suyama, T.L.; Engene, N.; Wingerd, J.S.; Matainaho, T.; Gerwick, W.H. Apratoxin D, a potent cytotoxic cyclodepsipeptide from papua new guinea collections of the marine cyanobacteria Lyngbya majuscule and Lyngbya sordida. *J. Nat. Prod.* **2008**, *71*, 1099–1103. [CrossRef]
21. Matthew, S.; Schupp, P.J.; Luesch, H. Apratoxin E, a cytotoxic peptolide from a Guamanian collection of the marine cyanobacterium Lyngbya bouillonii. *J. Nat. Prod.* **2008**, *71*, 1113–1116. [CrossRef]
22. Tidgewell, K.; Engene, N.; Byrum, T.; Media, J.; Doi, T.; Valeriote, F.A.; Gerwick, W.H. Evolved diversification of a modular natural product pathway: Apratoxins F and G, two cytotoxic cyclic depsipeptides from a Palmyra collection of Lyngbya bouillonii. *ChemBioChem* **2010**, *11*, 1458–1466. [CrossRef] [PubMed]
23. Thornburg, C.C.; Cowley, E.S.; Sikorska, J.; Shaala, L.A.; Ishmael, J.E.; Youssef, D.T.A.; McPhail, K.L. Apratoxin H and apratoxin A sulfoxide from the Red sea cyanobacterium Moorea producens. *J. Nat. Prod.* **2013**, *76*, 1781–1788. [CrossRef] [PubMed]
24. Kwan, J.C.; Ratnayake, R.; Abboud, K.A.; Paul, V.J.; Luesch, H. Grassypeptolides A−C, cytotoxic bis-thiazoline containing marine cyclodepsipeptides. *J. Org. Chem.* **2010**, *75*, 8012–8023. [CrossRef] [PubMed]
25. Thornburg, C.C.; Thimmaiah, M.; Shaala, L.A.; Hau, A.M.; Malmo, J.M.; Ishmael, J.E.; Youssef, D.T.A.; McPhail, K.L. Cyclic depsipeptides, grassypeptolides D, E and Ibu epidemethoxylyngbyastatin 3, from a Red sea Leptolyngbya cyanobacterium. *J. Nat. Prod.* **2011**, *74*, 1677–1685. [CrossRef] [PubMed]
26. Popplewell, W.L.; Ratnayake, R.; Wilson, J.A.; Beutler, J.A.; Colburn, N.H.; Henrich, C.J.; McMahon, J.B.; McKee, T.C. Grassypeptolides F and G, cyanobacterial peptides from Lyngbya majuscula. *J. Nat. Prod.* **2011**, *74*, 1686–1691. [CrossRef] [PubMed]
27. Luesch, H.; Yoshida, W.Y.; Moore, R.E.; Paul, V.J.; Mooberry, S.L. Isolation, Structure determination, and biological activity of lyngbyabellin A from the marine cyanobacterium Lyngbya majuscula. *J. Nat. Prod.* **2000**, *63*, 611–615. [CrossRef]
28. Han, B.; McPhail, K.L.; Gross, H.; Goeger, D.E.; Mooberry, S.L.; Gerwick, W.H. Isolation and structure of five lyngbyabellin derivatives from a Papua New Guinea collection of the marine cyanobacterium Lyngbya majuscula. *Tetrahedron* **2005**, *61*, 11723–11729. [CrossRef]
29. Choi, H.; Mevers, E.; Byrum, T.; Valeriote, F.A.; Gerwick, W.H. Lyngbyabellins K-N from two Palmyra Atoll collections of the marine cyanobacterium Moorea bouilloni. *Eur. J. Org. Chem.* **2012**, *2012*(27), 5141–5150. [CrossRef]
30. Matthew, S.; Salvador, L.A.; Schupp, P.J.; Paul, V.J.; Luesch, H. Cytotoxic halogenated macrolides and modified peptides from the apratoxin-producing marine cyanobacterium Lyngbya bouillonii from Guam. *J. Nat. Prod.* **2010**, *73*, 1544–1552. [CrossRef]
31. Soria-Mercado, I.E.; Pereira, A.; Cao, Z.; Murray, T.F.; Gerwick, W.H. Alotamide A, a novel neuropharmacological agent from the marine cyanobacterium Lyngbya bouillonii. *Org. Lett.* **2009**, *11*, 4704–4707. [CrossRef]

32. Admi, V.; Afek, U.; Carmeli, S. Raocyclamides A and B, novel cyclic hexapeptides isolated from the cyanobacterium Oscillatoria raoi. *J. Nat. Prod.* **1996**, *59*, 396–399. [CrossRef]
33. Portmann, C.; Sieber, S.; Wirthensohn, S.; Blom, J.F.; Da Silva, L.; Baudat, E.; Kaiser, M.; Brun, R.; Gademann, K. Balgacyclamides, antiplasmodial heterocyclic peptides from Microcystis aeruguinosa EAWAG 251. *J. Nat. Prod.* **2014**, *77*, 557–562. [CrossRef] [PubMed]
34. Linington, R.G.; González, J.; Ureña, L.-D.; Romero, L.I.; Ortega-Barría, E.; Gerwick, W.H. Venturamides A and B: Antimalarial constituents of the Panamanian marine cyanobacterium *Oscillatoria* sp. *J. Nat. Prod.* **2007**, *70*, 397–401. [CrossRef] [PubMed]
35. Ishida, K.; Nakagawa, H.; Murakami, M. Microcyclamide, a cytotoxic cyclic hexapeptide from the cyanobacterium Microcystis aeruginosa. *J. Nat. Prod.* **2000**, *63*, 1315–1317. [CrossRef]
36. Jüttner, F.; Todorova, A.K.; Walch, N.; von Philipsborn, W. Nostocyclamide M: A cyanobacterial cyclic peptide with allelopathic activity from Nostoc 31. *Phytochemistry* **2001**, *57*, 613–619. [CrossRef]
37. Portmann, C.; Blom, J.F.; Gademann, K.; Jüttner, F. Aerucyclamides A and B: Isolation and synthesis of toxic ribosomal heterocyclic peptides from the cyanobacterium Microcystis aeruginosa PCC 7806. *J. Nat. Prod.* **2008**, *71*, 1193–1196. [CrossRef]
38. Portmann, C.; Blom, J.F.; Kaiser, M.; Brun, R.; Jüttner, F.; Gademann, K. Isolation of aerucyclamides C and D and structure revision of microcyclamide 7806A: Heterocyclic ribosomal peptides from Microcystis aeruginosa PCC 7806 and their antiparasite evaluation. *J. Nat. Prod.* **2008**, *71*, 1891–1896. [CrossRef]
39. Chuang, P.-H.; Hsieh, P.-W.; Yang, Y.-L.; Hua, K.-F.; Chang, F.-R.; Shiea, J.; Wu, S.-H.; Wu, Y.-C. Cyclopeptides with anti-inflammatory activity from seeds of Annona montana. *J. Nat. Prod.* **2008**, *71*, 1365–1370. [CrossRef]
40. Ogino, J.; Moore, R.E.; Patterson, G.M.L.; Smith, C.D. Dendroamides, new cyclic hexapeptides from a blue-green alga. Multidrug-resistance reversing activity of dendroamide A. *J. Nat. Prod.* **1996**, *59*, 581–586. [CrossRef]
41. McDonald, L.A.; Foster, M.P.; Phillips, D.R.; Ireland, C.M.; Lee, A.Y.; Clardy, J. Tawicyclamides A and B, new cyclic peptides from the ascidian Lissoclinum patella: Studies on the solution- and solid-state conformations. *J. Org. Chem.* **1992**, *57*, 4616–4624. [CrossRef]
42. Arrault, A.; Witczak-Legrand, A.; Gonzalez, P.; Bontemps-Subielos, N.; Banaigs, B. Structure and total synthesis of cyclodidemnamide B, a cycloheptapeptide from the ascidian Didemnum molle. *Tetrahedron Lett.* **2002**, *43*, 4041–4044. [CrossRef]
43. Carroll, A.R.; Bowden, B.F.; Coll, J.C.; Hockless, D.C.R.; Skelton, B.W.; White, A.H. Studies of Australian ascidians. IV. Mollamide, a cytotoxic cyclic heptapeptide from the compound ascidian *Didemnum molle*. *Aust. J. Chem.* **1994**, *47*, 61–69. [CrossRef]
44. Carroll, A.R.; Coll, J.C.; Bourne, J.C.; MacLeod, J.K.; Zanriskie, T.M.; Ireland, C.M.; Bowden, B.F. Patellins 1-6 and trunkamide A: Novel cyclic hexa-, hepta- and octa-peptides from colonial ascidians, *Lissoclinum* sp. *Aust. J. Chem.* **1996**, *49*, 659–667. [CrossRef]
45. Rudi, A.; Aknin, M.; Gaydou, E.M.; Kashman, Y. Four new cytotoxic cyclic hexa- and heptapeptides from the marine ascidian Didemnum molle. *Tetrahedron* **1998**, *54*, 13203–13210. [CrossRef]
46. Donia, M.S.; Wang, B.; Dunbar, D.C.; Desai, P.V.; Patny, A.; Avery, M.; Hamann, M.T. Mollamides B and C, cyclic hexapeptides from the Indonesian tunicate Didemnum molle. *J. Nat. Prod.* **2008**, *71*, 941–945. [CrossRef]
47. Lu, Z.; Harper, M.K.; Pond, C.D.; Barrows, L.R.; Ireland, C.M.; Van Wagoner, R.M. Thiazoline peptides and a tris-phenethyl urea from Didemnum molle with anti-HIV activity. *J. Nat. Prod.* **2012**, *75*, 1436–1440. [CrossRef]
48. Rudi, A.; Chill, L.; Aknin, M.; Kashman, Y. Didmolamide A and B, two new cyclic hexapeptides from the marine ascidian Didemnum molle. *J. Nat. Prod.* **2003**, *66*, 575–577. [CrossRef]
49. Teruya, T.; Sasaki, H.; Suenaga, K. Hexamollamide, a hexapeptide from an Okinawan ascidian Didemnum molle. *Tetrahedron Lett.* **2008**, *49*, 5297–5299. [CrossRef]
50. Perez, L.J.; Faulkner, D.J. Bistratamides E-J, modified cyclic hexapeptides from the Philippines ascidian Lissoclinum bistratum. *J. Nat. Prod.* **2003**, *66*, 247–250. [CrossRef]
51. Fu, X.; Do, T.; Schmitz, F.J.; Andrusevich, V.; Engel, M.H. New cyclic peptides from the ascidian Lissoclinum patella. *J. Nat. Prod.* **1998**, *61*, 1547–1551. [CrossRef] [PubMed]

52. Morris, L.A.; Jantina Kettenes van den Bosch, J.; Versluis, K.; Thompson, G.S.; Jaspars, M. Structure determination and MS^n analysis of two new lissoclinamides isolated from the Indo-Pacific ascidian Lissoclinum patella: NOE restrained molecular dynamics confirms the absolute stereochemistry derived by degradative methods. *Tetrahedron* **2000**, *56*, 8345–8353. [CrossRef]
53. Ireland, C.; Scheuer, P.J. Ulicyclamide and ulithiacyclamide, two new small peptides from a marine tunicate. *J. Am. Chem. Soc.* **1980**, *102*, 5688–5691. [CrossRef]
54. Rashid, M.A.; Gustafson, K.R.; Cardellina II, J.H.; Boyd, M.R. Patellamide F, a new cytotoxic cyclic peptide from the colonial ascidian Lissoclinum patella. *J. Nat. Prod.* **1995**, *58*, 594–597. [CrossRef] [PubMed]
55. Hawkins, C.J.; Lavin, M.F.; Marshall, K.A.; Van den Brenk, A.L.; Watters, D.J. Structure-activity relationships of the lissoclinamides: Cytotoxic cyclic peptides from the ascidian Lissoclinum patella. *J. Med. Chem.* **1990**, *33*, 1634–1638. [CrossRef] [PubMed]
56. Degnan, B.M.; Hawkins, C.J.; Lavin, M.F.; McCaffrey, E.J.; Parry, D.L.; Van den Brenk, A.L.; Watters, D.J. New cyclic peptides with cytotoxic activity from the ascidian Lissoclinum patella. *J. Med. Chem.* **1989**, *32*, 1349–1354. [CrossRef] [PubMed]
57. Williams, D.E.; Moore, R.E. The structure of ulithiacyclamide B. Antitumor evaluation of cyclic peptides and macrolides from Lissoclinum patella. *J. Nat. Prod.* **1989**, *52*, 732–739. [CrossRef]
58. McDonald, L.A.; Ireland, C.M. Patellamide E: A new cyclic peptide from the ascidian Lissoclinum patella. *J. Nat. Prod.* **1992**, *55*, 376–379. [CrossRef]
59. Foster, M.P.; Concepcion, G.P.; Caraan, G.B.; Ireland, C.M. Bistratamides C and D. two new oxazole-containing cyclic hexapeptides isolated from a Philippine Lissoclinum bistratum ascidian. *J. Org. Chem.* **1992**, *57*, 6671–6675. [CrossRef]
60. Degnan, B.M.; Hawkins, C.J.; Lavin, M.F.; McCaffrey, E.J.; Parry, D.L.; Watters, D.J. Novel cytotoxic compounds from the ascidian Lissoclinum bistratum. *J. Med. Chem.* **1989**, *32*, 1354–1359. [CrossRef]
61. Urda, C.; Fernández, R.; Rodríguez, J.; Pérez, M.; Jiménez, C.; Cuevas, C. Bistratamides M and N, oxazole-thiazole containing cyclic hexapeptides isolated from Lissoclinum bistratum interaction of zinc (II) with bistratamide K. *Mar. Drugs* **2017**, *15*, 209. [CrossRef] [PubMed]
62. Toske, S.G.; Fenical, W. Cyclodidemnamide: A new cyclic heptapeptide from the marine ascidian Didemnum molle. *Tetrahedron Lett.* **1995**, *36*, 8355–8358. [CrossRef]
63. Rashid, M.A.; Gustafson, K.R.; Boswell, J.L.; Boyd, M.R. Haligramides A and B, two new cytotoxic hexapeptides from the marine sponge Haliclona nigra. *J. Nat. Prod.* **2000**, *63*, 956–959. [CrossRef] [PubMed]
64. Schmidt, E.W.; Raventos-Suarez, C.; Bifano, M.; Menendez, A.T.; Fairchild, C.R.; Faulkner, D.J. Scleritodermin A, a cytotoxic cyclic peptide from the Lithistid sponge Scleritoderma nodosum. *J. Nat. Prod.* **2004**, *67*, 475–478. [CrossRef]
65. Chill, L.; Kashman, Y.; Schleyer, M. Oriamide, a new cytotoxic cyclic peptide containing a novel amino acid from the marine sponge *Theonella* sp. *Tetrahedron* **1997**, *53*, 16147–16152. [CrossRef]
66. Mau, C.M.S.; Nakao, Y.; Yoshida, W.Y.; Scheuer, P.J. Waiakeamide, a cyclic hexapeptide from the sponge Ircinia dendroides. *J. Org. Chem.* **1996**, *61*, 6302–6304. [CrossRef]
67. Kobayashi, J.; Itagaki, F.; Shigemori, I.; Takao, T.; Shimonishi, Y. Keramamides E, G, H, and J, new cyclic peptides containing an oxazole or a thiazole ring from a Theonella sponge. *Tetrahedron* **1995**, *51*, 2525–2532. [CrossRef]
68. Issac, M.; Aknin, M.; Gauvin-Bialecki, A.; De Voogd, N.; Ledoux, A.; Frederich, M.; Kashman, Y.; Carmeli, S. Cyclotheonellazoles A–C, potent protease inhibitors from the marine sponge Theonella aff. swinhoei. *J. Nat. Prod.* **2017**, *80*, 1110–1116. [CrossRef]
69. Erickson, K.L.; Gustafson, K.R.; Milanowski, D.J.; Pannell, L.K.; Klose, J.R.; Boyd, M.R. Myriastramides A–C, new modified cyclic peptides from the Philippines marine sponge Myriastra clavosa. *Tetrahedron* **2003**, *59*, 10231–10238. [CrossRef]
70. Kehraus, S.; König, G.M.; Wright, A.D.; Woerheide, G. Leucamide A: A new cytotoxic heptapeptide from the Australian sponge Leucetta microraphis. *J. Org. Chem.* **2002**, *67*, 4989–4992. [CrossRef]
71. Tan, K.O.; Wakimoto, T.; Takada, K.; Ohtsuki, T.; Uchiyama, N.; Goda, Y.; Abe, I. Cycloforskamide, a cytotoxic macrocyclic peptide from the sea slug *Pleurobranchus forskalii*. *J. Nat. Prod.* **2013**, *76*, 1388–1391. [CrossRef] [PubMed]
72. Wesson, K.J.; Hamann, M.T. Keenamide A, a bioactive cyclic peptide from the marine mollusk Pleurobranchus forskalii. *J. Nat. Prod.* **1996**, *59*, 629–631. [CrossRef] [PubMed]

73. Dalisay, D.S.; Rogers, E.W.; Edison, A.S.; Molinski, T.F. Structure elucidation at the nanomole scale. 1. Trisoxazole macrolides and thiazole-containing cyclic peptides from the nudibranch Hexabranchus sanguineus. *J. Nat. Prod.* **2009**, *72*, 732–738. [CrossRef] [PubMed]
74. Zhou, X.; Huang, H.; Chen, Y.; Tan, J.; Song, Y.; Zou, J.; Tian, X.; Hua, Y.; Ju, J. Marthiapeptide A, an anti-infective and cytotoxic polythiazole cyclopeptide from a 60 L scale fermentation of the deep sea-derived Marinactinospora thermotolerans SCSIO 00652. *J. Nat. Prod.* **2012**, *75*, 2251–2255. [CrossRef]
75. Sone, H.; Kigoshi, H.; Yamada, K. Isolation and stereostructure of dolastatin I, a cytotoxic cyclic hexapeptide from the Japanese sea hare Dolabella auricularia. *Tetrahedron* **1997**, *53*, 8149–8154. [CrossRef]
76. Ojika, M.; Nemoto, T.; Nakamura, M.; Yamada, K. Dolastatin E, a new cyclic hexapeptide isolated from the sea hare Dolabella auricularia. *Tetrahedron Lett.* **1995**, *36*, 5057–5058. [CrossRef]
77. Tan, L.T.; Williamson, R.T.; Gerwick, W.H.; Watts, K.S.; McGough, K.; Jacobs, R. *cis, cis-* and *trans, trans*-Ceratospongamide, new bioactive cyclic heptapeptides from the Indonesian red alga *Ceratodictyon spongiosum* and symbiotic sponge *Sigmadocia symbiotica*. *J. Org. Chem.* **2000**, *65*, 419–425. [CrossRef]
78. Matsuo, Y.; Kanoh, K.; Yamori, T.; Kasai, H.; Katsuta, A.; Adachi, K.; Shin-ya, K.; Shizuri, Y. Urukthapelstatin A, a novel cytotoxic substance from marine-derived Mechercharimyces asporophorigenens YM11-542. *J. Antibiot.* **2007**, *60*, 251–255. [CrossRef]
79. Kanoh, K.; Matsuo, Y.; Adachi, K.; Imagawa, H.; Nishizawa, M.; Shizuri, Y. Mechercharmycins A and B, cytotoxic substances from marine-derived Thermoactinomyces sp. YM3-251. *J. Antibiot.* **2005**, *58*, 289–292. [CrossRef]
80. Itokawa, H.; Yun, Y.; Morita, H.; Takeya, K.; Yamada, K. Estrogen-like activity of cyclic peptides from Vaccaria segetalis extracts. *Planta Med.* **1995**, *61*, 561–562. [CrossRef]
81. Joo, S.H. Cyclic Peptides as therapeutic agents and biochemical tools. *Biomol. Ther. (Seoul)* **2012**, *20*, 19–26. [CrossRef] [PubMed]
82. Goodwin, D.; Simerska, P.; Toth, I. Peptides as therapeutics with enhanced bioactivity. *Curr. Med. Chem.* **2012**, *19*, 4451–4461. [CrossRef]
83. Pathak, D.; Dahiya, R. Cyclic peptides as novel antineoplastic agents: A review. *J. Sci. Pharm.* **2003**, *4*, 125–131.
84. Clark, W.D.; Corbett, T.; Valeriote, F.; Crews, P. Cyclocinamide A. An unusual cytotoxic halogenated hexapeptide from the marine sponge Psammocinia. *J. Am. Chem. Soc.* **1997**, *119*, 9285–9286. [CrossRef]
85. Laird, D.W.; LaBarbera, D.V.; Feng, X.; Bugni, T.S.; Harper, M.K.; Ireland, C.M. Halogenated cyclic peptides isolated from the sponge *Corticium* sp. *J. Nat. Prod.* **2007**, *70*, 741–746. [CrossRef] [PubMed]
86. Luesch, H.; Yoshida, W.Y.; Moore, R.E.; Paul, V.J. Isolation and structure of the cytotoxin Lyngbyabellin B and absolute configuration of Lyngbyapeptin A from the marine cyanobacterium Lyngbya majuscula. *J. Nat. Prod.* **2000**, *63*, 1437–1439. [CrossRef]
87. Kobayashi, L.; Sato, M.; Murayama, T.; Ishibashi, M.; Walchi, M.R.; Kanai, M.; Shoji, J.; Ohizumie, Y. Konbamide, a novel peptide with calmodulin antagonistic activity from the okinawan marine sponge Theonella sp. *J. Chem. Soc. Chem. Commun.* **1991**, 1050–1052. [CrossRef]
88. Gulavita, N.K.; Gunasekela, S.P.; Pomponi, S.A.; Robinson, E.V. Polydiscamide A: A new bioactive depsipeptide from the marine sponge Discodermia sp. *J. Org. Chem.* **1992**, *57*, 1767–1772. [CrossRef]
89. Jamison, M.T.; Molinski, T.F. Jamaicensamide A, a peptide containing β-amino-α-keto and thiazole-homologated η-amino acid residues from the sponge Plakina jamaicensis. *J. Nat. Prod.* **2016**, *79*, 2243–2249. [CrossRef]
90. Pettit, G.R.; Kamano, Y.; Holzapfel, C.W.; van Zyl, W.J.; Tuinman, A.A.; Herald, C.L.; Baczynskyj, L.; Schmidt, J.M. Antineoplastic agents. 150. The structure and synthesis of dolastatin 3. *J. Am. Chem. Soc.* **1987**, *109*, 7581–7582. [CrossRef]
91. Raveh, A.; Carmeli, S. Aeruginazole A, a novel thiazole-containing cyclopeptide from the cyanobacterium *Microcystis* sp. *Org. Lett.* **2010**, *12*, 3536–3539. [CrossRef] [PubMed]
92. Williams, P.G.; Yoshida, W.Y.; Moore, R.E.; Paul, V.J. Micromide and guamamide: Cytotoxic alkaloids from a species of the marine cyanobacterium Symploca. *J. Nat. Prod.* **2004**, *67*, 49–53. [CrossRef]
93. Poncet, J. The dolastatins, a family of promising antineoplastic agents. *Curr. Pharm. Des.* **1999**, *5*, 139–162. [PubMed]

94. Luesch, H.; Moore, R.E.; Paul, V.J.; Mooberry, S.L.; Corbett, T.H. Isolation of dolastatin 10 from the marine cyanobacterium Symploca species VP642 and total stereochemistry and biological evaluation of its analogue symplostatin 1. *J. Nat. Prod.* **2001**, *64*, 907–910. [CrossRef] [PubMed]
95. Harrigan, G.G.; Luesch, H.; Yoshida, W.Y.; Moore, R.E.; Nagle, D.G.; Paul, V.J.; Mooberry, S.L.; Corbett, T.H.; Valeriote, F.A. Symplostatin 1: A dolastatin 10 analogue from the marine cyanobacterium Symploca hydnoides. *J. Nat. Prod.* **1998**, *61*, 1075–1077. [CrossRef] [PubMed]
96. Pettit, G.R.; Xu, J.; Williams, M.D.; Hogan, F.; Schmidt, J.M.; Cerny, R.L. Antineoplastic agents 370. Isolation and structure of dolastatin 18. *Bioorg. Med. Cem. Lett.* **1997**, *7*, 827–832. [CrossRef]
97. Klein, D.; Braekman, J.-C.; Daloze, D.; Hoffmann, L.; Castillo, G.; Demoulin, V. Lyngbyapeptin A, a modified tetrapeptide from Lyngbya bouillonii (Cyanophyceae). *Tetrahedron Lett.* **1999**, *40*, 695–696. [CrossRef]
98. Luesch, H.; Yoshida, W.Y.; Moore, R.E.; Paul, V.J. Structurally diverse new alkaloids from Palauan collections of the apratoxin-producing marine cyanobacterium *Lyngbya* sp. *Tetrahedron* **2002**, *58*, 7959–7966. [CrossRef]
99. Tan, L.T. Marine Cyanobacteria: A Treasure Trove of Bioactive Secondary Metabolites for Drug Discovery. In *Studies in Natural Product Chemistry*, 1st ed.; Atta-ur-Rahman, Ed.; Elsevier: Amsterdam, The Netherlands, 2012; Volume 36, p. 80, Chapter 4.
100. Luesch, H.; Yoshida, W.Y.; Moore, R.E.; Paul, V.J. Apramides A–G, novel lipopeptides from the marine cyanobacterium Lyngbya majuscula. *J. Nat. Prod.* **2000**, *63*, 1106–1112. [CrossRef]
101. Sorek, H. Isolation, structure elucidation and biological activity of natural products from marine organisms. Ph.D. Thesis, Tel Aviv University, Tel Aviv, Israel, 2010.
102. Boden, C.; Pattenden, G. Total synthesis of lissoclinamide 5, a cytotoxic cyclic peptide from the tunicate Lissoclinum patella. *Tetrahedron Lett.* **1994**, *35*, 8271–8274. [CrossRef]
103. Wipf, P.; Fritch, P.C. Total synthesis and assignment of configuration of lissoclinamide 7. *J. Am. Chem. Soc.* **1996**, *118*, 12358–12367. [CrossRef]
104. Boden, C.D.J.; Pattenden, G. Total syntheses and re-assignment of configurations of the cyclopeptides lissoclinamide 4 and lissoclinamide 5 from Lissoclinum patella. *J. Chem. Soc. Perkin Trans. 1* **2000**, *6*, 875–882. [CrossRef]
105. Banker, R.; Carmeli, S. Tenuecyclamides A–D, cyclic hexapeptides from the cyanobacterium Nostoc spongiaeforme var. *tenue*. *J. Nat. Prod.* **1998**, *61*, 1248–1251. [CrossRef] [PubMed]
106. Hamamoto, Y.; Endo, M.; Nakagawa, M.; Nakanishi, T.; Mizukawa, K. A new cyclic peptide, ascidiacyclamide, isolated from ascidian. *J. Chem. Soc. Chem. Commun.* **1983**, *6*, 323–324. [CrossRef]
107. Todorova, A.K.; Juettner, F.; Linden, A.; Pluess, T.; von Philipsborn, W. Nostocyclamide: A new macrocyclic, thiazole-containing allelochemical from Nostoc sp. 31 (cyanobacteria). *J. Org. Chem.* **1995**, *60*, 7891–7895. [CrossRef]
108. Sera, Y.; Adachi, K.; Fujii, K.; Shizuri, Y. A new antifouling hexapeptide from a palauan sponge, *Haliclona* sp. *J. Nat. Prod.* **2003**, *66*, 719–721. [CrossRef]
109. Uemoto, H.; Yahiro, Y.; Shigemori, H.; Tsuda, M.; Takao, T.; Shimonishi, Y.; Kobayashi, J. Keramamides K and L, new cyclic peptides containing unusual tryptophan residue from Theonella sponge. *Tetrahedron* **1998**, *54*, 6719–6724. [CrossRef]
110. Kimura, M.; Wakimoto, T.; Egami, Y.; Tan, K.C.; Ise, Y.; Abe, I. Calyxamides A and B, cytotoxic cyclic peptides from the marine sponge Discodermia calyx. *J. Nat. Prod.* **2012**, *75*, 290–294. [CrossRef]
111. Just-Baringo, X.; Albericio, F.; Alvarez, M. Thiopeptide antibiotics: Retrospective and recent advances. *Mar. Drugs* **2014**, *12*, 317–351. [CrossRef]
112. Engelhardt, K.; Degnes, K.F.; Kemmler, M.; Bredholt, H.; Fjaervik, E.; Klinkenberg, G.; Sletta, H.; Ellingsen, T.E.; Zotchev, S.B. Production of a new thiopeptide antibiotic, TP-1161, by a marine Nocardiopsis species. *Appl. Environ. Microbiol.* **2010**, *76*, 4969–4976. [CrossRef]
113. Suzumura, K.; Yokoi, T.; Funatsu, M.; Nagai, K.; Tanaka, K.; Zhang, H.; Suzuki, K. YM-266183 and YM-266184, novel thiopeptide antibiotics produced by Bacillus cereus isolated from a marine sponge II. Structure elucidation. *J. Antibiot (Tokyo)* **2003**, *56*, 129–134. [CrossRef] [PubMed]
114. Palomo, S.; González, I.; de la Cruz, M.; Martín, J.; Tormo, J.R.; Anderson, M.; Hill, R.T.; Vicente, F.; Reyes, F.; Genilloud, O. Sponge-derived Kocuria and Micrococcus spp. as sources of the new thiazolyl peptide antibiotic kocurin. *Mar. Drugs* **2013**, *11*, 1071–1086. [CrossRef] [PubMed]

115. Just-Baringo, X.; Bruno, P.; Ottesen, L.K.; Cañedo, L.M.; Albericio, F.; Álvarez, M. Total synthesis and stereochemical assignment of baringolin. *Angew. Chem. Int. Ed. Engl.* **2013**, *52*, 7818–7821. [CrossRef] [PubMed]
116. Iniyan, A.M.; Sudarman, E.; Wink, J.; Kannan, R.R.; Vincent, S.G.P. Ala-geninthiocin, a new broad spectrum thiopeptide antibiotic, produced by a marine Streptomyces sp. ICN19. *J. Antibiot.* **2019**, *72*, 99–105. [CrossRef] [PubMed]
117. Ireland, C.M.; Durso, A.R.; Newman, R.A.; Hacker, M.P. Antineoplastic cyclic peptides from the marine tunicate Lissoclinum patella. *J. Org. Chem.* **1982**, *47*, 1807–1811. [CrossRef]
118. Bewley, C.A.; He, H.; Williams, D.H.; Faulkner, D.J. Aciculitins A–C: Cytotoxic and antifungal cyclic peptides from the lithistid sponge Aciculites orientalis. *J. Am. Chem. Soc.* **1996**, *118*, 4314–4321. [CrossRef]
119. Bewley, C.A.; Faulkner, D.J. Theonegramide, an antifungal glycopeptide from the Philippine lithistid sponge Theonella swinhoei. *J. Org. Chem.* **1994**, *59*, 4849–4852. [CrossRef]
120. Matsunaga, S.; Fusetani, N. Theonellamides A-E, cytotoxic bicyclic peptides, from a marine sponge Theonella sp. *J. Org. Chem.* **1995**, *60*, 1177–1181. [CrossRef]
121. Matsunaga, S.; Fusetani, N.; Hashimoto, K.; Walchli, M. Theonellamide, F. A novel antifungal bicyclic peptide from a marine sponge Theonella sp. *J. Am. Chem. Soc.* **1989**, *111*, 2582–2588. [CrossRef]
122. Morita, H.; Shimbo, K.; Shigemori, H.; Kobayashi, J. Antimitotic activity of moroidin, a bicyclic peptide from the seeds of Celosia argentea. *Bioorg. Med. Chem. Lett.* **2000**, *10*, 469–471. [CrossRef]
123. Kobayashi, J.; Suzuki, H.; Shimbo, K.; Takeya, K.; Morita, H. Celogentins A–C, new antimitotic bicyclic peptides from the seeds of Celosia argentea. *J. Org. Chem.* **2001**, *66*, 6626–6633. [CrossRef] [PubMed]
124. Rhodes, C.A.; Pei, D. Bicyclic Peptides as next-generation therapeutics. *Chemistry* **2017**, *23*, 12690–12703. [CrossRef] [PubMed]
125. Zhao, J.-C.; Yu, S.-M.; Liu, Y.; Yao, Z.-J. Biomimetic synthesis of ent-(−)-Azonazine and stereochemical reassignment of natural product. *Org. Lett.* **2013**, *15*, 4300–4303. [CrossRef] [PubMed]
126. Sun, P.; Maloney, K.N.; Nam, S.-J.; Haste, N.M.; Raju, R.; Aalbersberg, W.; Jensen, P.R.; Nizet, V.; Hensler, M.E.; Fenical, W. Fijimycins A–C, three antibacterial etamycin-class depsipeptides from a marine-derived *Streptomyces* sp. *Bioorg. Med. Chem.* **2011**, *19*, 6557–6562. [CrossRef]
127. Gala, F.; D'Auria, M.V.; De Marino, S.; Sepe, V.; Zollo, F.; Smith, C.D.; Keller, S.N.; Zampella, A. Jaspamides M–P: New tryptophan modified jaspamide derivatives from the sponge Jaspis splendans. *Tetrahedron* **2009**, *65*, 51–56. [CrossRef]
128. Tabudravu, J.; Morris, L.A.; Kettenes-van den Bosch, J.J.; Jaspars, M. Wainunuamide, a histidine-containing proline-rich cyclic heptapeptide isolated from the Fijian marine sponge Stylotella aurantium. *Tetrahedron Lett.* **2001**, *42*, 9273–9276. [CrossRef]
129. Um, S.; Kim, Y.-J.; Kwon, H.; Wen, H.; Kim, S.-H.; Kwon, H.C.; Park, S.; Shin, J.; Oh, D.-C. Sungsanpin, a lasso peptide from a deep-sea Streptomycete. *J. Nat. Prod.* **2013**, *76*, 873–879. [CrossRef]
130. Song, Y.; Li, Q.; Liu, X.; Chen, Y.; Zhang, Y.; Sun, A.; Zhang, W.; Zhang, J.; Ju, J. Cyclic hexapeptides from the deep South China sea-derived Streptomyces scopuliridis SCSIO ZJ46 active against pathogenic gram-positive bacteria. *J. Nat. Prod.* **2014**, *77*, 1937–1941. [CrossRef]
131. Zheng, J.; Zhu, H.; Hong, K.; Wang, Y.; Liu, P.; Wang, X.; Peng, X.; Zhu, W. Novel cyclic hexapeptides from marine-derived fungus, Aspergillus sclerotiorum PT06-1. *Org. Lett.* **2009**, *11*, 5262–5265. [CrossRef]
132. Mueller, L.K.; Baumruck, A.C.; Zhdanova, H.; Tietze, A.A. Challenges and perspectives in chemical synthesis of highly hydrophobic peptides. *Front. Bioeng. Biotechnol.* **2020**, *8*, 162. [CrossRef]
133. Dahiya, R.; Pathak, D. First total synthesis and biological evaluation of halolitoralin A. *J. Serb. Chem. Soc.* **2007**, *72*, 101–107. [CrossRef]
134. Dahiya, R.; Pathak, D. Synthesis, characterization and biological evaluation of halolitoralin B-A natural cyclic peptide. *Asian J. Chem.* **2007**, *19*, 1499–1505.
135. Dahiya, R.; Pathak, D. Synthetic studies on a natural cyclic tetrapeptide-halolitoralin C. *J. Pharm. Res.* **2006**, *5*, 69–73.
136. Dahiya, R.; Pathak, D.; Bhatt, S. Synthesis and biological evaluation of a novel series of 2-(2′-isopropyl-5′-methylphenoxy) acetyl amino acids and dipeptides. *Bull. Chem. Soc. Ethiop.* **2006**, *20*, 235–245. [CrossRef]
137. Dahiya, R.; Pathak, D. Synthetic studies on novel benzimidazolopeptides with antimicrobial, cytotoxic and anthelmintic potential. *Eur. J. Med. Chem.* **2007**, *42*, 772–798. [CrossRef]

138. Dahiya, R.; Kumar, A.; Yadav, R. Synthesis and biological activity of peptide derivatives of iodoquinazolinones/nitroimidazoles. *Molecules* **2008**, *13*, 958–976. [CrossRef]
139. Dahiya, R. Synthesis, characterization and antimicrobial studies on some newer imidazole analogs. *Sci. Pharm.* **2008**, *76*, 217–240. [CrossRef]
140. Rajiv, M.H.; Ramana, M.V. Synthesis of 6-nitrobenzimidazol-1-acetyl amino acids and peptides as potent anthelmintic agents. *Indian J. Heterocycl. Chem.* **2002**, *12*, 121–124.
141. Dahiya, R.; Mourya, R.; Agrawal, S.C. Synthesis and antimicrobial screening of peptidyl derivatives of bromocoumarins/methylimidazoles. *Afr. J. Pharma. Pharmacol.* **2010**, *4*, 214–225.
142. Dahiya, R.; Kumar, A. Synthesis, spectral and anthelmintic activity studies on some novel imidazole derivatives. *E-J. Chem.* **2008**, *5*, 1133–1143. [CrossRef]
143. Himaja, M.; Rajiv; Ramana, M.V.; Poojary, B.; Satyanarayana, D.; Subrahmanyam, E.V.; Bhat, K.I. Synthesis and biological activity of a novel series of 4-[2′-(6′-nitro) benzimidazolyl] benzoyl amino acids and peptides. *Boll. Chim. Farmac.* **2003**, *142*, 450–453.
144. Dahiya, R.; Kaur, R. Synthesis and anthelmintic potential of a novel series of 2-mercaptobenzimidazolopeptides. *Biosci. Biotech. Res. Asia* **2007**, *4*, 561–566.
145. Singh, A.P.; Ramadan, W.M.; Dahiya, R.; Sarpal, A.S.; Pathak, K. Product development studies of amino acid conjugate of aceclofenac. *Curr. Drug Deliv.* **2009**, *6*, 208–216. [CrossRef] [PubMed]
146. Dahiya, R.; Mourya, R. Synthesis of peptide analogs of 4-[2-(3-bromophenyl)-7-nitro-4-oxo-3,4-dihydro-3-quinazolinyl] benzoic acids as potent antifungal agents. *Indian J. Heterocycl. Chem.* **2013**, *22*, 407–412.
147. Dahiya, R.; Pathak, D. Synthesis of heterocyclic analogs of 5-(4-methylcarboxamidophenyl)-2- furoic acid as potent antimicrobial agents. *Indian J. Heterocycl. Chem.* **2006**, *16*, 53–56.
148. Dahiya, R.; Mourya, R. Synthetic studies on novel nitroquinazolinone analogs with antimicrobial potential. *Bull. Pharm. Res.* **2013**, *3*, 51–57.
149. Dahiya, R.; Kaur, R. Synthesis of some 1, 2, 5-trisubstituted benzimidazole analogs as possible anthelmintic and antimicrobial agents. *Int. J. Biol. Chem. Sci.* **2008**, *2*, 1–13. [CrossRef]
150. Dahiya, R.; Bansal, Y. Synthesis and antimicrobial potential of novel quinoxalinopeptide analogs. *Res. J. Chem. Environ.* **2008**, *12*, 52–58.
151. Dahiya, R. Synthesis of 4-(2-methyl-1*H*-5-imidazolyl) benzoyl amino acids and peptides as possible anthelmintic agents. *Ethiop. Pharm. J.* **2008**, *26*, 17–26. [CrossRef]
152. Dahiya, R.; Kumar, S.; Khokra, S.L.; Gupta, S.V.; Sutariya, V.B.; Bhatia, D.; Sharma, A.; Singh, S.; Maharaj, S. Toward the synthesis and improved biopotential of an *N*-methylated analog of a proline-rich cyclic tetrapeptide from marine bacteria. *Mar. Drugs* **2018**, *16*, 305. [CrossRef]
153. Dahiya, R.; Singh, S. Synthesis, characterization, and biological activity studies on fanlizhicyclopeptide A. *Iran. J. Pharm. Res.* **2017**, *16*, 1176–1184. [PubMed]
154. Dahiya, R.; Singh, S.; Sharma, A.; Chennupati, S.V.; Maharaj, S. First total synthesis and biological screening of a proline-rich cyclopeptide from a Caribbean marine sponge. *Mar. Drugs* **2016**, *14*, 228. [CrossRef] [PubMed]
155. Dahiya, R.; Gautam, H. Total synthesis and antimicrobial activity of a natural cycloheptapeptide of marine origin. *Mar. Drugs* **2010**, *8*, 2384–2394. [CrossRef] [PubMed]
156. Dahiya, R.; Kumar, A.; Gupta, R. Synthesis, cytotoxic and antimicrobial screening of a proline-rich cyclopolypeptide. *Chem. Pharm. Bull. (Tokyo)* **2009**, *57*, 214–217. [CrossRef]
157. Dahiya, R. Total synthesis and biological potential of psammosilenin A. *Arch. Pharm. (Weinheim)* **2008**, *341*, 502–509. [CrossRef]
158. Dahiya, R. Synthesis of a phenylalanine-rich peptide as potential anthelmintic and cytotoxic agent. *Acta Pol. Pharm.* **2007**, *64*, 509–516.
159. Dahiya, R. Synthetic and pharmacological studies on longicalycinin A. *Pak. J. Pharm. Sci.* **2007**, *20*, 317–323.
160. Dahiya, R.; Pathak, D.; Himaja, M.; Bhatt, S. First total synthesis and biological screening of hymenamide E. *Acta Pharm.* **2006**, *56*, 399–415.
161. Dahiya, R.; Gautam, H. Solution phase synthesis and bioevaluation of cordyheptapeptide B. *Bull. Pharm. Res.* **2011**, *1*, 1–10.
162. Dahiya, R. Synthesis, characterization and biological evaluation of a glycine-rich peptide-cherimolacyclopeptide E. *J. Chil. Chem. Soc.* **2007**, *52*, 1224–1229. [CrossRef]

163. Dahiya, R. Synthesis and in vitro cytotoxic activity of a natural peptide of plant origin. *J. Iran. Chem. Soc.* **2008**, *5*, 445–452. [CrossRef]
164. Dahiya, R. Synthesis, spectroscopic and biological investigation of cyclic octapeptide: Cherimolacyclopeptide G. *Turk. J. Chem.* **2008**, *32*, 205–215.
165. Dahiya, R.; Maheshwari, M.; Kumar, A. Toward the synthesis and biological evaluation of hirsutide. *Monatsh. Chem.* **2009**, *140*, 121–127. [CrossRef]
166. Dahiya, R. Synthesis and biological activity of a cyclic hexapeptide from *Dianthus superbus*. *Chem. Pap.* **2008**, *62*, 527–535. [CrossRef]
167. Dahiya, R.; Gautam, H. Synthesis and pharmacological studies on a cyclooligopeptide from marine bacteria. *Chin. J. Chem.* **2011**, *29*, 1911–1916.
168. Dahiya, R.; Singh, S.; Kaur, K.; Kaur, R. Total synthesis of a natural cyclooligopeptide from fruits of sugar-apples. *Bull. Pharm. Res.* **2017**, *7*, 151.
169. Dahiya, R.; Singh, S. First total synthesis and biological potential of a heptacyclopeptide of plant origin. *Chin. J. Chem.* **2016**, *34*, 1158–1164. [CrossRef]
170. Bruno, P.; Peña, S.; Just-Baringo, X.; Albericio, F.; Álvarez, M. Total synthesis of aeruginazole A. *Org. Lett.* **2011**, *13*, 4648–4651. [CrossRef]
171. You, S.-L.; Kelly, J.W. Total synthesis of didmolamides A and B. *Tetrahedron Lett.* **2005**, *46*, 2567–2570. [CrossRef]
172. Zhou, W.; Nie, X.-D.; Zhang, Y.; Si, C.-M.; Zhou, Z.; Sun, X.; Wei, B.-G. A practical approach to asymmetric synthesis of dolastatin 10. *Org. Biomol. Chem.* **2017**, *15*, 6119–6131. [CrossRef]
173. Sellanes, D.; Manta, E.; Serra, G. Toward the total synthesis of scleritodermin A: Preparation of the C_1–N_{15} fragment. *Tetrahedron Lett.* **2007**, *48*, 1827–1830. [CrossRef] [PubMed]
174. Zhang, W.; Ma, Z.-H.; Mei, D.; Li, C.-X.; Zhang, X.-L.; Li, Y.-X. Total synthesis and reassignment of stereochemistry of obyanamide. *Tetrahedron* **2006**, *62*, 9966–9972. [CrossRef]
175. Zhang, W.; Ding, N.; Li, Y. Synthesis and biological evaluation of analogues of the marine cyclic depsipeptide obyanamide. *J. Pept. Sci.* **2011**, *17*, 533–539. [CrossRef] [PubMed]
176. Zhang, Y.; Islam, M.A.; McAlpine, S.R. Synthesis of the natural product marthiapeptide A. *Org. Lett.* **2015**, *17*, 5149–5151. [CrossRef] [PubMed]
177. Dahiya, R.; Singh, S.; Varghese Gupta, S.; Sutariya, V.B.; Bhatia, D.; Mourya, R.; Chennupati, S.V.; Sharma, A. First total synthesis and pharmacological potential of a plant based hexacyclopeptide. *Iran. J. Pharm. Res.* **2019**, *18*, 938–947.
178. Dahiya, R.; Singh, S. Synthesis, characterization and biological screening of diandrine A. *Acta Pol. Pharm.* **2017**, *74*, 873–880.
179. Dahiya, R.; Kumar, A. Synthetic and biological studies on a cyclopolypeptide of plant origin. *J. Zhejiang Univ. Sci. B* **2008**, *9*, 391–400. [CrossRef]
180. Dahiya, R.; Kaur, K. Synthesis and pharmacological investigation of segetalin C as a novel antifungal and cytotoxic agent. *Arzneimittelforschung* **2008**, *58*, 29–34. [CrossRef]
181. Dahiya, R.; Kaur, K. Synthetic and biological studies on natural cyclic heptapeptide: Segetalin E. *Arch. Pharm. Res.* **2007**, *30*, 1380–1386. [CrossRef]
182. Dahiya, R.; Maheshwari, M.; Yadav, R. Synthetic and cytotoxic and antimicrobial activity studies on annomuricatin B. *Z. Naturforsch. B* **2009**, *64*, 237–244. [CrossRef]
183. Dahiya, R.; Gautam, H. Toward the first total synthesis of gypsin D: A natural cyclopolypeptide from Gypsophila arabica. *Am. J. Sci. Res.* **2010**, *11*, 150–158.
184. Wipf, P.; Fritch, P.C.; Geib, S.J.; Sefler, A.M. Conformational studies and structure–activity analysis of lissoclinamide 7 and related cyclopeptide alkaloids. *J. Am. Chem. Soc.* **1998**, *120*, 4105–4112. [CrossRef]
185. Fennell, B.J.; Carolan, S.; Pettit, G.R.; Bell, A. Effects of the antimitotic natural product dolastatin 10, and related peptides, on the human malarial parasite Plasmodium falciparum. *J. Antimicrb. Chemother.* **2003**, *51*, 833–841. [CrossRef] [PubMed]
186. Mooberry, S.L.; Leal, R.M.; Tinley, T.L.; Luesch, H.; Moore, R.E.; Corbett, T.H. The molecular pharmacology of symplostatin 1: A new antimitotic dolastatin 10 analog. *Int. J. Cancer* **2003**, *104*, 512–521. [CrossRef] [PubMed]

187. Liu, Y.; Salvador, L.A.; Byeon, S.; Ying, Y.; Kwan, J.C.; Law, B.K.; Hong, J.; Luesch, H. Anticolon cancer activity of largazole, a marine-derived tunable histone deacetylase inhibitor. *J. Pharmacol. Exp. Ther.* **2010**, *335*, 351–361. [CrossRef]
188. Kang, H.K.; Choi, M.C.; Seo, C.H.; Park, Y. Therapeutic properties and biological benefits of marine-derived anticancer peptides. *Int. J. Mol. Sci.* **2018**, *19*, 919. [CrossRef]
189. Espiritu, R.A.; Cornelio, K.; Kinoshita, M.; Matsumori, N.; Murata, M.; Nishimura, S.; Kakeya, H.; Yoshida, M.; Matsunaga, S. Marine sponge cyclic peptide theonellamide A disrupts lipid bilayer integrity without forming distinct membrane pores. *Biochim. Biophys. Acta* **2016**, *1858*, 1373–1379. [CrossRef]
190. Mahaffy, R.E.; Pollard, T.D. Influence of phalloidin on the formation of actin filament branches by Arp2/3 Complex. *Biochemistry* **2008**, *47*, 6460–6467. [CrossRef]
191. Odaka, C.; Sanders, M.L.; Crews, P. Jasplakinolide induces apoptosis in various transformed cell lines by a caspase-3-like protease-dependent pathway. *Clin. Diagn. Lab. Immun.* **2000**, *7*, 947–952. [CrossRef]
192. Wu, Q.-X.; Crews, M.S.; Draskovic, M.; Sohn, J.; Johnson, T.A.; Tenney, K.; Valeriote, F.A.; Yao, X.-J.; Bjeldanes, L.F.; Crews, P. Azonazine, a novel dipeptide from a Hawaiian marine sediment-derived fungus, Aspergillus insulicola. *Org. Lett.* **2010**, *12*, 4458–4461. [CrossRef]
193. Dahiya, S.; Pathak, K. Physicochemical characterization and dissolution enhancement of aceclofenac-hydroxypropyl beta-cyclodextrin binary systems. *PDA J. Pharm. Sci. Technol.* **2006**, *60*, 378–388. [PubMed]
194. Dahiya, S.; Pathak, K. Influence of amorphous cyclodextrin derivatives on aceclofenac release from directly compressible tablets. *Pharmazie* **2007**, *62*, 278–283. [PubMed]
195. Dahiya, S.; Kaushik, A.; Pathak, K. improved pharmacokinetics of aceclofenac immediate release tablets incorporating its inclusion complex with hydroxypropyl-β-cyclodextrin. *Sci. Pharm.* **2015**, *83*, 501–510. [CrossRef]
196. Dahiya, S. Studies on formulation development of a poorly water-soluble drug through solid dispersion technique. *Thai J. Pharm. Sci.* **2010**, *34*, 77–87.
197. Dahiya, S.; Kaushik, A. Effect of water soluble carriers on dissolution enhancement of aceclofenac. *Asian J. Pharm.* **2010**, *4*, 34–40. [CrossRef]
198. Dahiya, S.; Tayde, P. Binary and ternary solid systems of carvedilol. *Bull. Pharm. Res.* **2013**, *3*, 128–134.
199. Dahiya, R.; Dahiya, S. Ocular delivery of peptides and proteins. In *Drug Delivery for the Retina and Posterior Segment Disease*; Patel, J.K., Sutariya, V., Kanwar, J.R., Pathak, Y.V., Eds.; Springer: Cham, Switzerland, 2018; pp. 411–437, Chapter 24.
200. Dahiya, S.; Dahiya, R. Recent nanotechnological advancements in delivery of peptide and protein macromolecules. In *Nanotechnology in Biology and Medicine: Research Advancements and Future Perspectives*, 1st ed.; Rauta, P.R., Mohanta, Y.K., Nayak, D., Eds.; CRC Press, Taylor & Francis Group: Boca Raton, FL, USA, 2019; pp. 143–157, Chapter 11.
201. Otvos, L., Jr.; Wade, J.D. Current challenges in peptide-based drug discovery. *Front Chem.* **2014**, *2*, 62. [CrossRef]
202. Ayoub, M.; Scheidegger, D. Peptide drugs, overcoming the challenges, a growing business. *Chim. Oggi.* **2006**, *24*, 46–48.
203. Usmani, S.S.; Bedi, G.; Samuel, J.S.; Singh, S.; Kalra, S.; Kumar, P.; Ahuja, A.A.; Sharma, M.; Gautam, A.; Raghava, G.P.S. THPdb: Database of FDA-approved peptide and protein therapeutics. *PLoS ONE* **2017**, *12*, e0181748. [CrossRef]
204. Perez, E.A.; Hillman, D.W.; Fishkin, P.A.; Krook, J.E.; Tan, W.W.; Kuriakose, P.A.; Alberts, S.R.; Dakhil, S.R. Phase II trial of dolastatin-10 in patients with advanced breast cancer. *Investig. New Drugs* **2005**, *23*, 257–261. [CrossRef]
205. Mita, A.C.; Hammond, L.A.; Bonate, P.L.; Weiss, G.; McCreery, H.; Syed, S.; Garrison, M.; Chu, Q.S.; DeBono, J.S.; Jones, C.B.; et al. Phase I and pharmacokinetic study of tasidotin hydrochloride (ILX651), a third-generation dolastatin-15 analogue, administered weekly for 3 weeks every 28 days in patients with advanced solid tumors. *Clin. Cancer Res.* **2006**, *12*, 5207–5215. [CrossRef] [PubMed]
206. Smyth, J.; Boneterre, M.E.; Schellens, J.; Calvert, H.; Greim, G.; Wanders, J.; Hanauske, A. Activity of the dolastatin analogue, LU103793, in malignant melanoma. *Ann. Oncol.* **2001**, *12*, 509–511. [CrossRef] [PubMed]

207. Riely, G.J.; Gadgeel, S.; Rothman, I.; Saidman, B.; Sabbath, K.; Feit, K.; Kris, M.G.; Rizvi, N.A. A phase 2 study of TZT-1027, administered weekly to patients with advanced non-small cell lung cancer following treatment with platinum-based chemotherapy. *Lung Cancer* **2007**, *55*, 181–185. [CrossRef] [PubMed]
208. Ebbinghaus, S.; Hersh, E.; Cunningham, C.C.; O'Day, S.; McDermott, D.; Stephenson, J.; Richards, D.A.; Eckardt, J.; Haider, O.L.; Hammond, L.A. Phase II study of synthadotin (SYN-D.; ILX651) administered daily for 5 consecutive days once every 3 weeks (qdx5q3w) in patients (Pts) with inoperable locally advanced or metastatic melanoma. *J. Clin. Oncol.* **2004**, *22*, 7530. [CrossRef]
209. Supko, J.G.; Lynch, T.J.; Clark, J.W.; Fram, R.; Allen, L.F.; Velagapudi, R.; Kufe, D.W.; Eder, J.P., Jr. A phase I clinical and pharmacokinetic study of the dolastatin analogue cemadotin administered as a 5-day continuous intravenous infusion. *Cancer Chemother. Pharmacol.* **2000**, *46*, 319–328. [CrossRef] [PubMed]
210. Giddings, L.A.; Newman, D.J. Microbial natural products: Molecular blueprints for antitumor drugs. *J. Ind. Microbiol. Biotechnol.* **2013**, *40*, 1181–1210. [CrossRef]
211. Newman, D.J.; Cragg, G.M. Current status of marine-derived compounds as warheads in anti-tumor drug candidates. *Mar. Drugs* **2017**, *15*, 99. [CrossRef]

MDPI
St. Alban-Anlage 66
4052 Basel
Switzerland
Tel. +41 61 683 77 34
Fax +41 61 302 89 18
www.mdpi.com

Marine Drugs Editorial Office
E-mail: marinedrugs@mdpi.com
www.mdpi.com/journal/marinedrugs

www.ingramcontent.com/pod-product-compliance
Lightning Source LLC
LaVergne TN
LVHW070555100526
838202LV00012B/472
* 9 7 8 3 0 3 6 5 2 7 5 2 9 *

About the Editors

Michael Chourdakis is an Associate Professor of Medical Nutrition–Hygiene at the School of Medicine of the Aristotle University of Thessaloniki, Greece. He has a strong interest in clinical trials (e.g., Principal Investigator of MIntS, NCT02383329, European Coordinator for the RE-ENERGIZE Study, NCT00985205) and is also the co-author of over 85 original publications, is the editor of three books on Clinical Nutrition (including the Greek version of the ESPEN Blue book) and of several chapters in clinical nutrition books in Greek, English, and German. He is a reviewer for over 12 peer-reviewed journals and serves as an assistant editor of two peer-reviewed journals. He is a member of various national and international societies, currently serving as the President of the Hellenic Society for Clinical Nutrition and Metabolism (GrESPEN) and was the IT-Officer of the European Society for Clinical Nutrition and Metabolism (ESPEN) between 2012–2017. He currently serves as the Guidelines' Officer for ESPEN (2020–24). He was a member of various national and international organizing and scientific congress committees and was the Chairman of the 1st Clinical Nutrition Congress held in Greece and the 24th ESPEN Course of Clinical Nutrition, which was held for the first time in Greece in 2017. He has participated as a lecturer and/or speaker in numerous national and international congresses/workshops/courses/LLL in more than 15 countries on 4 continents. Finally, he has been multi-awarded in 2017 and 2018 from the Faculty of Health Sciences of the Aristoteles University of Thessaloniki for his outstanding performance in various domains such as publishing, funds gathering, etc.

Emmanuella Magriplis is an Assistant Professor in Nutritional Epidemiology & Public Health at the Agricultural University of Athens (AUA), Greece. She has a strong interest in large epidemiological studies that investigate nutrition and health related diseases, mostly chronic diseases. She is the lead data analyst of the Hellenic National Nutrition & Health Survey (HNNHS). She has also collaborated on two other major studies including the European ATHLOS and an umbrella project PROgnostic Factor Evaluation—Systematic Searches, repOrting & Reviewing (PROFESSOR study). She simultaneously collaborates with the Hellenic Food Authority on public health prevention. Emmanuella Magriplis is a coauthor of 56 publications in peer-reviewed scientific journals, has contributed to the scientific editing and translation of five books, and has written three book chapters—all related to nutritional methodology, epidemiology, education, and public health nutrition. She is also a reviewer for more than 20 peer-reviewed journals and serves as a reviewing editor in two journals and has been a guest editor in over three journal-specific Special Issues. She completed her basic degree in Nutrition and Dietetics (BSc, McGill University) during which she received eight major scholarships and awards, one of which was from the Government of Canada (Natural Sciences and Engineering Research Council, NSERC), for academic excellence, having completed her studies at the top 15% of Canadian students in her field. She continued in the field of Epidemiology (MSc, University of London, LSHTM) gaining great expertise in Nutritional Epidemiology (PhD, Agricultural University of Athens, AUA).

Emmanuella Magriplis is currently affiliated with three universities other than the Agricultural University of Athens (AUA): Harokopio University, Aristoteles University of Thessaloniki, and United Arab Emirates University. For 3 years she was also affiliated with the University of Oxford (Centre for Statistics in Medicine, CSM) and worked on developing optimal methodological approaches for Systematic Review and Meta-analysis data extraction. A specific research project based on this work was published, with regard to heart failure, in a peer-reviewed journal. Emmanuella Magriplis is also currently the course coordinator and lecturer of Nutritional Epidemiology and Nutrition Education for undergraduate students. She also teaches Public Health Nutrition at the undergraduate and postgraduate level at AUA. She is also responsible for monitoring methodological and statistical research aspects for 5 Masters and 4 PhD students. Emmanuella Magriplis acts as a nutritional consultant for one of the largest Greek food manufacturing companies and is a member of the Hellenic Atherosclerosis Society and a board member of the Hellenic Nutrition Society. Emmanuella Magriplis has been recently elected as the vice president of a working group of the Hellenic Atherosclerosis Society, entitled "Epidemiology & Atherosclerosis Prevention" and has been also chosen to represent Greece at the European Commission Task Force responsible for setting Maximum Amounts of Vitamins & Minerals in Food Supplements and Fortified Foods.

nutrients MDPI

Editorial

Special Issue "Mediterranean Diet and Metabolic Diseases"

Emmanuella Magriplis [1,*] and Michail Chourdakis [2,*]

1 Department of Food Science and Human Nutrition, Agricultural University of Athens, Iera Odos 75, 11855 Athens, Greece
2 Laboratory of Hygiene, Social and Preventive Medicine and Medical Statistics, School of Medicine, Faculty of Health Sciences, Aristotle University of Thessaloniki, 54124 Thessaloniki, Greece
* Correspondence: emagriplis@aua.gr (E.M.); mhourd@gapps.auth.gr (M.C.)

Citation: Magriplis, E.; Chourdakis, M. Special Issue "Mediterranean Diet and Metabolic Diseases". *Nutrients* **2021**, *13*, 2680. https://doi.org/10.3390/nu13082680

Received: 14 July 2021
Accepted: 27 July 2021
Published: 1 August 2021

The Mediterranean diet (MD) has been considered among the healthiest dietary patterns since a little over 50 years ago, Ancel Keys—as the key figure—provided evidence for the beneficial effects of the MD. Furthermore, MD is recognized by UNESCO as an "Intangible Cultural Heritage of Humanity" since it is an integral part of tradition and heritage as well as one of the healthiest and most sustainable dietary patterns due to the fact that its baseline is plant-based foods, non-refined grains and cereals, and of course extra virgin olive oil. The MD has been inversely associated with various chronic and metabolic diseases, including cardiovascular disease and obesity, as well as with further metabolic factors. However, in past decades studies have shown that countries in the Mediterranean basin are drifting away from this prudent pattern and are adopting a more Westernized diet. This drift is due to many multidimensional and region-specific influences, including socioeconomic, sociodemographic, environmental and cultural/ethnic, as well as factors that interfere with food preferences/dislikes, with accessibility to foods and with religious beliefs.

If present trends persist, it is expected that non-communicable diseases (NCD) will have a growing incidence, making the studies included in the present Special Issue (SI) imperative, since despite the first ecological and population-based data, the aspects of the MD that may promote health in respect to other lifestyle variables remain under investigation, as Balakoudi and colleagues concluded following a systematic review [1]. This SI contains multifaceted research articles and a systematic review, which have addressed these issues both in healthy individuals and in those with specifically defined disease states or risk factors. Specifically, this SI contains research that has been carried out in not only the general population, but also among patients with Type 1 diabetes mellitus (T1DM) [2] or dyslipidemia [3–5], as well as among firefighters who are proxy to healthy and physically fit individuals [6,7], adding valuable information to the pre-stated gap in knowledge.

A very interesting paper that has been included in the present SI examines MD adherence during the COVID-19 pandemic by Polish women diagnosed with T1DM2. The authors performed an online case control study during the peak of the second COVID-19 pandemic wave and used the Mediterranean Diet Adherence Screener (MEDAS) to assess the level of adherence to the MD. Overall, the authors found that the majority of participants had a moderate adherence and found that significantly more women with T1DM compared to healthy women adhered to olive oil, fruit and fish and seafood intake. However, a significantly larger percentage also exceeded butter consumption per day and did not adhere to red meat recommendations, indicating a higher saturated fat intake, a factor in contrast to the American Diabetes Association guidelines [8,9]. This is of importance considering the adverse effects of the COVID-19 virus on health, especially on individuals who are already at high risk, such as individuals with diabetes mellitus.

In another study, Formisano and her colleagues helped to address gaps among individuals with dyslipidemia. another risk factor for metabolic diseases, especially atherosclerotic cardiovascular disease. They aimed to evaluate how adherence to the MD affects the lipid profile in patients with dyslipidemia, using a retrospective design [3]. Elevated levels of low-density lipoprotein cholesterol (LDL-c) and triglycerides (TG), with low levels of high-density lipoprotein cholesterol (HDL-c), represent the most atherogenic dyslipidemic profile, which has been shown to be potentially ameliorated from a higher MD adherence. The authors reported the beneficial effects of a higher MD adherence on both HDL-c and TG levels, the latter coinciding with more frequent olive oil intake, the main denominator of the MD. Results on HDL-c were in agreement with a cross-sectional study [7] and an intervention study [6] on healthy volunteers also included in the issue [6], and results on HDL-c and TG are in agreement with the systematic review published on metabolic syndrome specific risk factors [1]. The authors found that nutritional counselling improved adherence, as was also suggested by Grabia and colleagues in their study on T1DM women [2]. The authors also addressed the main conflicting issue today with regard to recommended intakes of total saturated fats, and based on their findings they suggested that foods containing saturated fats may need to be distinguished when researched. This suggestion pertains to investigating the whole food instead of specific macronutrients, in order to consider interactions, instead of the nutrient alone.

Four of the studies included in this issue have been carried out in healthy volunteers [4–7]. Romanidou and colleagues reported that for a unitary increase in MD adherence, the ratio of total cholesterol to HDL-c decreased by 0.03 and HDL-c increased by 0.25 mg/dL in 460 firefighters, after adjusting for multiple confounders [7]. Two of the studies examined adults residing in the United Arab Emirates (UAE), one of the countries that makes up the Gulf Cooperation Council that has seen a rapid improvement in socio-economic status and a simultaneous dietary transition. This dietary transition, characterized by an increase in processed food and meat intake—both regarded as factors that act as a mediator to overweight and obesity, metabolic syndrome and other risk factors—has contributed to the estimated high mortality from NCD's in these regions in total (65–68%); in UAE, CVD accounts for 25% of all deaths, a value that reaches 29% in Abu Dhabi.

Jarrar and his colleagues evaluated urinary sodium excretion using 24-h urine samples, the ideal methodology for evaluating sodium intake from food and added salt during cooking or at the table [4]. Sodium is the mineral that has received great attention in past years, and it is widely accepted that intakes above 2300 mg increase the risk of hypertension. Sodium, other than salt, is found in high concentrations in processed foods and meat—foods that characterize Western-type diets—whereas it is low in fruit, vegetables, and legumes—foods that prevail in the MD. The authors reported that 67.4% of the population that was assessed exceeded the recommended intake of 5–6 g of salt per day, with an average of 10.4 g per day, although only 45.5% reported always adding salt to their food and only 20% were aware of their overconsumption.

These results in combination with the unhealthy dietary patterns reported by Ismail and colleagues in UAE adults [5] reveal the extent of the problem in this region. The authors performed an online study to assess dietary habits and other behaviors during the COVID-19 lockdown. This was imperative since such measures may affect food accessibility and may also trigger stress leading to a more frequent consumption of "comfort foods". Results showed that during the lockdown, almost half of the respondents consumed sweets, 1/5 also had sweetened drinks in their diet, over 1/3 of the population consumed salty snacks, and a little over 60% consumed animal protein at least once a day. These results underline that in addition to the dietary transition seen the past decades in this region, the pandemic has further triggered unhealthy dietary choices that may further increase metabolic diseases, and the authors agree with Grabia and colleagues [2] and recommend dietary counseling to increase fruits, vegetables, and other foods close to the MD pattern. Moreover, the importance of dietary counseling on the lipid profile in healthy [6,7] and dyslipidemic individuals [3] was evident by intervention studies included in the present SI.

Metabolic Syndrome is one among many metabolic diseases with a dramatic rise in the past years. It has been closely linked with the transition to a more Westernized diet and is inversely associated with the MD. In this SI, this relationship was examined by Balakoudi and colleagues through a systematic review that assessed the impact of MD adherence on various parameters of the metabolic syndrome as defined by NCEP-ATP III criteria1. These parameters included waist circumference (WC), blood pressure, fasting blood glucose, HDL-c and TG, with a total of 41 observational studies included, summing to 74,058 adults. In total, 23 studies evaluated the level of MD adherence on WC with a significantly inverse pooled effect being found. HDL-c was assessed by 39 studies (N = 31,800 individuals) and the pooled effect showed increased levels with higher MD adherence, while TG were found significantly lower, in agreement with other studies included in the Special Issue [3,6,7].

It has to be mentioned at this point that to date there is no specific value that can be used to define the ideal level for high MD adherence, an aspect that needs to be further investigated, especially following results from the 6-month intervention study performed by Sotos-Prieto and colleagues, which resulted in favorable changes in lipid profile, even with a non-significant slight increase to the MD adherence [6].

The intervention study included in this SI addressed how it can ameliorate adherence to the MD diet and how this improvement, if any, affects specific metabolic biomarkers and other anthropometrics related to CVD in firefighters [6,7]. The authors concluded that the MD may promote beneficial changes in specific lipid species, including HDL-c, all LDL-c sizes, TG, total cholesterol and ApoA/ApoB ratio, due to the high content of mono- and polyunsaturated fatty acid found in this dietary pattern [6].

Collectively, this SI includes an array of studies from various countries that address directly or indirectly the effects of MD on health and additionally address the influence of the COVID-19 pandemic, the new challenge of the decade. It effectively summarizes not only effects of specific nutrients, such as sodium and saturated fats, but also of whole foods as well, on specific risk factors and biochemical indices, as well as to end-points of diseases. Finally, it highlights the importance of addressing the best way of defining high/low adherence to the MD and the need for population-specific interventions and potentially developing new and innovative uniform tools that will lead to an increase of adherence and preserve the MD pattern.

Conflicts of Interest: The authors declare no conflict of interest.

References

1. Bakaloudi, D.R.; Chrysoula, L.; Kotzakioulafi, E.; Theodoridis, X.; Chourdakis, M. Impact of the Level of Adherence to Mediterranean Diet on the Parameters of Metabolic Syndrome: A Systematic Review and Meta-Analysis of Observational Studies. *Nutrients* **2021**, *13*, 1514. [CrossRef] [PubMed]
2. Grabia, M.; Puścion-Jakubik, A.; Markiewicz-Żukowska, R.; Bielecka, J.; Mielech, A.; Nowakowski, P.; Socha, K. Adherence to Mediterranean Diet and Selected Lifestyle Elements among Young Women with Type 1 Diabetes Mellitus from Northeast Poland: A Case-Control COVID-19 Survey. *Nutrients* **2021**, *13*, 1173. [CrossRef] [PubMed]
3. Formisano, E.; Pasta, A.; Cremonini, A.L.; Di Lorenzo, I.; Sukkar, S.G.; Pisciotta, L. Effects of a Mediterranean Diet, Dairy, and Meat Products on Different Phenotypes of Dyslipidemia: A Preliminary Retrospective Analysis. *Nutrients* **2021**, *13*, 1161. [CrossRef] [PubMed]
4. Jarrar, A.H.; Stojanovska, L.; Apostolopoulos, V.; Cheikh Ismail, L.; Feehan, J.; Ohuma, E.O.; Ahmad, A.Z.; Alnoaimi, A.A.; Al Khaili, L.S.; Allowch, N.H.; et al. Assessment of Sodium Knowledge and Urinary Sodium Excretion among Regions of the United Arab Emirates: A Cross-Sectional Study. *Nutrients* **2020**, *12*, 2747. [CrossRef] [PubMed]
5. Cheikh Ismail, L.; Osaili, T.M.; Mohamad, M.N.; Al Marzouqi, A.; Jarrar, A.H.; Abu Jamous, D.O.; Magriplis, E.; Ali, H.I.; Sabbah, H.A.; Hasan, H.; et al. Eating Habits and Lifestyle during COVID-19 Lockdown in the United Arab Emirates: A Cross-Sectional Study. *Nutrients* **2020**, *12*, 3314. [CrossRef] [PubMed]
6. Sotos-Prieto, M.; Ruiz-Canela, M.; Song, Y.; Christophi, C.; Mofatt, S.; Rodriguez-Artalejo, F.; Kales, S.N. The Effects of a Mediterranean Diet Intervention on Targeted Plasma Metabolic Biomarkers among US Firefighters: A Pilot Cluster-Randomized Trial. *Nutrients* **2020**, *12*, 3610. [CrossRef] [PubMed]
7. Romanidou, M.; Tripsianis, G.; Hershey, M.S.; Sotos-Prieto, M.; Christophi, C.; Moffatt, S.; Constantinidis, T.C.; Kales, S.N. Association of the Modified Mediterranean Diet Score (mMDS) with Anthropometric and Biochemical Indices in US Career Firefighters. *Nutrients* **2020**, *12*, 3693. [CrossRef] [PubMed]

8. Gaforio, J.J.; Visioli, F.; Alarcón-de-la-Lastra, C.; Castañer, O.; Delgado-Rodríguez, M.; Fitó, M.; Hernández, A.F.; Huertas, J.R.; Martínez-González, M.A.; Menendez, J.A.; et al. Virgin Olive Oil and Health: Summary of the III International Conference on Virgin Olive Oil and Health Consensus Report, JAEN (Spain) 2018. *Nutrients* **2019**, *11*, 2039. [CrossRef] [PubMed]
9. Association, A.D. 4. Comprehensive Medical Evaluation and Assessment of Comorbidities: Standards of Medical Care in Diabetes-2021. *Diabetes Care* **2021**, *44*, S40–S52. [CrossRef] [PubMed]

nutrients

MDPI

Article

The Effects of a Mediterranean Diet Intervention on Targeted Plasma Metabolic Biomarkers among US Firefighters: A Pilot Cluster-Randomized Trial

Mercedes Sotos-Prieto [1,2,3,*], Miguel Ruiz-Canela [4,5], Yiqing Song [6], Costas Christophi [3,7], Steven Mofatt [8], Fernando Rodriguez-Artalejo [1,2,9] and Stefanos N. Kales [3,10]

1 Department of Preventive Medicine and Public Health, School of Medicine, Universidad Autónoma de Madrid, IdiPaz (Instituto de Investigación Sanitaria Hospital Universitario La Paz), Calle del Arzobispo Morcillo 4, 28029 Madrid, Spain; fernando.artalejo@uam.es
2 Biomedical Research Network Centre of Epidemiology and Public Health (CIBERESP), Carlos III Health Institute, 28029 Madrid, Spain
3 Department of Environmental Health, Harvard T.H. Chan School of Public Health, Boston, MA 02115, USA; costas.christophi@cut.ac.cy (C.C.); stefokali@aol.com (S.N.K.)
4 Department of Preventive Medicine and Public Health, IdiSNA, University of Navarra, 31009 Pamplona, Spain; mcanela@unav.es
5 Biomedical Research Network Centre for Pathophysiology of Obesity and Nutrition (CIBEROBN), Carlos III Health Institute, 28029 Madrid, Spain
6 Department of Epidemiology, Richard M. Fairbanks School of Public Health, Indiana University, Indianapolis, IN 46202, USA; yiqsong@iu.edu
7 Cyprus International Institute for Environmental and Public Health, Cyprus University of Technology, 30 Archbishop Kyprianou Str., 3036 Lemesos, Cyprus
8 National Institute for Public Safety Health, Indianapolis, IN 46204, USA; steven.mofatt@ascension.org
9 IMDEA-Food Institute, CEI UAM+CSIC, 28049 Madrid, Spain
10 Department of Occupational Medicine, Cambridge Health Alliance, Harvard Medical School, Cambridge, MA 02145, USA
* Correspondence: mercedes.sotos@uam.es; Tel.: +34-914975441

Received: 22 September 2020; Accepted: 18 November 2020; Published: 24 November 2020

Abstract: Metabolomics is improving the understanding of the mechanisms of the health effects of diet. Previous research has identified several metabolites associated with the Mediterranean Diet (MedDiet), but knowledge about longitudinal changes in metabolic biomarkers after a MedDiet intervention is scarce. A subsample of 48 firefighters from a cluster-randomized trial at Indianapolis fire stations was randomly selected for the metabolomics study at 12 months of follow up (time point 1), where Group 1 (n = 24) continued for another 6 months in a self-sustained MedDiet intervention, and Group 2 (n = 24), the control group at that time, started with an active MedDiet intervention for 6 months (time point 2). A total of 225 metabolites were assessed at the two time points by using a targeted NMR platform. The MedDiet score improved slightly but changes were non-significant (intervention: 24.2 vs. 26.0 points and control group: 26.1 vs. 26.5 points). The MedDiet intervention led to favorable changes in biomarkers related to lipid metabolism, including lower LDL-C, ApoB/ApoA1 ratio, remnant cholesterol, M-VLDL-CE; and higher HDL-C, and better lipoprotein composition. This MedDiet intervention induces only modest changes in adherence to the MedDiet and consequently in metabolic biomarkers. Further research should confirm these results based on larger study samples in workplace interventions with powerful study designs.

Keywords: Mediterranean Diet; metabolites; clinical trial; lipoprotein composition; biomarkers

1. Introduction

Currently, the understanding of diet-health relationships has gradually shifted from individual dietary components to overall dietary patterns that beneficially modulate metabolic physiology [1]. In this regard, several epidemiological and clinical studies have shown that the traditional Mediterranean-style eating pattern (characterized by high intake of fruits and vegetables, olive oil, legumes, whole grains, and fish and moderate consumption of white meat, dairy and wine during meals) has many health benefits [2,3], including beneficial changes in biomarkers of CVD risk [4,5] and lower risk of cardiovascular disease (CVD) [6–8].

However, the exact mechanisms of the benefits of the Mediterranean-style dietary pattern have yet to be understood. The application of metabolomics to measure changes in biological variables in response to dietary interventions has been proposed as a potential tool to discover biomarkers associated with healthier eating [9–13]. There is observational epidemiological evidence that acylcarnitines, Trimethylamine N-oxide (TMAO), some amino acids such as phenylalanine, glutamate as well as several lipid classes are associated with CVD risk [14]. While the effects of individual dietary ingredients on metabolome have been reported [15–20], only a few studies have focused on overall dietary patterns [21–26]. Some cross-sectional studies such as the Whitehall II study showed that a healthy diet was associated with specific fatty acids that reduced the risk of CVD [27]. In a British population, the association between the adherence to the MedDiet and cardiometabolic outcomes was mediated by baseline levels of acylcarnitines, sphingolipids, and phospholipids [24]. In the Supplementation en Vitamines et Mineraux Antioxydants (SU.VI.MAX) study, some metabolites were also cross-sectionally associated with dietary recommendations [28]. More recently, a metabolic signature of the Mediterranean Diet has been consistently identified in two large cohorts [26].

Importantly, studies analyzing changes in metabolites levels in response to MedDiet interventions are still scarce and inconclusive. In the Metabolic Syndrome Reduction in Navarra (RESMENA)study, after 2 months of an energy restricted MedDiet intervention, some significant changes in metabolites were shown but they were no longer observed after 6 months [22]. Additional evidence comes from the Prevention with Mediterranean Diet (PREDIMED) study, where several a priori-designed analyses found that the MedDiet may reduce the deleterious effect on cardiovascular or type-2 diabetes risk associated with 1 year changes in branched-chain amino acids [29,30], carnitines [31] and other metabolites. However, in most of these analyses, the 1 year metabolite changes were similar between the intervention and the control group, suggesting that the observed protective effect of the MedDiet could be due to other mechanisms.

Therefore, the objective of this study is to identify changes in plasma metabolic biomarkers associated with a MedDiet intervention within a subsample of a cluster-randomized controlled trial (Feeding America's Bravest) among firefighters. We hypothesize that the MedDiet intervention induces changes in metabolites within clinically relevant pathways.

2. Materials and Methods

2.1. Study Design and Participants

The overall study design, intervention strategies and primary outcomes of the Feeding America's Bravest trial have been previously reported [32]. Briefly, Feeding America's Bravest is a step-wedge cluster-randomized controlled trial within the 44 stations of Indianapolis Fire Department, which aims to compare a MedDiet Nutritional Intervention vs. an ad libitum Midwestern-style diet (control or no intervention) during 12 months. Group 1 (or the intervention group for 12 months) continued under a self-sustained continuation phase for another 12 months. Group 2 (initially controls) crossed over (at 12 months) to receive the active Mediterranean Diet Nutritional Intervention for 6 months followed by another 6 months of a self-sustained intervention phase. For this nested study, we randomly selected a sub-group of participants ($n = 48$) whose fire stations had been assigned to the MedDiet intervention ($n = 24$) or the control group ($n = 24$) for the previous 12 months. At that time (time point 1 for our study and 12 months follow up of the parent study), the intervention group (Group 1) continued under a self-sustained phase for another 6 months (time point 2 for our study or 18 months of the parent study) and the control group underwent the active MedDiet intervention for 6 months. Plasma metabolic biomarkers were analyzed at the two time points (Figure 1). The overarching Feeding America's Bravest protocol was approved by the Harvard Institutional Review Board (IRB16-0170) and is registered at Clinical Trials (NCT02941757). All participants provided informed consent for participation.

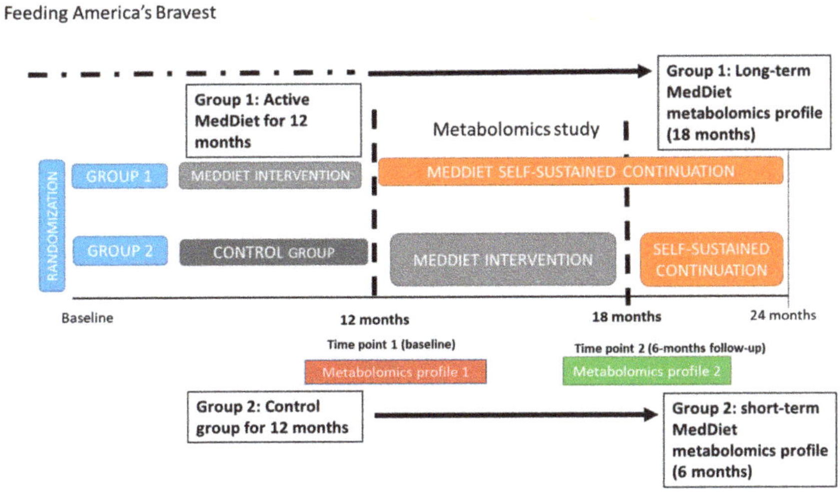

Figure 1. Study design and timeline of the metabolomics study within Feeding America´s Bravest parent study (step-wedge cluster-randomized control trial).

2.2. Mediterranean Diet Intervention

At the two time points of this study, data on sociodemographic characteristics, physical activity, sleep behaviors (a modified Pittsburgh Sleep Quality Index, where on a scale from 0 to 7 participants were asked to identify the statement which option best described their habitual level of physical activity over the past month [33]), food consumption based on a self- reported validated food frequency questionnaire [34] and a modified Mediterranean Diet scale [35], and anthropometric and clinical variables were assessed.

The MedDiet intervention has been described in detail elsewhere [32]. Briefly, it consisted of educational sessions and videos created by a certified nutritionist, leaflet and recommendations about the Mediterranean Dietand lifestyle, firefighter-tailored Mediterranean recipes (by modifying Firefighters´ favorite recipes according to the MedDiet principles by a chef and a nutritionist), in-site chef cooking demonstration, a firefighters' food pyramid, Mediterranean food samples and discount coupons to a large supermarket chain for specific Mediterranean Diet-compatible foods [32].

Adherence to the MedDiet was assessed by the validated modified Mediterranean Diet Score (mMDS) [35,36] and the PREDIMED score. (36) The mMDS range from 0 (lowest) to 51 (highest conformity to the MedDiet) [36] and consists of 13 domains including consumption of fast food, fruits, vegetables, legumes, nuts, sweet desserts, fried foods, ocean fish, breads and starches (consumed at home and the fire station), the type and frequency of alcoholic beverages, non-alcoholic beverages (consumed at home and the fire station) and the type of cooking oil or fat (consumed at home and the fire station). Each component ranged from 0 (less adherence) to 4 points (better adherence) except the type of alcohol (wine; 0–2 points) and the type of cooking oil or fat (0–5 points). Weighted scores was considered for domains evaluated at both the homes and fire stations based on the percentage of meals consumed at each location [36].

The PREDIMED score [37] consists of 14 questions; 12 of them are about food consumption frequency (olive oil consumption, vegetables, fruits, red/processed meats, butter/margarine, soda drinks, wine, legumes, fish/seafood, nuts, commercial sweets, sofrito consumption), and another two about food intake habits considered characteristic of the Spanish Mediterranean Diet (preference of poultry consumption instead of red meats, use of olive oil as main culinary fat). Each question was scored 0 or 1, with a total possible range of 0 to 14; higher scores indicate greater adherence to the MedDiet.

2.3. Collection of Plasma Samples

In this nested study, 12 h fasting blood samples were collected at time point 1 (baseline for this metabolomics study and 12 months for the trial) and time point 2 (6 months follow up for this metabolomics study and 18 months for the trial) of follow up; samples were kept cold and immediately processed to separate the plasma with a refrigerated centrifuge. Next, the 200 μL cryovials were placed at −80 °C.

2.4. Plasma Biomarkers Measurements

Metabolites were quantified in plasma samples from 83 individuals that had optimal values using high-throughput proton Nuclear Magnetic Resonance (NMR) metabolomics (Nightingale Health Ltd., Helsinki, Finland). This method provides simultaneous quantification of routine lipids, lipoprotein subclass profiling with lipid concentrations within 14 subclasses, fatty acid composition, and various low-molecular metabolites including amino acids, ketone bodies and glycolysis-related metabolites. Details of the experimentation and applications of the NMR metabolomics platform have been described previously [38]. All measured metabolites fall in the range of detection; representative coefficients of variations (CVs) for the metabolic biomarkers were published previously [39,40].

2.5. Statistical Analysis

Differences in baseline characteristics between the two groups were examined by *t*-test ANOVA for continuous variables (means ± standard deviation [SD]) or Chi-square for categorical data (percentages). Statistical analyses of the metabolites were performed on log-transformed data that were scaled to SD units to facilitate comparisons across metabolites. The effect of the MedDiet intervention between point 1 and point 2 in this analysis (6 months) was assessed using a linear mixed-effects model adjusted for age and sex. As many of the metabolites are biologically correlated, applying a multiple testing correction using all the 225 biomarkers would be too strict. Thus, account for multiple testing, Bonferroni correction was applied with significance level defined as 0.05/21 = 0.002, with 21 being the number of principal components that explained 99% of the variation in the NMR data.

Cross-sectional linear associations between the adherence to the mMDS score and metabolite concentrations at both time points for both the MedDiet intervention and control groups were obtained using a linear regression model adjusted for age and sex. The analyses were performed using ggforestplot R package (version 0.0.2) and the linear mixed-effects model was fitted with the nlme R package (version 3.1.-144).

3. Results

3.1. Participant Characteristics

Characteristics of the 48 participants at time point 1, and changes after 6 months follow up (time point 2), are summarized in Table 1. Of the 48 participants at time point 1, 44 (92%) were followed up and provided dietary information and anthropometric measures at time point 2. Information for the plasma metabolites were available for n = 47 at baseline and n = 36 at the end of follow up (Supplementary Materials Figure S1). There were no statistically significant differences in the adherence to the mMDS or PREDIMED score at time 1 and after the 6 months follow up within and between groups. Similarly, no differences were seen for age or sex (Table 1).

Table 1. Characteristics of the firefighters participating in the Feeding America's Bravest intervention study.

	Time Point 1 (n = 48)			Time Point 2 (n = 44 *)				
	12 Months MedDiet Intervention (n = 24)	Control Group (n = 24)	p-Value	18 Months MedDiet Intervention (n = 22)	Control Group After a 6 Months of Active MedDiet Intervention (n = 22)	p-Value	p-Value (Follow Up-Baseline) Intervention Group	p-Value (Follow Up-Baseline) Control Group
Sex, male (%)	91.7	95.8	0.55	84.6	94.1	0.39	N/A	N/A
Age (years)	47.5 (6.7)	47.6 (8.6)	0.95	45.9 (6.7)	49.9 (8.4)	0.17	N/A	N/A
PREDIMED score (0–14 points)	6.1 (2.1)	6.6 (2.1)	0.31	6.4 (1.9)	6.7 (1.9)	0.64	0.48	0.64
mMDs score (0–51 points)	24.2 (6.5)	26.1 (4.9)	0.27	26.0 (6.5)	26.5 (5.6)	0.81	0.23	0.52
Fast food consumption (0–4 points)	2.8 (0.94)	3 (0.61)	0.47	2.76 (0.83)	2.69 (0.63)	0.79	0.06	0.13
Fruit (0–4 points)	1.56 (0.61)	1.65 (0.79)	0.70	1.62 (0.56)	1.71 (0.69)	0.693	0.62	0.71
Vegetable (0–4 points)	1.8 (0.93)	2.11 (0.69)	0.314	1.70 (0.85)	2.06 (0.56)	0.16	0.07	0.11
Sweet desserts (0–4 points)	1 (0.69)	1.24 (0.75)	0.340	0.85 (0.69)	1.35 (0.61)	0.04	0.05	0.84
Cooking oil or fat use at home (0–5 points)	3.0 (2.20)	2.88 (1.99)	0.57	3.85 (1.77)	3.59 (1.87)	0.70	0.07	0.56
Fried food consumption (0–4 points)	0.12 (0.47)	0.35 (0.78)	0.27	0.46 (0.88)	0.71 (0.98)	0.49	0.33	0.33
Breads and starches at home (0–4 points)	2.70 (1.82)	2.39 (1.97)	0.63	1.15 (1.80)	1.41 (1.62)	0.92	0.07	0.21
Ocean fish (0–4 points)	0.78 (0.88)	0.53 (0.72)	0.37	0.39 (0.87)	0.65 (0.86)	0.42	0.09	0.33
Non-alcoholic beverage at home	2.61 (1.72)	3.06 (1.39)	0.41	2.85 (1.41)	3.11 (1.45)	0.61	0.12	0.38
Alcoholic beverages (0–4 points)	1.06 (1.26)	0.94 (1.14)	0.78	1.31 (1.43)	1.12 (1.22)	0.61	1.0	0.58
Wine (0–2 points)	1.58 (0.51)	1.89 (0.31)	0.03	1.61 (0.51)	1.82 (0.39)	0.22	0.35	0.33
Legumes (0–4 points)	3.05 (0.87)	3.06 (0.87)	0.99	3.15 (1.28)	2.53 (1.12)	0.17	0.04	0.04
Nuts (0–4 points)	2.40 (1.09)	2.6 (0.9)	0.57	2.69 (1.11)	2.47 (0.71)	0.61	0.09	0.29

Pairwise comparisons over time include only those participants with complete information at baseline and at the end of follow up (n = 23). * At the end of follow up, 44 participants provided information about diet, n = 36 plasma serum and diet information, and 30 participants were assessed for anthropometric and other cardiovascular risk factors (Figure S1). Thus, mMDS and PREDIMED included n = 44 for the analysis at the end of follow up and for the comparisons.

3.2. The 6 Month Effect of the MedDiet Intervention

Figure 2 shows the 6 months effects of the intervention in the most relevant metabolites pathways. Data on the effect of the intervention in all the metabolites studied by group are presented in Table S1. The main subgroups affected by the intervention were the lipids and lipoproteins. Specifically, we observed a reduction in LDL-C, ApoB/ApoA1 ratio, remnant cholesterol, and higher HDL-C, and other subfractions such as lower cholesterol in L-VLDL-C, S-VLDL-C, L-LDL-C, M-LDL-C, S-LDL-C lipoproteins, and the composition of the lipoproteins after 6 months of intervention. Of note, these associations did not reach statistical significance after correcting the *p*-values for multiple testing (except for a decrease in M-VLDL-CE and an increase in lactate).

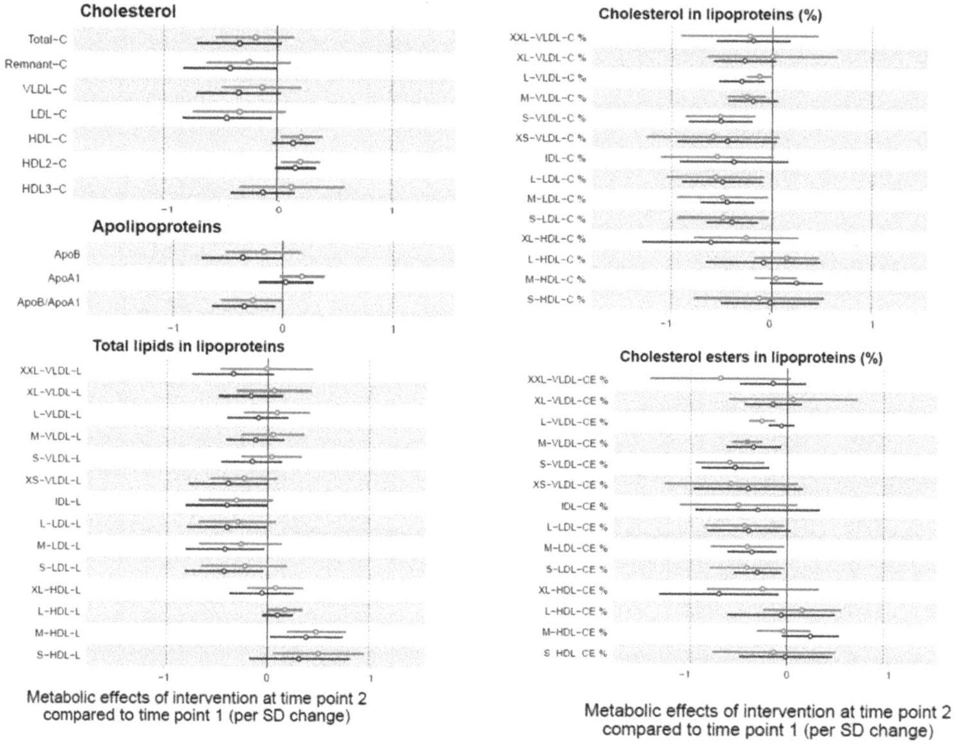

Figure 2. Metabolic effects of the intervention after 6 months follow up (time point 2) compared to baseline (time point 1) (linear mixed models adjusted by age and sex). Results show changes by SD in each metabolite per unit change in mMDS score and are displayed by hollow points. Only those significant results (after correction of multiple testing) are indicated by filled points along with their 95% confidence intervals. In black is shown Group 1 (the intervention group for 12 months) that continued under a self-sustained continuation phase for another 6 months. In red is shown Group 2 (control) that received the active Mediterranean Diet Nutritional Intervention for 6 months.

3.3. Cross-Sectional Association between Mediterranean Diet Adherence and Biomarkers

We also examined the cross-sectional linear association between biomarkers and adherence to the MedDiet at point 1 and 2 of this study, regardless of the participant's group at baseline and follow up. Results were similar at both time points, although somewhat higher effect sizes where observed at time 2 where all participants had received at least 6 months of the MedDiet intervention (Figure 3). A 1 unit difference in mMDS score was associated with lower total lipids in lipoproteins of different sizes (VLDL, LDL) and ApoB/ApoA1 ratio, lower concentrations of a marker of inflammation (Glyc A), lower concentrations of branched chain amino acids and higher polyunsaturated fatty acids (PUFAs) and Docosahexaenoic acid (DHA) (Figure 3). We further included all the participants grouped together and analyzed the association between unit changes in the MedDiet score and SD changes in metabolic markers. We found a similar pattern in the results, but not significant, with a tendency to higher lipoprotein particle size with higher MedDiet scores (Figure S2).

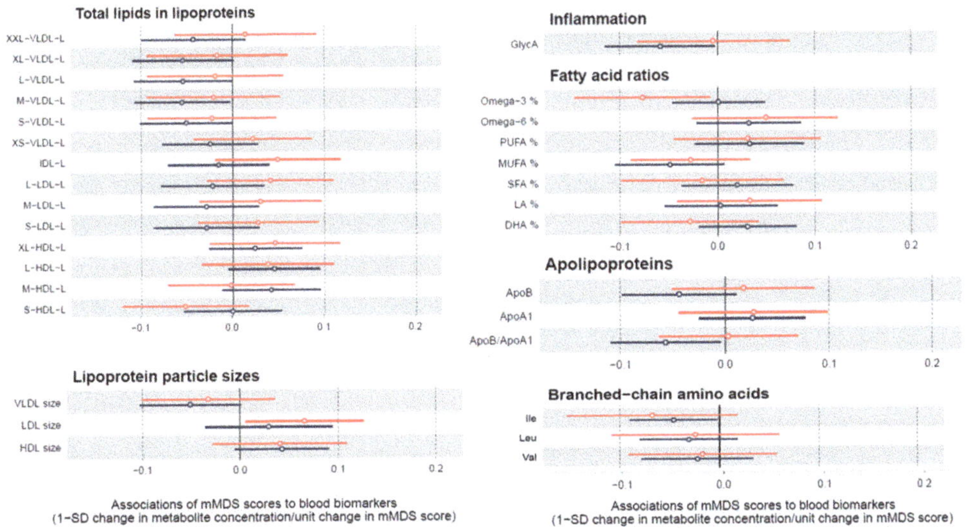

Figure 3. Cross-sectional association between biomarkers and adherence to the MedDiet for all participants at time point 1 and time point 2. Red lines show the results for the participants at baseline and black lines for the participants at follow up. Results show changes by SD in each biomarker per unit change in mMDS score and are displayed by hollow points along with their 95% confidence intervals.

Similar results were found when we used the PREDIMED score instead of the mMDS (Figure S3).

4. Discussion

In this sub-study of firefighters in Indianapolis participating in a cluster-randomized MedDiet intervention trial, we found that the MedDiet intervention was associated with favorable changes in markers of cardiovascular risk, specifically those related to the lipid metabolism (cholesterol, lipid composition, or cholesterol esters in the VLDL, IDL, and LDL lipoprotein subclasses, and ApoB/ApoA ratio) that were non-significant after correcting for multiple testing (except for a decrease in M-VLDL-CE). When the adherence to the MedDiet was measured with a self-reported scale (mMDS), the direction of the association with metabolites was similar at both time points (baseline and 6 months after the follow up).

Our results highlighting the changes in plasma metabolites related to lipid metabolism are in line with other studies [20,26]. A recent investigation that identified a metabolic signature of adherence to the MedDiet showed that out of 67 metabolites, 45 were lipids followed by 19 amino acids, 2 vitamins and 1 xenobiotic [26]. Although we used a different methodology and a different set of biomarkers, and thus we could not replicate this metabolic signature, our results support that the MedDiet may induce changes in relevant lipid species and subclasses related to atherogenic risk. In fact, the MedDiet is high in healthy fats (>35–40% of the total energy) mostly from monounsaturated fatty acids (MUFAs) (olive oil mostly) and PUFAs (from nuts and fish), and therefore the results are not surprising. In the firefighter population, we previously reported good correlation between nutrient intake from the food frequency questionnaire and the corresponding plasma biomarkers (omega-3, Eicosapentaenoic acid (EPA), and DHA) [36]. In line with these results, we found that changes in the MedDiet scores showed some tendency to be associated with fatty acids (an increase in PUFA% specifically DHA% in the expense of MUFA%). Although olive oil is a main component of the MedDiet, previous research found that higher consumption of this oil was linked to changes in omega 3, but not MUFA concentrations [36,41,42]. In addition, the average olive oil consumption in the firefighters is only approximately 0.5 tbsp/day, which is similar to other US cohorts [43] but much lower than in a Spanish cohort (4 tbsp/day) [44]. Nonetheless, it looks like changes in omega 3 to fatty acid ratio, PUFA to FA ratio and DHA to FA ratio increase with changes in the adherence to the MedDiet. This is in line with other studies [20,36], and suggests that those biomarkers could serve as indicators of adherence to the MedDiet.

We found that the MedDiet intervention induced a decrease in total cholesterol, remnant-C, VLDL-C and LDL-C and an increase in HDL-C and HDL2-C. Many studies have already demonstrated the effect of the MedDiet on total lipid metabolism, especially reducing total cholesterol and increasing HDL-C [45]. For example, the PREDIMED study, a randomized control trial, found that those in the MedDiet intervention (with olive oil or nuts) over 6 months had an increase in HDL-C but not a reduction in LDL-C [45]. Other studies support that replacing dietary saturated fatty acids (SFAs) with PUFA reduces the plasma LDL-C and subsequently the risk of cardiovascular disease [46–48].

In our study, we also observed a decrease in large, medium and small LDL fractions such as total lipids, cholesterol, particle concentration or cholesterol esters. Similarly, the MedDiet intervention decreased total cholesterol and cholesterol esters in the large, medium and small VLDL. Literature shows that VLDL concentrations are related directly or indirectly in the development of atherosclerosis [49]; for example the fatty acid composition of VLDL is critical for the activity of lipoprotein lipase and the formation of proatherogenic LDL and VLDL remnants [50]. In the FINRISK cohort, increased risk of cardiovascular disease was associated with all VLDL, IDL, and LDL subclasses, while the L- and M-HDL subclasses were associated with lower risk [51]. Despite the evidence of the role of these metabolites in CVD development, few studies have studied the effect of a MedDiet intervention in different lipids composition of lipoproteins or its subfractions. Interestingly, our results on lipid subfractions agree with a recent publication using the same metabolomic approach, where 47 participants were randomized to a SFA-rich diet, a MUFA-rich diet or a MED diet for 8 weeks. Additionally, in another study, compared to the control group, those participants that replaced SFAs with PUFAs reduced the lipoprotein particle concentration [52]. Finally, olive oil consumption modifies the lipid composition of VLDL [53] as well as the lipoprotein subfractions [54].

In our study, the effect was consistently shown in both groups, usually being stronger in the group undergoing a longer MedDiet intervention/exposure (MedDiet intervention + a self-sustained continuation phase), suggesting that the MedDiet induces favorable changes in metabolites related to CVD disease while the adherence to the MedDiet is sustained. For example, in our study, the ApoB/ApoA1 ratio was decreased in both groups after the intervention and also by adherence to the mMDS, which agrees with other short-term randomized trial with the MedDiet supplemented with olive oil, suggesting that these ratios may predict CVD beyond conventional lipid measures [55]. Finally, we found a significant association with lactate, a metabolite that was previously shown to increase the diabetes risk in the PREDIMED study [56]. However, we found that it occurs in the opposite direction.

Study Limitations

This was a pilot study with a small sample size. Possibly because of this, most associations lost statistical significance after correcting for multiple testing. However, results were in line with previous research, suggesting that a larger sample size would have retrieved significant results. In addition, the fact that we did not find differences in the mMDS adherence between groups may reflect selection bias since this is a sub-study within 400 firefighters participating in the Feeding America's Bravest trial, and participants willing to participate could potentially be healthier and more health conscious. Moreover, the control group had higher scores of mMDS at baseline and their scores were slightly improved during the intervention; however, the results were consistent in the cross-sectional analysis. We only adjusted for age and sex, since it was a randomized study with no significant differences between this sub-study and the parent study for the rest of the variables which suggests the need to perform a study that includes larger metabolites. In addition, we did not analyze other metabolites included in other studies nor at baseline for the parent study. In this pilot trial, Group 2 could be considered as the intervention group but Group 1 was not a pure control group because they already finished an active MedDiet intervention and began their self-sustained MedDiet phase. The changes in biomarkers in Group 1 (between time point 1 and 2) are more likely to reflect both residual effects of the MedDiet and continued effects from self-sustained diet intervention. Additionally, most of our participants were male and thus generalizability should be explored. In any case, the results in this study should be corroborated in larger clinical studies with longer follow up due to the pilot study nature and with a powerful study design.

5. Conclusions

This MedDiet intervention induces only modest changes in adherence to the MedDiet and consequently in metabolic biomarkers related to lipid metabolism. Further research should confirm these results based on larger study samples in workplace interventions with powerful study designs.

Supplementary Materials: The following are available online at http://www.mdpi.com/2072-6643/12/12/3610/s1, Figure S1: Flowchart of participants at time point 1 and 2 of the Feeding America's Bravest trial, Figure S2: Associations of unit changes in mMDS score by SD changes in plasma biomarkers between month 6 (time point 2) and baseline (time point 1) in all participants grouped together, Figure S3: Association between biomarkers and the PREDIMED score adherence (cross-sectional analysis), Table S1: The 6 months effect of the Mediterranean Diet intervention on metabolic biomarkers (linear mixed model analysis with *p*-values corrected for multiple testing).

Author Contributions: All authors have participated sufficiently and meaningfully to the research study and the preparation of this manuscript. M.S.-P. formulated the study question and design, interpreted the results, and drafted the manuscript. M.S.-P. and M.R.-C. were involved in statistical modeling. M.S.-P., S.N.K., Y.S. and S.M. contributed to the conception and design of the study and acquisition of the data. All authors contributed to the interpretation of data and critical revision of the manuscript and approved the final version. M.S.P., M.R.-C. and S.N.K. share primary responsibility for the final content. All authors have read and agreed to the published version of the manuscript.

Funding: This research was funded by EMW-2014-FP-00612, US Department of Homeland Security, a Ohio University OURC grant and a CHSP Research Innovation grant, and the 2018 Southeast Center for Integrated Metabolomics Pilot & Feasibility Project. M.S.-P. holds a Ramón y Cajal contract (RYC-2018-025069-I) from the Ministry of Science, Innovation and Universities and FEDER/FSE and FIS grant PI20/00896. The funding agencies had no role in study design, data collection and analysis, interpretation of results, manuscript preparation or in the decision to submit this manuscript for publication

Acknowledgments: We appreciate the participation of the Indianapolis Fire Departments as well as the firefighters and their spouses. We also thank Noora Kanerva and Heli Julkunen for their help with data analysis, as well as the Indiana Clinical and Translational Science Institute for helping with sample processing, the Kroger Company (coupons and customer loyalty discounts), Barilla America (Barilla Plus Products), Arianna Trading Company, Innoliva and Molino de Zafra, Spain (extra virgin olive oil samples and discounts) and the Almond Board of California (free samples of roasted unsalted almonds) for study support. The sponsors had no involvement in the overall study design; collection, analysis and interpretation of data; writing of the report; or the decision to submit the report for publication.

Conflicts of Interest: The authors declare no conflict of interest.

References

1. Cespedes, E.M.; Hu, F.B. Dietary patterns: From nutritional epidemiologic analysis to national guidelines. *Am. J. Clin. Nutr.* **2015**, *101*, 899–900. [CrossRef] [PubMed]
2. Martínez-González, M.A.; Gea, A.; Ruiz-Canela, M. The Mediterranean Diet and Cardiovascular Health. *Circ. Res.* **2019**, *124*, 779–798. [CrossRef]

3. Dinu, M.; Pagliai, G.; Casini, A.; Sofi, F. Mediterranean diet and multiple health outcomes: An umbrella review of meta-analyses of observational studies and randomised trials. *Eur. J. Clin. Nutr.* **2017**. [CrossRef]
4. Godos, J.; Zappala, G.; Bernardini, S.; Giambini, I.; Bes-Rastrollo, M.; Martinez-Gonzalez, M. Adherence to the Mediterranean diet is inversely associated with metabolic syndrome occurrence: A meta-analysis of observational studies. *Int. J. Food Sci. Nutr.* **2017**, *68*, 138–148. [CrossRef] [PubMed]
5. Mattei, J.; Sotos-Prieto, M.; Bigornia, S.J.; Noel, S.E.; Tucker, K.L. The Mediterranean Diet Score Is More Strongly Associated with Favorable Cardiometabolic Risk Factors over 2 Years Than Other Diet Quality Indexes in Puerto Rican Adults. *J. Nutr.* **2017**, *147*, 661–669. [CrossRef]
6. Rosato, V.; Temple, N.J.; La Vecchia, C.; Castellan, G.; Tavani, A.; Guercio, V. Mediterranean diet and cardiovascular disease: A systematic review and meta-analysis of observational studies. *Eur. J. Nutr.* **2017**. [CrossRef]
7. Sotos-Prieto, M.; Bhupathiraju, S.N.; Mattei, J.; Fung, T.T.; Li, Y.; Pan, A.; Willett, W.C.; Rimm, E.B.; Hu, F.B. Changes in Diet Quality Scores and Risk of Cardiovascular Disease Among US Men and Women. *Circulation* **2015**, *132*, 2212–2219. [CrossRef]
8. Sotos-Prieto, M.; Bhupathiraju, S.N.; Mattei, J.; Fung, T.T.; Li, Y.; Pan, A.; Willett, W.C.; Rimm, E.B.; Hu, F.B. Association of Changes in Diet Quality with Total and Cause-Specific Mortality. *N. Engl. J. Med.* **2017**, *377*, 143–153. [CrossRef]
9. Guasch-Ferré, M.; Bhupathiraju, S.N.; Hu, F.B. Use of Metabolomics in Improving Assessment of Dietary Intake. *Clin. Chem.* **2018**, *64*, 82–98. [CrossRef]
10. Brennan, L.; Hu, F.B. Metabolomics Based Dietary Biomarkers in Nutritional Epidemiology-Current Status and Future Opportunities. *Mol. Nutr. Food Res.* **2018**, 1701064. [CrossRef]
11. Hardin, D.S. Validating dietary intake with biochemical markers. *J. Am. Diet. Assoc.* **2009**, *109*, 1698–1699. [CrossRef] [PubMed]
12. Garcia-Perez, I.; Posma, J.M.; Gibson, R.; Chambers, E.S.; Hansen, T.H.; Vestergaard, H.; Hansen, T.; Beckmann, M.; Pedersen, O.; Elliott, P.; et al. Objective assessment of dietary patterns by use of metabolic phenotyping: A randomised, controlled, crossover trial. *Lancet Diabetes Endocrinol.* **2017**, *5*, 184–195. [CrossRef]
13. Scalbert, A.; Brennan, L.; Manach, C.; Andres-Lacueva, C.; Dragsted, L.O.; Draper, J.; Rappaport, S.M.; van der Hooft, J.J.; Wishart, D.S. The food metabolome: A window over dietary exposure. *Am. J. Clin. Nutr.* **2014**, *99*, 1286–1308. [CrossRef] [PubMed]
14. Ruiz-Canela, M.; Hruby, A.; Clish, C.B.; Liang, L.; Martinez-Gonzalez, M.A.; Hu, F.B. Comprehensive Metabolomic Profiling and Incident Cardiovascular Disease: A Systematic Review. *J. Am. Heart Assoc.* **2017**, *6*. [CrossRef] [PubMed]
15. Cheung, W.; Keski-Rahkonen, P.; Assi, N.; Ferrari, P.; Freisling, H.; Rinaldi, S.; Slimani, N.; Zamora-Ros, R.; Rundle, M.; Frost, G.; et al. A metabolomic study of biomarkers of meat and fish intake. *Am. J. Clin. Nutr.* **2017**, *105*, 600–608. [CrossRef]
16. Papandreou, C.; Hernández-Alonso, P.; Bulló, M.; Ruiz-Canela, M.; Yu, E.; Guasch-Ferré, M.; Toledo, E.; Dennis, C.; Deik, A.; Clish, C.; et al. Plasma Metabolites Associated with Coffee Consumption: A Metabolomic Approach within the PREDIMED Study. *Nutrients* **2019**, *11*, 32. [CrossRef] [PubMed]
17. Hernández-Alonso, P.; Papandreou, C.; Bulló, M.; Ruiz-Canela, M.; Dennis, C.; Deik, A.; Wang, D.D.; Guasch-Ferré, M.; Yu, E.; Toledo, E.; et al. Plasma Metabolites Associated with Frequent Red Wine Consumption: A Metabolomics Approach within the PREDIMED Study. *Mol. Nutr. Food Res.* **2019**, *63*, e1900140. [CrossRef] [PubMed]
18. Schmidt, J.A.; Rinaldi, S.; Ferrari, P.; Carayol, M.; Achaintre, D.; Scalbert, A.; Cross, A.J.; Gunter, M.J.; Fensom, G.K.; Appleby, P.N.; et al. Metabolic profiles of male meat eaters, fish eaters, vegetarians, and vegans from the EPIC-Oxford cohort. *Am. J. Clin. Nutr.* **2015**, *102*, 1518–1526. [CrossRef]
19. Edmands, W.M.B.; Beckonert, O.P.; Stella, C.; Campbell, A.; Lake, B.G.; Lindon, J.C.; Holmes, E.; Gooderham, N.J. Identification of human urinary biomarkers of cruciferous vegetable consumption by metabonomic profiling. *J. Proteome Res.* **2011**, *10*, 4513–4521. [CrossRef]
20. Michielsen, C.C.J.R.; Hangelbroek, R.W.J.; Feskens, E.J.M.; Afman, L.A. Disentangling the Effects of Monounsaturated Fatty Acids from Other Components of a Mediterranean Diet on Serum Metabolite Profiles: A Randomized Fully Controlled Dietary Intervention in Healthy Subjects at Risk of the Metabolic Syndrome. *Mol. Nutr. Food Res.* **2019**, *63*, e1801095. [CrossRef]

21. Jin, Q.; Black, A.; Kales, S.N.; Vattem, D.; Ruiz-Canela, M.; Sotos-Prieto, M. Metabolomics and Microbiomes as Potential Tools to Evaluate the Effects of the Mediterranean Diet. *Nutrients* **2019**, *11*, 207. [CrossRef] [PubMed]
22. Bondia-Pons, I.; Martinez, J.A.; de la Iglesia, R.; Lopez-Legarrea, P.; Poutanen, K.; Hanhineva, K.; Zulet, M.d.l.Á. Effects of short- and long-term Mediterranean-based dietary treatment on plasma LC-QTOF/MS metabolic profiling of subjects with metabolic syndrome features: The Metabolic Syndrome Reduction in Navarra (RESMENA) randomized controlled trial. *Mol. Nutr. Food Res.* **2015**, *59*, 711–728. [CrossRef]
23. Playdon, M.C.; Moore, S.C.; Derkach, A.; Reedy, J.; Subar, A.F.; Sampson, J.N.; Albanes, D.; Gu, F.; Kontto, J.; Lassale, C.; et al. Identifying biomarkers of dietary patterns by using metabolomics. *Am. J. Clin. Nutr.* **2017**, *105*, 450–465. [CrossRef] [PubMed]
24. Tong, T.Y.N.; Koulman, A.; Griffin, J.L.; Wareham, N.J.; Forouhi, N.G.; Imamura, F. A Combination of Metabolites Predicts Adherence to the Mediterranean Diet Pattern and Its Associations with Insulin Sensitivity and Lipid Homeostasis in the General Population: The Fenland Study, United Kingdom. *J. Nutr.* **2020**, *150*, 568–578. [CrossRef] [PubMed]
25. Rebholz, C.M.; Lichtenstein, A.H.; Zheng, Z.; Appel, L.J.; Coresh, J. Serum untargeted metabolomic profile of the Dietary Approaches to Stop Hypertension (DASH) dietary pattern. *Am. J. Clin. Nutr.* **2018**, *108*, 243–255. [CrossRef] [PubMed]
26. Li, J.; Guasch-Ferré, M.; Chung, W.; Ruiz-Canela, M.; Toledo, E.; Corella, D.; Bhupathiraju, S.N.; Tobias, D.K.; Tabung, F.K.; Hu, J.; et al. The Mediterranean diet, plasma metabolome, and cardiovascular disease risk. *Eur. Heart J.* **2020**. [CrossRef] [PubMed]
27. Akbaraly, T.; Würtz, P.; Singh-Manoux, A.; Shipley, M.J.; Haapakoski, R.; Lehto, M.; Desrumaux, C.; Kähönen, M.; Lehtimäki, T.; Mikkilä, V.; et al. Association of circulating metabolites with healthy diet and risk of cardiovascular disease: Analysis of two cohort studies. *Sci. Rep.* **2018**, *8*, 8620. [CrossRef]
28. Lécuyer, L.; Dalle, C.; Micheau, P.; Pétéra, M.; Centeno, D.; Lyan, B.; Lagree, M.; Galan, P.; Hercberg, S.; Rossary, A.; et al. Untargeted plasma metabolomic profiles associated with overall diet in women from the SU.VI.MAX cohort. *Eur. J. Nutr.* **2020**. [CrossRef]
29. Ruiz-Canela, M.; Guasch-Ferré, M.; Toledo, E.; Clish, C.B.; Razquin, C.; Liang, L.; Wang, D.D.; Corella, D.; Estruch, R.; Hernáez, Á.; et al. Plasma branched chain/aromatic amino acids, enriched Mediterranean diet and risk of type 2 diabetes: Case-cohort study within the PREDIMED Trial. *Diabetologia* **2018**, *61*, 1560–1571. [CrossRef]
30. Ruiz-Canela, M.; Toledo, E.; Clish, C.B.; Hruby, A.; Liang, L.; Salas-Salvadó, J.; Razquin, C.; Corella, D.; Estruch, R.; Ros, E.; et al. Plasma Branched-Chain Amino Acids and Incident Cardiovascular Disease in the PREDIMED Trial. *Clin. Chem.* **2016**, *62*, 582–592. [CrossRef]
31. Guasch-Ferré, M.; Ruiz-Canela, M.; Li, J.; Zheng, Y.; Bulló, M.; Wang, D.D.; Toledo, E.; Clish, C.; Corella, D.; Estruch, R.; et al. Plasma Acylcarnitines and Risk of Type 2 Diabetes in a Mediterranean Population at High Cardiovascular Risk. *J. Clin. Endocrinol. Metab.* **2019**, *104*, 1508–1519. [CrossRef] [PubMed]
32. Sotos-Prieto, M.; Cash, S.B.; Christophi, C.A.; Folta, S.; Moffatt, S.; Muegge, C.; Korre, M.; Mozaffarian, D.; Kales, S.N. Rationale and design of feeding America's bravest: Mediterranean diet-based intervention to change firefighters' eating habits and improve cardiovascular risk profiles. *Contemp. Clin. Trials* **2017**, *61*, 101–107. [CrossRef] [PubMed]
33. Jackson, A.S.; Blair, S.N.; Mahar, M.T.; Wier, L.T.; Ross, R.M.; Stuteville, J.E. Prediction of functional aerobic capacity without exercise testing. *Med. Sci. Sport. Exerc.* **1990**, *22*, 863–870. [CrossRef] [PubMed]
34. Salvini, S.; Hunter, D.J.; Sampson, L.; Stampfer, M.J.; Colditz, G.A.; Rosner, B.; Willett, W.C. Food-based validation of a dietary questionnaire: The effects of week-to-week variation in food consumption. *Int. J. Epidemiol.* **1989**, *18*, 858–867. [CrossRef] [PubMed]
35. Gong, Y.; Yang, J.; Farioli, A.; Korre, M.; Kales, S.N. Modified Mediterranean Diet Score and Cardiovascular Risk in a North American Working Population. *PLoS ONE* **2014**, *9*, e87539. [CrossRef]
36. Sotos-Prieto, M.; Christophi, C.; Black, A.; Furtado, J.D.; Song, Y.; Magiatis, P.; Papakonstantinou, A.; Melliou, E.; Moffatt, S.; Kales, S.N. Assessing Validity of Self-Reported Dietary Intake within a Mediterranean Diet Cluster Randomized Controlled Trial among US Firefighters. *Nutrients* **2019**, *11*, 2250. [CrossRef]
37. Schroder, H.; Fito, M.; Estruch, R.; Martinez-Gonzalez, M.A.; Corella, D.; Salas-Salvado, J.; Lamuela-Raventos, R.; Ros, E.; Salaverria, I.; Fiol, M.; et al. A short screener is valid for assessing Mediterranean diet adherence among older Spanish men and women. *J. Nutr.* **2011**, *141*, 1140–1145. [CrossRef]

38. Soininen, P.; Kangas, A.J.; Würtz, P.; Suna, T.; Ala-Korpela, M. Quantitative serum nuclear magnetic resonance metabolomics in cardiovascular epidemiology and genetics. *Circ. Cardiovasc. Genet.* **2015**, *8*, 192–206. [CrossRef]
39. Kettunen, J.; Demirkan, A.; Würtz, P.; Draisma, H.H.M.; Haller, T.; Rawal, R.; Vaarhorst, A.; Kangas, A.J.; Lyytikäinen, L.-P.; Pirinen, M.; et al. Genome-wide study for circulating metabolites identifies 62 loci and reveals novel systemic effects of LPA. *Nat. Commun.* **2016**, *7*, 11122. [CrossRef]
40. Würtz, P.; Kangas, A.J.; Soininen, P.; Lawlor, D.A.; Davey Smith, G.; Ala-Korpela, M. Quantitative Serum Nuclear Magnetic Resonance Metabolomics in Large-Scale Epidemiology: A Primer on -Omic Technologies. *Am. J. Epidemiol.* **2017**, *186*, 1084–1096. [CrossRef]
41. Hebestreit, K.; Yahiaoui-Doktor, M.; Engel, C.; Vetter, W.; Siniatchkin, M.; Erickson, N.; Halle, M.; Kiechle, M.; Bischoff, S.C. Validation of the German version of the Mediterranean Diet Adherence Screener (MEDAS) questionnaire. *BMC Cancer* **2017**, *17*, 341. [CrossRef] [PubMed]
42. Barceló, F.; Perona, J.S.; Prades, J.; Funari, S.S.; Gomez-Gracia, E.; Conde, M.; Estruch, R.; Ruiz-Gutiérrez, V. Mediterranean-style diet effect on the structural properties of the erythrocyte cell membrane of hypertensive patients: The Prevencion con Dieta Mediterranea Study. *Hypertension* **2009**, *54*, 1143–1150. [CrossRef] [PubMed]
43. Guasch-Ferré, M.; Hu, F.B.; Martínez-González, M.A.; Fitó, M.; Bulló, M.; Estruch, R.; Ros, E.; Corella, D.; Recondo, J.; Gómez-Gracia, E.; et al. Olive oil intake and risk of cardiovascular disease and mortality in the PREDIMED Study. *BMC Med.* **2014**, *12*, 78. [CrossRef] [PubMed]
44. Guasch-Ferré, M.; Liu, G.; Li, Y.; Sampson, L.; Manson, J.E.; Salas-Salvadó, J.; Martínez-González, M.A.; Stampfer, M.J.; Willett, W.C.; Sun, Q.; et al. Olive Oil Consumption and Cardiovascular Risk in U.S. Adults. *J. Am. Coll. Cardiol.* **2020**, *75*, 1729–1739. [CrossRef]
45. Estruch, R.; Martínez-González, M.A.; Corella, D.; Salas-Salvadó, J.; Ruiz-Gutiérrez, V.; Covas, M.I.; Fiol, M.; Gómez-Gracia, E.; López-Sabater, M.C.; Vinyoles, E.; et al. Effects of a Mediterranean-style diet on cardiovascular risk factors: A randomized trial. *Ann. Intern. Med.* **2006**, *145*, 1–11. [CrossRef]
46. Mensink, R.P.; Zock, P.L.; Kester, A.D.M.; Katan, M.B. Effects of dietary fatty acids and carbohydrates on the ratio of serum total to HDL cholesterol and on serum lipids and apolipoproteins: A meta-analysis of 60 controlled trials. *Am. J. Clin. Nutr.* **2003**, *77*, 1146–1155. [CrossRef]
47. Sacks, F.M.; Lichtenstein, A.H.; Wu, J.H.Y.; Appel, L.J.; Creager, M.A.; Kris-Etherton, P.M.; Miller, M.; Rimm, E.B.; Rudel, L.L.; Robinson, J.G.; et al. Dietary Fats and Cardiovascular Disease: A Presidential Advisory From the American Heart Association. *Circulation* **2017**, *136*, e1–e23. [CrossRef]
48. Stone, N.J.; Robinson, J.G.; Lichtenstein, A.H.; Bairey Merz, C.N.; Blum, C.B.; Eckel, R.H.; Goldberg, A.C.; Gordon, D.; Levy, D.; Lloyd-Jones, D.M.; et al. 2013 ACC/AHA guideline on the treatment of blood cholesterol to reduce atherosclerotic cardiovascular risk in adults: A report of the American College of Cardiology/American Heart Association Task Force on Practice Guidelines. *J. Am. Coll. Cardiol.* **2014**, *63*, 2889–2934. [CrossRef]
49. Wilhelm, M.G.; Cooper, A.D. Induction of atherosclerosis by human chylomicron remnants: A hypothesis. *J. Atheroscler. Thromb.* **2003**, *10*, 132–139. [CrossRef]
50. Liu, J.; Sempos, C.T.; Donahue, R.P.; Dorn, J.; Trevisan, M.; Grundy, S.M. Non-high-density lipoprotein and very-low-density lipoprotein cholesterol and their risk predictive values in coronary heart disease. *Am. J. Cardiol.* **2006**, *98*, 1363–1368. [CrossRef]
51. Metabolite Profiling and Cardiovascular Event Risk: A Prospective Study of 3 Population-Based Cohorts—PubMed. Available online: https://pubmed.ncbi.nlm.nih.gov/25573147/?from_single_result=Metabolite+profiling+and+cardiovascular+event+risk%3A+a+prospective+study+of+3+population-based+cohorts (accessed on 3 June 2020).
52. Ulven, S.M.; Christensen, J.J.; Nygård, O.; Svardal, A.; Leder, L.; Ottestad, I.; Lysne, V.; Laupsa-Borge, J.; Ueland, P.M.; Midttun, Ø.; et al. Using metabolic profiling and gene expression analyses to explore molecular effects of replacing saturated fat with polyunsaturated fat-a randomized controlled dietary intervention study. *Am. J. Clin. Nutr.* **2019**, *109*, 1239–1250. [CrossRef] [PubMed]
53. Perona, J.S.; Cañizares, J.; Montero, E.; Sánchez-Domínguez, J.M.; Pacheco, Y.M.; Ruiz-Gutierrez, V. Dietary virgin olive oil triacylglycerols as an independent determinant of very low-density lipoprotein composition. *Nutrition* **2004**, *20*, 509–514. [CrossRef]

54. Damasceno, N.R.T.; Sala-Vila, A.; Cofán, M.; Pérez-Heras, A.M.; Fitó, M.; Ruiz-Gutiérrez, V.; Martínez-González, M.-Á.; Corella, D.; Arós, F.; Estruch, R.; et al. Mediterranean diet supplemented with nuts reduces waist circumference and shifts lipoprotein subfractions to a less atherogenic pattern in subjects at high cardiovascular risk. *Atherosclerosis* **2013**, *230*, 347–353. [CrossRef] [PubMed]
55. Solá, R.; Fitó, M.; Estruch, R.; Salas-Salvadó, J.; Corella, D.; de La Torre, R.; Muñoz, M.A.; López-Sabater, M.d.C.; Martínez-González, M.-A.; Arós, F.; et al. Effect of a traditional Mediterranean diet on apolipoproteins B, A-I, and their ratio: A randomized, controlled trial. *Atherosclerosis* **2011**, *218*, 174–180. [CrossRef] [PubMed]
56. Guasch-Ferré, M.; Santos, J.L.; Martínez-González, M.A.; Clish, C.B.; Razquin, C.; Wang, D.; Liang, L.; Li, J.; Dennis, C.; Corella, D.; et al. Glycolysis/gluconeogenesis- and tricarboxylic acid cycle-related metabolites, Mediterranean diet, and type 2 diabetes. *Am. J. Clin. Nutr.* **2020**, *111*, 835–844. [CrossRef] [PubMed]

Publisher's Note: MDPI stays neutral with regard to jurisdictional claims in published maps and institutional affiliations.

nutrients

MDPI

Article

Association of the Modified Mediterranean Diet Score (mMDS) with Anthropometric and Biochemical Indices in US Career Firefighters

Maria Romanidou [1,*], Grigorios Tripsianis [1], Maria Soledad Hershey [2], Mercedes Sotos-Prieto [3,4,5], Costas Christophi [3,6], Steven Moffatt [7], Theodoros C. Constantinidis [8] and Stefanos N. Kales [3,9]

1 Department of Medical Statistics, Medical Faculty, Democritus University of Thrace, 68100 Alexandroupolis, Greece; gtryps@med.duth.gr
2 Department of Preventive Medicine and Public Health, Navarra Institute for Health Research, University of Navarra, 31008 Pamplona, Spain; mhershey@alumni.unav.es
3 Department of Environmental Health, T.H. Chan School of Public Health, Harvard University, Boston, MA 02215, USA; msotosp@hsph.harvard.edu or Mercedes.sotos@uam.es (M.S.-P.); costas.christophi@cut.ac.cy (C.C.); skales@hsph.harvard.edu (S.N.K.)
4 Department of Preventive Medicine and Public Health, School of Medicine, Universidad Autónoma de Madrid, IdiPaz (Instituto de Investigación Sanitaria Hospital Universitario La Paz), Calle del Arzobispo Morcillo 4, 28029 Madrid, Spain
5 Biomedical Research Network Centre of Epidemiology and Public Health (CIBERESP), Carlos III Health Institute, 28029 Madrid, Spain
6 Cyprus International Institute for Environmental and Public Health, Cyprus University of Technology, 30 Archbishop Kyprianou Str., Lemesos 3036, Cyprus
7 National Institute for Public Safety Health, IN 324 E New York Street, Indianapolis, IN 46204, USA; steven.moffatt@ascension.org
8 Laboratory of Hygiene and Environmental Protection, Medical School, Democritus University of Thrace, 68100 Alexandroupolis, Greece; tconstan@med.duth.gr
9 Occupational Medicine, Cambridge Health Alliance/Harvard Medical School, Cambridge, MA 02319, USA
* Correspondence: mromanid@med.duth.gr

Received: 6 November 2020; Accepted: 27 November 2020; Published: 30 November 2020

Abstract: The Mediterranean diet is associated with multiple health benefits, and the modified Mediterranean Diet Score (mMDS) has been previously validated as a measure of Mediterranean diet adherence. The aim of this study was to examine associations between the mMDS and anthropometric indices, blood pressure, and biochemical parameters in a sample of career firefighters. The participants were from Indiana Fire Departments, taking part in the "Feeding America's Bravest" study, a cluster-randomized controlled trial that aimed to assess the efficacy of a Mediterranean diet intervention. We measured Mediterranean diet adherence using the mMDS. Anthropometric, blood pressure, and biochemical measurements were also collected. Univariate and multivariate linear regression models were used. In unadjusted analyses, many expected favorable associations between the mMDS and cardiovascular disease risk factors were found among the 460 firefighters. After adjustment for age, gender, ethnicity, physical activity, and smoking, a unitary increase in the mMDS remained associated with a decrease of the total cholesterol/HDL ratio (β-coefficient −0.028, $p = 0.002$) and an increase of HDL-cholesterol (β-coefficient 0.254, $p = 0.004$). In conclusion, greater adherence to the Mediterranean diet was associated with markers of decreased cardiometabolic risk. The mMDS score is a valid instrument for measuring adherence to the Mediterranean diet and may have additional utility in research and clinical practice.

Keywords: Mediterranean diet; Mediterranean diet scores; anthropometrics; lipids; cardiometabolic risk

---

1. Introduction

Obesity, metabolic syndrome, and cardiovascular disease (CVD) have major impacts on US emergency responders, such as firefighters. These non-communicable, lifestyle-influenced conditions can put firefighters' career and life at risk [1–6]. The hazardous working environment, with risks of burns and physical trauma, air pollutants, physical and emotional stress, and shiftwork, causes additional stress to the cardiovascular system and may put firefighters at a higher cardiovascular disease risk with respect to the general population [7,8]. In fact, among US firefighters, sudden cardiac death is the leading cause of on-duty death, is, in most cases, due to underlying coronary heart disease and cardiomegaly, and is responsible for over 40% of duty-related deaths [9,10].

The number and proportion of CVD fatalities have remained relatively similar over the years, which suggests the need for more aggressive lifestyle-related interventions [11]. A recent study in older firefighters suggested that wellness programs can improve the cardiorespiratory function [12]. The eating and lifestyle patterns of firefighters often lead to obesity and have negative impacts on society by contributing to an increased rate of sick leave and increased healthcare expenses [13,14]. On the other hand, firefighters who follow a healthy lifestyle by exercising and maintaining a healthy weight are more likely to maintain high levels of cardiorespiratory fitness during aging [15].

The Mediterranean diet has been shown to reduce the risk of CVD and promote longevity in a variety of international settings [16–18]. There is also an increasing trend to introduce the Mediterranean diet at work as an intervention to prevent non-communicable diseases [19]. The existing evidence also suggests that adherence to the Mediterranean diet not only improves the physical health and wellbeing of workers but also may reduce work stress and blood pressure [20–22]. In two recent meta-analyses of Randomized Control Trials (RCT), the Mediterranean diet, also in combination with physical activity, was the only eating pattern which showed significant and beneficial effects on weight, body mass index (BMI) waist circumference, total cholesterol, high-density lipoprotein (HDL)-cholesterol, glucose, and blood pressure, without any evidence of adverse associations [23,24].

Various Mediterranean diet scores have been developed worldwide to quantify adherence to the Mediterranean diet [25–29]. In the ATTICA intervention in Greece, adherence was measured with the MedDietScore (0–55 items) [30,31], while the European Prospective Investigation into Cancer Nutrition (EPIC) group used the MED score (0–9 scale) [32,33]. Other adaptations include the Italian alternative Mediterranean diet score aMED (0–9 scale) [34] and the I-MEDAS from Israel (17-item questionnaire) [35]. The PREDIMED score, which is based on 14 items from the Prevención con Dieta Mediterránea in Spain, is also widely used [36,37]. However, the use of these scores in different populations, cultures, and ethnicities has been questioned, as they may not be directly adaptable to different ethnic and social groups [38].

In the US, a Mediterranean diet score was constructed specifically to measure adherence to the Mediterranean diet in career firefighters and is known as the modified Mediterranean Diet Score (mMDS) [39].

"Feeding America's Bravest" is a cluster-randomized-controlled trial that aimed to assess the efficacy of a Mediterranean Diet intervention in 60 fire stations in two Indiana (USA) Fire Departments [40]. To assess Mediterranean diet adherence, the aforementioned mMDS was used. Its validity versus previously validated questionnaires [41,42] was established using a sample of firefighters participating in "Feeding America's Bravest" [43]. The aim of the present study was to further corroborate the validity of the mMDS as a measure of Mediterranean diet adherence by examining its cross-sectional associations with anthropometric indices, blood pressure, and biochemical parameters in participants of the "Feeding America's Bravest" study.

2. Materials and Methods

2.1. Study Population

In this cross-sectional study, we used baseline nutrition surveys to calculate the mMDS from a total study base of 486 career firefighters (428 firefighters were recruited from the Indianapolis Fire Department's 44 stations and 58 from the Fishers, Indiana Fire Department's 6 stations) who consented to and enrolled in the ongoing study "Feeding America's Bravest": Mediterranean Diet-Based Interventions to change Firefighters' Eating Habits and Improve Cardiovascular Risk Profiles between 28 November 2016 and 16 April 2018 [34,39]. We excluded firefighters who did not complete baseline anthropometric measurements or if their biomarker indices were missing (Figure 1). Recruitment, consent, and study procedures were carried out by trained staff of the National Institute for Public Safety Health, who work regularly with both or the respective fire departments.

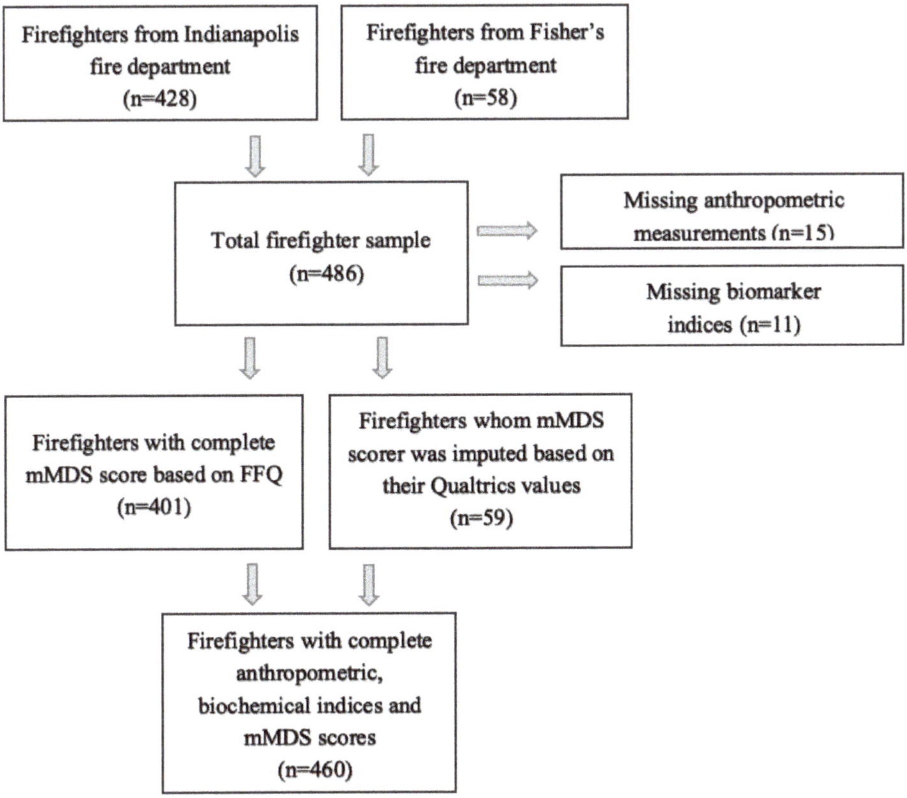

Figure 1. Flow chart for firefighters' sample selection. mMDS: modified Mediterranean Diet Score, FFQ: Food Frequency Questionnaire.

2.2. Dietary Assessment

A validated 131-item semi-quantitative Food Frequency Questionnaire (FFQ) [41] and the mMDS score [39] were used to quantify the firefighters' dietary intake patterns at baseline. The FFQ is a questionnaire previously developed by Yang et al. [39]. Two additional domains were added to the mMDS (nuts and legume consumption), and the score ranged between 0 = minimum adherence to the Mediterranean diet and 51 = maximum adherence to the Mediterranean diet. Because we had previously validated the mMDS in a Qualtrics survey with the Harvard FFQ [43] and more initial Indianapolis participants had complete FFQs, we calculated their mMDS score based on the FFQ and used a scaled value of the directly derived Qualtrics score for the Fishers firefighters who had not done an FFQ.

2.3. Physical Activity

Physical activity was calculated based on a 0–7 scale through a validated self-report scale (Self-Report of Physical Activity (SRPA)) embedded into our study questionnaire [44]. At baseline, the firefighters were asked to describe their physical activity levels over the past month using the following options: 0 = avoid walking or exertion (e.g., always use elevator, drive whenever possible instead of walking, biking, or rollerblading); 1 = walk for pleasure, routinely use stairs, occasionally exercise sufficiently to cause heavy breathing or perspiration; 2 = 10 to 60 min per week; 3 = over one hour per week; 4 = run less than 1 mile per week or spend less than 30 min per week in comparable physical activity; 5 = run 1 to 5 miles per week or spend 30 to 60 min per week in comparable physical activity; 6 = run 5 to 10 miles per week or spend 1 to 3 h per week in comparable physical activity; and 7 = run over 10 miles per week or spend over 3 h per week in comparable physical activity.

2.4. Outcome Assessments

At baseline recruitment, the participants underwent blood pressure and anthropometric assessments as part of the initial study visit. Resting blood pressure was measured using an appropriately sized cuff in seated position for each firefighter. BMI was recorded for all study subjects in kg/m^2 from measured height and weight. Body fat (%) was estimated by a Bioelectrical Impedance Analyzer (BIA) [40,45].

Separately, the firefighters had biochemical indices assessed at fire department-sponsored medical examinations. We used the biochemical measurements gathered at the closest date from the date of study consent within the same 12-month period. Blood samples were also collected after an overnight fast at baseline and at follow-up. Using EDTA collection tubes, up to 15 mL of blood was collected. Plasma and serum were aliquoted, frozen at −80 °C, stored, and run in batches. Automated high-throughput enzymatic analysis was used to determine the blood lipid profiles of the firefighters. This analysis achieved coefficients of variation ≤3% for cholesterol and ≤5% for triglycerides, using a cholesterol assay kit and reagents (Ref:7D62–21) and triglyceride assay kit and reagents (Ref:7D74–21) by the ARCHITECT c System, Abbott Laboratories, IL, USA. The lipid measures included total cholesterol, triglycerides, total cholesterol/HDL ratio, HDL-cholesterol, and low-density lipoprotein (LDL)-cholesterol.

2.5. Covariate Assessment

We collected sociodemographic characteristics, medical history, lifestyle habits, and dietary intake from the study's comprehensive lifestyle questionnaire [40].

2.6. Statistical Analysis

Statistical analysis was performed using IBM Statistical Package for the Social Sciences (SPSS), version 19.0 (IBM Corp., Armonk, NY, USA). The normality of the quantitative variables was tested with the Kolmogorov-Smirnov test. The quantitative variables were expressed as mean ± standard deviation (SD) or as median (Q1, Q3), as appropriate. The qualitative variables were expressed as absolute and relative (%) frequencies.

Multivariable linear regression models were used to examine the association of mMDS with anthropometric, blood pressure, and biochemical variables, after adjusting for age, gender, race, physical activity, and smoking. Beta coefficients were reported with the corresponding standard errors (SE) and p values. Component items of the mMDS were compared between firefighters with high and low values of biochemical parameters using the chi-square test.

All tests were two-tailed, and statistical significance was considered for p values < 0.05.

2.7. Ethics Statement

The overarching "Feeding America's Bravest" protocol was approved by the Harvard Institutional Review Board (IRB16-0170) ethics committee and is registered at Clinical Trials (NCT02941757). All participants provided signed informed consent for participation. The participants who met the criteria for enrollment in the intervention were all informed about their right to decline participation to the intervention or to withdraw at any time as per the Declaration of Helsinki, and the participants who decided to enroll gave full informed consent as per the protocol of the research [40].

3. Results

3.1. Sampling Procedure and Outcome

A sample of 460 firefighters from the two fire departments had complete data for analysis in the current study and represented 95% of all participants who consented to the parent clinical trial (Figure 1).

3.2. General Characteristics of the Firefighters

The majority of the firefighters were males (94.4%), with a mean age of 46.7 years (SD 8.3 years). Firefighters' personal characteristics are shown in Table 1. The mean mMDS in the study population was 21.88 (SD 6.68). The majority of the firefighters were overweight/obese, with an average body fat percentage of 28.10% (SD 6.55%).

Table 1. Characteristics of the participants.

Characteristic	*N*	
Male gender, *n* (%)	448	423 (94.4)
Age (years), mean (SD)	460	46.7 (8.3)
Race, *n* (%)	311	
Caucasian		266 (85.5)
African American		39 (12.5)
Other		6 (1.9)
Currently smoking, *n* (%)	314	15 (4.8)
Physical activity *, *n* (%)	307	
Low		39 (12.7)
Medium		65 (21.2)
High		203 (66.1)
Hours sitting per week, median (Q1–Q3)	300	15 (10–24)
Number of meals at the firehouse, median (Q1–Q3)	309	3 (2–3)
FFQ mMDS, mean (SD)	460	21.88 (6.68)
Anthropometric variables		
BMI (kg/m^2), mean (SD)	460	30.01 (4.39)
Normal weight	74	16%
Overweight	156	34%
Obese	230	50%
Waist circumference (cm), mean (SD)	459	99.7 (12.5)
Body fat percentage (%), mean (SD)	458	28.10 (6.55)
Blood pressure variables		
Resting SBP (mmHg), mean (SD)	460	125.5 (11.2)
Resting DBP (mmHg), mean (SD)	460	79.1 (6.8)

Table 1. *Cont.*

Characteristic	N	
Biochemical variables		
Total Cholesterol (mg/dL), mean (SD)	460	197.1 (37.7)
HDL-Cholesterol (mg/dL), mean (SD)	460	48.5 (11.4)
LDL-Cholesterol (mg/dL), mean (SD)	452	123.5 (32.6)
Total Cholesterol/HDL ratio, mean (SD)	460	4.26 (1.32)
Triglycerides (mg/dL), mean (SD)	459	126.0 (76.6)
Glucose (mg/dL), mean (SD)	460	99.5 (19.6)

* Physical activity. Low: did not participate regularly in programmed recreation, sport, or heavy physical activity. Medium: participated regularly in recreation requiring modest physical activity, such as golf, horseback riding, calisthenics, gymnastics, table tennis, bowling, weight-lifting, yard work. High: participated regularly in heavy physical exercise such as running or jogging, swimming, rowing, skipping rope, running in place, or engaging in vigorous aerobic activity such as tennis. basketball, or handball. FFQ: Food Frequency questionnaire, mMDS: modified Mediterranean Diet Score, SD: Standard Deviation, BMI: body mass index, SBP: systolic blood pressure, DBP: diastolic blood pressure, HDL: high-density lipoprotein, LDL: low-density lipoprotein.

3.3. *Association of the Modified Mediterranean Diet Score with Anthropometric and Biochemical Indices*

The association of mMDS with the participants' anthropometric measures, blood pressure, and biochemical variables is shown in Table 2. When the mMDS scores were categorized into quartiles, multivariate analysis adjusted for age and gender revealed statistically significant inverse associations of mMDS quartiles with BMI (p = 0.030), waist circumference (p = 0.002), body fat percentage (p = 0.002), and total cholesterol/HDL ratio (p = 0.007), whereas there was a positive association with HDL-cholesterol (p = 0.002).

Table 2. Association of the mMDS (categorized into quartiles) with anthropometric measures, blood pressure, and biochemical variables.

	mMDS						
Risk Factor	**1st Quartile**	**2nd Quartile**	**3rd Quartile**	**4th Quartile**	***P* Trend ***	***P* Trend †**	***P* Trend ‡**
Number of subjects	106	122	118	114			
Anthropometric variables							
BMI (kg/m^2)	30.59 (4.06)	30.14 (4.82)	30.17 (4.70)	29.16 (3.77)	0.023	0.030	0.914
Waist circumference (cm)	102.0 (11.6)	100.6 (13.6)	99.3 (12.9)	96.8 (11.0)	0.001	0.002	0.685
Body fat percentage (%)	28.96 (5.64)	28.61 (6.38)	28.42 (7.06)	26.42 (6.75)	0.005	0.002	0.886
Blood pressure variables							
Resting SBP (mmHg)	125.7 (10.8)	124.7 (11.4)	126.6 (12.7)	125.1 (9.5)	0.980	0.836	0.515
Resting DBP (mmHg)	79.6 (7.2)	78.8 (6.7)	79.3 (6.3)	78.6 (7.1)	0.418	0.522	0.927
Biochemical variables							
Total Cholesterol (mg/dL)	200.2 (36.6)	193.1 (37.0)	198.2 (41.4)	197.5 (35.4)	0.894	0.876	0.742
HDL-Cholesterol (mg/dL)	45.6 (10.1)	48.6 (11.9)	48.7 (11.5)	50.9 (11.4)	0.001	0.002	0.022
LDL-Cholesterol (mg/dL)	127.3 (32.7)	119.5 (30.1)	124.4 (35.3)	123.6 (32.2)	0.703	0.690	0.587
Total Cholesterol/HDL ratio	4.60 (1.31)	4.19 (1.58)	4.27 (1.28)	4.03 (0.96)	0.004	0.007	0.020
Triglycerides (mg/dL)	140.8 (85.9)	118.4 (62.7)	129.2 (88.4)	116.9 (65.7)	0.071	0.107	0.364
Glucose (mg/dL)	99.9 (14.3)	100.9 (23.2)	98.6 (20.5)	98.6 (18.9)	0.450	0.594	0.770

* unadjusted; † adjusted for gender and age; ‡ adjusted for age, gender, race, physical activity, and smoking.

After further adjustment for subjects' ethnicity, physical activity, and smoking (Table 2), being in a higher mMDS quartile remained significantly inversely associated with the total cholesterol/HDL ratio ($p = 0.020$) and positively associated with HDL-cholesterol ($p = 0.022$).

3.4. Effects of a Unitary Increase in the Modified Mediteranean Score on Anthropometric Measures, Blood Pressure, and Biochemical Indices

The association of mMDS with subjects' anthropometric measures, blood pressure, and biochemical variables, as a continuous variable, was further analyzed using linear regression models (Table 3).

Table 3. Effect of a unitary increase in the mMDS on anthropometric measures, blood pressure, and biochemical variables.

	Linear Regression Models					
	Adjusted by Gender and Age			Adjusted by Age, Gender, Race, Physical Activity, and Smoking		
Risk Factor	B Coefficient	SE	*p* Value	B Coefficient	SE	*p* Value
Anthropometric variables						
BMI (kg/m^2)	−0.080	0.030	0.008	−0.026	0.038	0.490
Waist circumference (in)	−0.114	0.031	<0.001	−0.045	0.039	0.241
Body fat percentage (%)	−0.141	0.043	0.001	−0.028	0.057	0.627
Blood pressure variables						
Resting SBP (mmHg)	−0.041	0.076	0.590	0.004	0.107	0.969
Resting DBP (mmHg)	−0.056	0.046	0.223	−0.037	0.062	0.552
Biochemical variables						
Total Cholesterol (mg/dL)	−0.160	0.264	0.546	−0.289	0.332	0.385
HDL Cholesterol (mg/dL)	0.254	0.075	<0.001	0.286	0.100	0.004
LDL Cholesterol (mg/dL)	−0.193	0.230	0.402	−0.341	0.300	0.256
Total cholesterol-HDL ratio	−0.028	0.009	0.002	−0.030	0.010	0.002
Triglycerides (mg/dL)	−1.010	0.532	0.058	−0.909	0.644	0.159
Glucose (mg/dL)	−0.137	0.135	0.313	−0.155	0.186	0.404

SD, standard deviation; B, unstandardized Beta coefficient; SE, standard error.

Multivariate linear regression analysis, adjusting for subjects' age and gender, revealed that a unitary increase in the mMDS was significantly inversely associated with BMI (β-coefficient −0.080, $p = 0.008$), waist circumference (β-coefficient −0.114, $p < 0.001$), body fat percentage (β-coefficient −0.141, $p = 0.001$), and total cholesterol/HDL ratio (β-coefficient −0.028, $p = 0.002$), whereas it was positively associated with HDL-cholesterol (β-coefficient 0.254, $p < 0.001$). After further adjustment for subjects' ethnicity, physical activity, and smoking, mMDS was significantly associated with a lower total cholesterol/HDL ratio (β-coefficient −0.030, $p = 0.002$), whereas there was a positive association of mMDS with HDL-cholesterol (β-coefficient 0.286, $p = 0.004$).

3.5. Effects of Single Components of the Modified Mediteranean Score on Anthropometric Measures, Blood Pressure, and Biochemical Indices

Examining component food items of the mMDS and total cholesterol/HDL ratio, total cholesterol-HDL ratio, and blood glucose, fast-food consumption was positively associated with a total cholesterol/HDL ratio >6 ($p = 0.003$) and with triglycerides levels ≥150 mg/dL ($p < 0.001$). Sweet desserts consumption was associated with a total cholesterol/HDL ratio >6 ($p = 0.004$) and with triglycerides levels ≥150 mg/dL ($p = 0.002$), while lower consumption of fruits and vegetables was associated with a total cholesterol/HDL ratio >6 ($p = 0.049$). Fried food consumption was associated with a total cholesterol/HDL ratio >6 ($p = 0.004$) and with triglycerides levels ≥150 mg/dL ($p = 0.037$), and consumption of non-alcoholic beverages at home was associated with glucose levels ≥100 mg/dL ($p = 0.036$). No other statistically significant associations were observed (Appendix A Table A1).

4. Discussion

Our study shows that greater adherence to a Mediterranean diet, as measured by higher mMDS, was favorably associated, as expected, with various anthropometric and biochemical parameters after adjustment by age and gender. After further adjustment for ethnicity, physical activity, and smoking, a higher mMDS remained associated with a lower total cholesterol/HDL ratio and increased HDL-cholesterol. These results are generally in agreement with those of our previous larger study in a different Midwest firefighter cohort of 780 career male firefighters. The study sample was representative, as the participants had similar demographics, anthropometrics, and dietary habits to those of their entire fire departments and other mid-Western firefighters [39]. In our former cross-sectional study, the results indicated that a higher mMDS was associated with HDL-cholesterol and with lower LDL-cholesterol when adjusted for age, BMI, and physical activity and that the firefighters who adhere the most to the Mediterranean diet had a 35% lower risk of prevalent metabolic syndrome [39]. Taken together, our findings are biologically plausible based on previous research and lend additional credibility and validity to the mMDS. The PREDIMED study also found similar results for the Mediterranean diet arms of the intervention, where a reduction of carbohydrates and the increase of monounsaturated dietary fatty acids (MUFA) resulted in lower cholesterol levels and increased HDL cholesterol levels [46]. Similar results were reported from another recent randomized control trial from Italy [47]. In summary, the present study is consistent with past research demonstrating that the Mediterranean diet has cardioprotective effects by improving HDL-cholesterol levels and the total cholesterol/HDL ratio [19,23,48].

Regarding anthropometrics, our results adjusted for age and gender were consistent with previous findings associating the Mediterranean diet with BMI, waist circumference, and weight loss [19,34,49–52]. However, we found no statistically significant associations, after further adjusting for ethnicity, physical activity, and smoking status. Similarly, several other scores such as the Mediterranean Diet Scale (MDScale), Mediterranean Food Pattern (MFP), MD Score (MDS), Short Mediterranean Diet Questionnaire (SMDQ), and MedDiet score were also not significantly associated with BMI [51,52]. The difference between our unadjusted and adjusted models may indicate an insufficient sample size in the current study.

In our study, there was no statistically significant association between the mMDS and glucose levels, consistent with previous research and the most recent RCT meta-analysis studies [23,24,53], although we did find that high consumption of non-alcoholic sugar-sweetened beverages at home was associated with higher glucose levels, as has been shown elsewhere [54,55]. Sweet desserts consumption was associated with a total cholesterol/HDL ratio >6 and with triglycerides levels ≥150 mg/dL. Firefighters with low fruit consumption were more likely to have a total cholesterol/HDL ratio >6. On average, the firefighters were consuming three servings of fruits and vegetables per day, in contrast with the recommendations of five or more daily servings of fruits and vegetables of the American Heart Association (AHA) [56]. Thus, our results highlight the need to increase the consumption of fruits and vegetables, because of their cardioprotective role, as an integral part of the Mediterranean diet [48,57,58]. In a recent study based on how the American population can adopt the Mediterranean diet, it was recommended that the American population should replace their usual desserts such us cookies, ice creams, pies, and sweet and creamy desserts with fresh fruits to optimize their health [59]. Increased fried food consumption was also associated with a total cholesterol/HDL ratio >6 and with triglycerides levels ≥150 mg/dL. It is well documented that the quality of fried food depends on the type of the oil used for frying [60]. Even though the scores for cooking with oils or fats at home and at work were not associated with any of the indices, these scores were below 4, indicating that the consumed fat or oils were mostly oils and spreads other than olive oil (e.g., margarine, corn or vegetable oil, and other spreads). Because at baseline the firefighters were unlikely to use olive oil for cooking, their olive oil consumption was reduced, and they were missing a basic component of the Mediterranean diet which is very important for its anti-inflammatory and antioxidant benefits [61–63].

The major limitation of this study is its cross-sectional nature, which does not allow us to infer causation. Another limitation of our study is that the firefighters were mainly men (94.4%). However, this reflects the current demographic of the US career fire service. Our study was also subject to a degree of non-response bias, as the lifestyle questionnaires were completed online by firefighters and not during the face-to-face study visits.

One of our study's strengths is that the firefighters' anthropometrics included their body fat percentage and waist circumference, not only their BMI. In fact, BMI may cause some false positives due to the increased muscle mass of some firefighters [64]. Another strength is that all our data were collected using standardized procedures, which limits bias. Also, the mMDS was created so to cover the eating habits of the firefighters at work and at home for better accuracy [39]. Finally, one of the strengths of our study is that the previously validated instrument [43] we used to examine Mediterranean diet adherence was created for the American firefighters, based on their lifestyle, eating habits, nature of work (meals at home and at work), type of drinks, and alcohol consumption and therefore is a good-quality validated instrument for this population, as it is known that the quality of Mediterranean diet scores has been questioned in different populations [38].

5. Conclusions

In conclusion, greater adherence to a Mediterranean diet, as measured by a higher mMDS, was favorably associated with lower measures of cardiometabolic risk. In fully adjusted models including physical activity level and smoking, the associations of a higher mMDS with a lower total cholesterol/HDL ratio and increased HDL-cholesterol remained robust. The mMDS has now evidence of validity with respect to more established questionnaires and has been determined in relation to additional biologically plausible associations from two different and independent mid-western (US) firefighter cohorts. Therefore, the mMDS should be a valid tool for assessing the outcome of cluster-randomized controlled trials of Mediterranean lifestyle interventions in this population and similar ones. It may also have further utility not only in research but also in clinical practice.

Author Contributions: Conceptualization, M.R., G.T., T.C.C., and S.N.K.; methodology, M.R., M.S.H., M.S.-P., S.N.K., G.T., C.C., formal analysis, M.R. and G.T.; resources and analysis of the samples S.M., M.R., G.T.,M.S.-P.; data curation, G.T., C.C.; writing—original draft preparation, M.R.; writing—review and editing, M.R., M.S.-P., C.C., S.N.K., G.T., M.S.H., T.C.C.; supervision, S.N.K., G.T., T.C.C.; project administration, S.M. and S.N.K.; funding acquisition, S.N.K and M.S.-P. All authors contributed to the interpretation of data and critical revision of the manuscript and approved the final version. All authors have read and agreed to the published version of the manuscript.

Funding: This research was funded by EMW-2014-FP-00612, US Department of Homeland Security. Ohio University Ohio University OURC grant, CHSP Research Innovation Grant and Boston Nutrition Obesity Research Center small grant. M.S.-P. holds a Ramón y Cajal contract (RYC-2018-025069-I) from the Ministry of Science, Innovation and Universities and FEDER/FSE and FIS grant PI20/00896. The funding agencies had no role in study design, data collection and analysis, interpretation of results, manuscript preparation or in the decision to submit this manuscript for publication.

Acknowledgments: We want to acknowledge the participation of the Indianapolis Fire Departments, the firefighters, and their spouses. We also thank Indiana Clinical and Translational Science Institute for the help with sample processing, Kroger Company (coupons and customer loyalty discounts), Barilla America (Barilla Plus Products), Arianna Trading Company, Innoliva and Molino de Zafra, Spain (extra virgin olive oil samples and discounts), and the Almond Board of California (free samples of roasted unsalted almonds). The sponsors have had no involvement in the overall study design; collection, analysis and interpretation of data; writing of the report; or the decision to submit the report for publication.

Conflicts of Interest: Maria Romanidou, Grigorios Tripsianis, Mercedes Sotos-Prieto, Maria Soledad Hershey, Costas Christophi, Theodoros Constantinidis, and Steven Moffatt declare no conflict of interest. Kales reports non-financial support from Barilla America, non-financial support from California Almond Board, non-financial support from Arianna Trading Company, non-financial support from Innoliva/Molina de Zafra, during the conduct of the study; personal fees from Medicolegal Consulting, personal fees from the Mediterranean Diet Roundtable, outside the submitted work.

Appendix A

Table A1. Comparison of the single items of the modified Mediterranean diet scores (mMDS) according to biochemical indices.

	Total Cholesterol-HDL Ratio > 6					Triglycerides ≥ 150 mg/dL					Glucose ≥ 100 mg/dL				
	No (*N* = 374)		Yes (*N* = 27)		*p*	No (*N* = 300)		Yes (*N* = 100)		*p*	No (*N* = 243)		Yes (*N* = 158)		*p*
	Mean	SD	Mean	SD	Value	Mean	SD	Mean	SD	Value	Mean	SD	Mean	SD	Value
Total mMDS	22.23	6.80	18.19	6.63	0.003	22.47	6.80	20.44	6.86	0.010	22.12	6.67	21.70	7.15	0.549
Single item mMDS															
Fast food consumption *	1.57	0.95	1.00	0.83	0.003	1.66	0.93	1.14	0.92	<.001	1.51	0.97	1.56	0.93	0.634
Fruit consumption	1.57	0.90	1.22	0.70	0.049	1.58	0.91	1.44	0.82	0.163	1.58	0.94	1.49	0.80	0.270
Vegetable consumption	2.56	1.06	2.44	0.93	0.586	2.53	1.05	2.63	1.08	0.396	2.56	1.07	2.54	1.03	0.841
Sweet desserts consumption	1.85	1.57	0.96	1.22	0.004	1.93	1.57	1.37	1.50	0.002	1.76	1.57	1.84	1.56	0.625
Cooking oil or fat use at home	2.12	1.85	1.63	1.74	0.185	2.12	1.86	1.99	1.84	0.554	2.22	1.83	1.88	1.86	0.073
Fried food consumption	1.56	1.18	0.89	0.93	0.004	1.58	1.19	1.30	1.10	0.037	1.47	1.18	1.58	1.17	0.374
Breads or starches consumed at home	1.75	1.48	1.67	1.52	0.782	1.82	1.47	1.50	1.51	0.062	1.73	1.49	1.77	1.48	0.805
Ocean fish consumption	1.64	1.14	1.70	0.99	0.765	1.67	1.13	1.57	1.12	0.459	1.66	1.07	1.61	1.21	0.700
Non-alcoholic beverages at home	2.66	1.13	2.44	1.37	0.339	2.69	1.14	2.50	1.17	0.144	2.74	1.12	2.50	1.18	0.036
Alcoholic beverages	2.09	1.57	1.78	1.48	0.317	2.02	1.60	2.24	1.44	0.224	2.03	1.59	2.13	1.54	0.516
Wine consumption	0.81	0.98	0.89	1.01	0.679	0.81	0.98	0.82	0.99	0.953	0.83	0.99	0.78	0.98	0.645
Legumes consumption	0.67	1.26	0.74	1.29	0.791	0.66	1.26	0.74	1.29	0.585	0.71	1.29	0.63	1.23	0.510
Nuts consumption	1.39	1.62	0.81	1.44	0.073	1.40	1.62	1.20	1.61	0.277	1.32	1.59	1.41	1.66	0.612

* Fast-food consumption per week (score 0–4), i.e., frequency of choosing options such as McDonalds, Burger King, Kentucky Fried Chicken, etc.

References

1. Soares, E.M.K.V.K.; Smith, D.; Porto, L.G.G. Worldwide prevalence of obesity among firefighters: A systematic review protocol. *BMJ Open* **2020**, *10*, e031282. [CrossRef] [PubMed]
2. Tsismenakis, A.J.; Christophi, C.A.; Burress, J.W.; Kinney, A.M.; Kim, M.; Kales, S.N. The obesity epidemic and future emergency responders. *Obesity* **2009**, *17*, 1648–1650. [CrossRef] [PubMed]
3. Lavie, C.J.; Milani, R.V.; Ventura, H.O. Obesity and cardiovascular disease. risk factor, paradox, and impact of weight loss. *J. Am. Coll. Cardiol.* **2009**, *53*, 1925–1932. [CrossRef] [PubMed]
4. Dunlay, S.M.; Givertz, M.M.; Aguilar, D.; Allen, L.A.; Chan, M.; Desai, A.S.; Deswal, A.; Dickson, V.V.; Kosiborod, M.N.; Lekavich, C.L.; et al. Type 2 diabetes mellitus and heart failure, a scientific statement from the American Heart Association and Heart Failure Society of America. *J. Card. Fail.* **2019**, *25*, 584–619. [CrossRef] [PubMed]
5. Donovan, R.; Nelson, T.; Peel, J.; Lipsey, T.; Voyles, W.; Israel, R.G. Cardiorespiratory fitness and the metabolic syndrome in firefighters. *Occup. Med.* **2009**, *59*, 487–492. [CrossRef]
6. Soteriades, E.S.; Hauser, R.; Kawachi, I.; Liarokapis, D.; Christiani, D.C.; Kales, S.N. Obesity and cardiovascular disease risk factors in firefighters: A prospective cohort study. *Obes. Res.* **2005**, *13*, 1756–1763. [CrossRef]
7. Navarro, K.M.; Kleinman, M.T.; Mackay, C.E.; Reinhardt, T.E.; Balmes, J.R.; Broyles, G.A.; Ottmar, R.D.; Naher, L.P.; Domitrovich, J.W. Wildland firefighter smoke exposure and risk of lung cancer and cardiovascular disease mortality. *Environ. Res.* **2019**, *173*, 462–468. [CrossRef]
8. Kales, S.; Smith, D.L. Firefighting and the heart. *Circulation* **2017**, *135*, 1296–1299. [CrossRef]
9. Smith, D.L.; Haller, J.M.; Korre, M.; Fehling, P.C.; Sampani, K.; Porto, L.G.G.; Christophi, C.A.; Kales, S.N. Pathoanatomic findings associated with duty-related cardiac death in US firefighters: A case-control study. *J. Am. Heart Assoc.* **2018**, *7*, e009446. [CrossRef]
10. Smith, D.L.; Haller, J.M.; Korre, M.; Sampani, K.; Porto, L.G.G.; Fehling, P.C.; Christophi, C.A.; Kales, S.N. The relation of emergency duties to cardiac death among US firefighters. *Am. J. Cardiol.* **2019**, *123*, 736–741. [CrossRef]
11. Kahn, S.A.; Leonard, C.; Siordia, C. Firefighter fatalities: Crude mortality rates and risk factors for line of duty injury and death. *J. Burn Care Res.* **2018**, *40*, 196–201. [CrossRef] [PubMed]
12. Gao, X.; Deming, N.J.; Moore, K.; Alam, T. Cardiorespiratory fitness decline in aging firefighters. *Am. J. Public Health* **2020**, *110*, E1. [CrossRef] [PubMed]
13. Neovius, M.; Kark, M.; Rasmussen, F. Association between obesity status in young adulthood and disability pension. *Int. J. Obes.* **2008**, *32*, 1319–1326. [CrossRef] [PubMed]
14. Linde, J.A.; Andrade, K.; MacLehose, R.F.; Mitchell, N.R.; Harnack, L.; Cousins, J.M.; Graham, D.J.; Jeffery, R.W. HealthWorks: Results of a multi-component group-randomized worksite environmental intervention trial for weight gain prevention. *Int. J. Behav. Nutr. Phys. Act.* **2012**, *9*, 14. [CrossRef]
15. Baur, D.M.; Christophi, C.A.; Cook, E.F.; Kales, S. Age-Related decline in cardiorespiratory fitness among career firefighters: Modification by physical activity and adiposity. *J. Obes.* **2012**, *2012*, 1–6. [CrossRef]
16. Eleftheriou, D.; Benetou, V.; Trichopoulou, A.; La Vecchia, C.; Bamia, C. Mediterranean diet and its components in relation to all-cause mortality: Meta-analysis. *Br. J. Nutr.* **2018**, *120*, 1081–1097. [CrossRef]
17. Barbagallo, M.; Barbagallo, M. Mediterranean diet and longevity. *Eur. J. Cancer Prev.* **2004**, *13*, 453–456. [CrossRef]
18. Bo, S.; Ponzo, V.; Goitre, I.; Fadda, M.; Pezzana, A.; Beccuti, G.; Gambino, R.; Cassader, M.; Soldati, L.; Broglio, F. Predictive role of the Mediterranean diet on mortality in individuals at low cardiovascular risk: A 12-year follow-up population-based cohort study. *J. Transl. Med.* **2016**, *14*, 91. [CrossRef]
19. Korre, M.; Tsoukas, M.A.; Frantzeskou, E.; Yang, J.; Kales, S. Mediterranean diet and workplace health promotion. *Curr. Cardiovasc. Risk Rep.* **2014**, *8*, 1–7. [CrossRef]
20. Nissensohn, M.; Román-Viñas, B.; Sánchez-Villegas, A.; Piscopo, S.; Serra-Majem, L. The Effect of the Mediterranean diet on hypertension: A systematic review and meta-analysis. *J. Nutr. Educ. Behav.* **2016**, *48*, 42–53.e1. [CrossRef]
21. Korre, M.; Sotos-Prieto, M.; Kales, S. Survival Mediterranean style: Lifestyle changes to improve the health of the US fire service. *Front. Public Health* **2017**, *5*, 7–13. [CrossRef]

22. Benhammou, S.; Heras-González, L.; Ibáñez-Peinado, D.; Barceló, C.; Hamdan, M.; Rivas, A.; Mariscal-Arcas, M.; Olea-Serrano, F.; Monteagudo, C. Comparison of Mediterranean diet compliance between European and non-European populations in the Mediterranean basin. *Appetite* **2016**, *107*, 521–526. [CrossRef] [PubMed]
23. Dinu, M.; Pagliai, G.; Casini, A.; Sofi, F. Mediterranean diet and multiple health outcomes: An umbrella review of meta-analyses of observational studies and randomised trials. *Eur. J. Clin. Nutr.* **2018**, *72*, 30–43. [CrossRef]
24. Malakou, E.; Linardakis, M.; Armstrong, M.E.; Zannidi, D.; Foster, C.; Johnson, L.; Papadaki, A. The combined effect of promoting the Mediterranean diet and physical activity on metabolic risk factors in adults: A systematic review and meta-analysis of randomised controlled trials. *Nutrients* **2018**, *10*, 1577. [CrossRef] [PubMed]
25. Sotos-Prieto, M.; Moreno-Franco, B.; Ordovás, J.M.; León, M.; Casasnovas, J.A.; Peñalvo, J.L. Design and development of an instrument to measure overall lifestyle habits for epidemiological research: The Mediterranean Lifestyle (MEDLIFE) index. *Public Health Nutr.* **2015**, *18*, 959–967. [CrossRef] [PubMed]
26. Della Corte, C.; Mosca, A.; Vania, A.; Alterio, A.; Iasevoli, S.; Nobili, V. Good adherence to the Mediterranean diet reduces the risk for NASH and diabetes in pediatric patients with obesity: The results of an Italian Study. *Nutrition* **2017**, *39–40*, 8–14. [CrossRef] [PubMed]
27. Serra-Majem, L.; Román-Viñas, B.; Sanchez-Villegas, A.; Guasch-Ferré, M.; Corella, D.; La Vecchia, C. Benefits of the Mediterranean diet: Epidemiological and molecular aspects. *Mol. Asp. Med.* **2019**, *67*, 1–55. [CrossRef]
28. Foscolou, A.; Magriplis, E.; Tyrovolas, S.; Soulis, G.; Bountziouka, V.; Mariolis, A.; Piscopo, S.; Valacchi, G.; Anastasiou, F.; Gotsis, E.; et al. Lifestyle determinants of healthy ageing in a Mediterranean population: The multinational MEDIS study. *Exp. Gerontol.* **2018**, *110*, 35–41. [CrossRef]
29. Izadi, V.; Tehrani, H.; Haghighatdoost, F.; Dehghan, A.; Surkan, P.J.; Azadbakht, L. Adherence to the DASH and Mediterranean diets is associated with decreased risk for gestational diabetes mellitus. *Nutrition* **2016**, *32*, 1092–1096. [CrossRef]
30. Panagiotakos, D.B.; Georgousopoulou, E.N.; Pitsavos, C.; Chrysohoou, C.; Metaxa, V.; Georgiopoulos, G.; Kalogeropoulou, K.; Tousoulis, D.; Stefanadis, C. Ten-Year (2002–2012) cardiovascular disease incidence and all-cause mortality, in urban Greek population: The ATTICA Study. *Int. J. Cardiol.* **2015**, *180*, 178–184. [CrossRef]
31. Panagiotakos, D.B.; Pitsavos, C.; Stefanadis, C. Dietary patterns: A Mediterranean diet score and its relation to clinical and biological markers of cardiovascular disease risk. *Nutr. Metab. Cardiovasc. Dis.* **2006**, *16*, 559–568. [CrossRef] [PubMed]
32. Trichopoulos, D. Adherence to a Mediterranean diet and survival in a Greek population. *N. Engl. J. Med.* **2003**, 2599–2608. [CrossRef] [PubMed]
33. Naska, A.; Trichopoulou, A. Back to the future: The Mediterranean diet paradigm. *Nutr. Metab. Cardiovasc. Dis.* **2014**, *24*, 216–219. [CrossRef] [PubMed]
34. Gnagnarella, P.; Dragà, D.; Misotti, A.M.; Sieri, S.; Spaggiari, L.; Cassano, E.; Baldini, F.; Soldati, L.; Maisonneuve, P. Validation of a short questionnaire to record adherence to the Mediterranean diet: An Italian experience. *Nutr. Metab. Cardiovasc. Dis.* **2018**, *28*, 1140–1147. [CrossRef] [PubMed]
35. Abu-Saad, K.; Endevelt, R.; Goldsmith, R.; Shimony, T.; Nitsan, L.; Shahar, D.R.; Keinan-Boker, L.; Ziv, A.; Kalter-Leibovici, O. Adaptation and predictive utility of a Mediterranean diet screener score. *Clin. Nutr.* **2019**, *38*, 2928–2935. [CrossRef] [PubMed]
36. Guasch-Ferré, M.; Salas-Salvadó, J.; Ros, E.; Estruch, R.; Corella, D.; Fitó, M.; Martinez-Gonzalez, M.; Arós Borau, F.; Gómez-Gracia, E.; Fiol, M.; et al. The PREDIMED trial, Mediterranean diet and health outcomes: How strong is the evidence? *Nutr. Metab. Cardiovasc. Dis.* **2017**, *27*, 624–632. [CrossRef]
37. Martínez-González, M.Á.; García-Arellano, A.; Toledo, E.; Salas-Salvadó, J.; Buil-Cosiales, P.; Corella, D.; Covas, M.I.; Schröder, H.; Arós, F.; Gómez-Gracia, E.; et al. A 14-Item Mediterranean diet assessment tool and obesity indexes among high-risk subjects: The PREDIMED Trial. *PLoS ONE* **2012**, *7*, e43134. [CrossRef]
38. Zaragoza-Martí, A.; Cabañero-Martínez, M.J.; Hurtado-Sánchez, J.A.; Laguna-Pérez, A.; Ferrer-Cascales, R. Evaluation of Mediterranean diet adherence scores: A systematic review. *BMJ Open* **2018**, *8*, 1–8. [CrossRef]
39. Yang, J.; Farioli, A.; Korre, M.; Kales, S.N. Modified Mediterranean Diet score and cardiovascular risk in a north American working population. *PLoS ONE* **2014**, *9*, e87539. [CrossRef]

40. Sotos-Prieto, M.; Cash, S.B.; Christophi, C.; Folta, S.C.; Moffatt, S.; Muegge, C.M.; Korre, M.; Mozaffarian, D.; Kales, S.N. Rationale and design of feeding America's bravest: Mediterranean diet-based intervention to change firefighters' eating habits and improve cardiovascular risk profiles. *Contemp. Clin. Trials* **2017**, *61*, 101–107. [CrossRef]
41. Willett, W.C.; Sampson, L.; Stampfer, M.J.; Rosner, B.; Bain, C.; Witschi, J.; Hennekens, C.H.; Speizer, F.E. Reproducibility and validity of a semiquantitative food frequency questionnaire. *Am. J. Epidemiol.* **1985**, *122*, 51–65. [CrossRef] [PubMed]
42. Salvini, S.; Hunter, D.J.; Sampson, L.; Stampfer, M.J.; Colditz, G.A.; Rosner, B.; Willett, W.C. Food-Based validation of a dietary questionnaire: The effects of week-to-week variation in food consumption. *Int. J. Epidemiol.* **1989**, *18*, 858–867. [CrossRef] [PubMed]
43. Sotos-Prieto, M.; Christophi, C.; Black, A.; Furtado, J.D.; Song, Y.; Magiatis, P.; Papakonstantinou, A.; Melliou, E.; Moffatt, S.; Kales, S.N. Assessing validity of self-reported dietary intake within a Mediterranean diet cluster randomized controlled trial among US firefighters. *Nutrients* **2019**, *11*, 2250. [CrossRef]
44. Jackson, A.S.; Blair, S.N.; Mahar, M.T.; Wier, L.T.; Ross, R.M.; Stuteville, J.E. Prediction of functional aerobic capacity without exercise testing. *Med. Sci. Sports Exerc.* **1990**, *22*, 863–870. [CrossRef] [PubMed]
45. Hershey, M.S.; Sotos-Prieto, M.; Ruiz-Canela, M.; Martínez-González, M.Á.; Cassidy, A.; Moffatt, S.; Kales, S. Anthocyanin intake and physical activity: Associations with the lipid profile of a US working population. *Molecules* **2020**, *25*, 4398. [CrossRef] [PubMed]
46. Estruch, R. Anti-Inflammatory effects of the Mediterranean diet: The experience of the PREDIMED study. *Proc. Nutr. Soc.* **2010**, *69*, 333–340. [CrossRef] [PubMed]
47. Amato, M.; Bonomi, A.; Laguzzi, F.; Veglia, F.; Tremoli, E.; Werba, J.P.; Giroli, M.G. Overall dietary variety and adherence to the Mediterranean diet show additive protective effects against coronary heart disease. *Nutr. Metab. Cardiovasc. Dis.* **2020**, *30*, 1315–1321. [CrossRef]
48. Merino, J.; Kones, R.; Ros, E. Effects of Mediterranean diet on endothelial function. In *Endothelium and Cardiovascular Diseases*; Academic Press: Cambridge, MA, USA, 2018; pp. 363–389.
49. Romaguera, D.; Norat, T.; Mouw, T.; May, A.M.; Bamia, C.; Slimani, N.; Travier, N.; Besson, H.; Luan, J.; Wareham, N.; et al. Adherence to the Mediterranean Diet is associated with lower abdominal adiposity in European men and women. *J. Nutr.* **2009**, *139*, 1728–1737. [CrossRef]
50. Mattei, J.; Sotos-Prieto, M.; Bigornia, S.J.; Noel, S.E.; Tucker, K.L. The Mediterranean diet score is more strongly associated with favorable cardiometabolic risk factors over 2 years than other diet quality indexes in puerto rican adults. *J. Nutr.* **2017**, *147*, 661–669. [CrossRef]
51. Aoun, C.; Papazian, T.; Helou, K.; El Osta, N.; Khabbaz, L.R. Comparison of five international indices of adherence to the Mediterranean diet among healthy adults: Similarities and differences. *Nutr. Res. Pract.* **2019**, *13*, 333–343. [CrossRef]
52. Trichopoulou, A.; Naska, A.; Orfanos, P.; Trichopoulos, D. Mediterranean diet in relation to body mass index and waist-to-hip ratio: The Greek European prospective investigation into cancer and nutrition study. *Am. J. Clin. Nutr.* **2005**, *82*, 935–940. [CrossRef] [PubMed]
53. Estruch, R.; Martínez-González, M.A.; Corella, D.; Salas-Salvadó, J.; Ruiz-Gutiérrez, V.; Covas, M.I.; Fiol, M.; Gómez-Gracia, E.; López-Sabater, M.C.; Vinyoles, E.; et al. Effects of a Mediterranean-style diet on cardiovascular risk factors a randomized trial. *Ann. Intern. Med.* **2006**, *145*, 1–11. [CrossRef] [PubMed]
54. Estruch, R.; Ros, E.; Salas-Salvadó, J.; Covas, M.-I.; Corella, D.; Arós, F.; Gómez-Gracia, E.; Ruiz-Gutiérrez, V.; Fiol, M.; Lapetra, J.; et al. Primary prevention of cardiovascular disease with a Mediterranean diet. *N. Engl. J. Med.* **2013**, *368*, 1279–1290. [CrossRef] [PubMed]
55. Sahingoz, S.A.; Sanlier, N. Compliance with Mediterranean Diet Quality Index (KIDMED) and nutrition knowledge levels in adolescents. A case study from Turkey. *Appetite* **2011**, *57*, 272–277. [CrossRef] [PubMed]
56. Krauss, R.M.; Eckel, R.H.; Howard, B.; Appel, L.J.; Daniels, S.R.; Deckelbaum, R.J.; Erdman, J.W.; Kris-Etherton, P.; Goldberg, I.J.; Kotchen, T.A.; et al. AHA Dietary Guidelines: Revision 2000: A statement for healthcare professionals from the Nutrition Committee of the American Heart Association. *Circulation* **2000**, *102*, 2284–2299. [CrossRef]
57. Willett, W.C. The Mediterranean diet: Science and practice. *Public Health Nutr.* **2006**, *9*, 105–110. [CrossRef]
58. Mozaffarian, D. Dietary and policy priorities for cardiovascular disease, diabetes, and obesity. *Circulation* **2016**, *133*, 187–225. [CrossRef]

59. Martínez-González, M.A.; Hershey, M.S.; Zazpe, I.; Trichopoulou, A. Transferability of the Mediterranean diet to non-mediterranean countries. What is and what is not the Mediterranean diet. *Nutrients* **2017**, *9*, 1226. [CrossRef]
60. Soriguer, F.; Rojo-Martínez, G.; Dobarganes, M.C.; Almeida, J.M.G.; Esteva, I.; Beltrán, M.; De Adana, M.S.R.; Tinahones, F.; Gómez-Zumaquero, J.M.; García-Fuentes, E.; et al. Hypertension is related to the degradation of dietary frying oils. *Am. J. Clin. Nutr.* **2003**, *78*, 1092–1097. [CrossRef]
61. Godos, J.; Rapisarda, G.; Marventano, S.; Galvano, F.; Mistretta, A.; Grosso, G. Association between polyphenol intake and adherence to the Mediterranean diet in Sicily, southern Italy. *NFS J.* **2017**, *8*, 1–7. [CrossRef]
62. Pérez-Martínez, P.; Mikhailidis, D.P.; Athyros, V.G.; Bullo, M.; Couture, P.; Covas, M.I.; De Koning, L.; Delgado-Lista, J.; Díaz-López, A.; Drevon, C.A.; et al. Lifestyle recommendations for the prevention and management of metabolic syndrome: An international panel recommendation. *Nutr. Rev.* **2017**, *75*, 307–326. [CrossRef] [PubMed]
63. Morin, S.J.; Gaziano, J.M.; Djoussé, L. Relation between plasma phospholipid oleic acid and risk of heart failure. *Eur. J. Nutr.* **2017**, *57*, 2937–2942. [CrossRef] [PubMed]
64. Gurevich, K.; Poston, W.S.C.; Anders, B.; Ivkina, M.A.; Archangelskaya, A.; Jitnarin, N.; Starodubov, V.I. Obesity prevalence and accuracy of BMI-defined obesity in Russian firefighters. *Occup. Med.* **2016**, *67*, 61–63. [CrossRef] [PubMed]

Publisher's Note: MDPI stays neutral with regard to jurisdictional claims in published maps and institutional affiliations.

nutrients

MDPI

Article

Effects of a Mediterranean Diet, Dairy, and Meat Products on Different Phenotypes of Dyslipidemia: A Preliminary Retrospective Analysis

Elena Formisano [1], Andrea Pasta [2], Anna Laura Cremonini [3], Ilaria Di Lorenzo [2], Samir Giuseppe Sukkar [3] and Livia Pisciotta [2,3,*]

1 Nutritional Unit ASL-1 Imperiese, Giovanni Borea Civil Hospital, 18038 Sanremo, Italy; formisano.elena@gmail.com

2 Department of Internal Medicine, University of Genoa, 16132 Genoa, Italy; andreapasta93@gmail.com (A.P.); ilariadilorenzo25@libero.it (I.D.L.)

3 Dietetics and Clinical Nutrition Unit, IRCCS Policlinic Hospital San Martino, 16132 Genoa, Italy; annalauracremonini@gmail.com (A.L.C.); samir.sukkar@hsanmartino.it (S.G.S.)

* Correspondence: livia.pisciotta@unige.it; Tel.: +39-0103-538-689

Abstract: Background: Dyslipidemia is one of the major causes of atherosclerotic cardiovascular disease (ASCVD) and a Mediterranean Diet (MD) is recommended for its prevention. The objectives of this study were to evaluate adherence to an MD at baseline and follow-up, in a cohort of dyslipidemic patients, and to evaluate how different food intakes can influence lipid profile, especially how different sources of saturated fatty acids impact lipid phenotype. Methods: A retrospective analysis was conducted on 106 dyslipidemic patients. Clinical characteristics, lipid profile, and food habits data were collected at baseline and after three months of follow-up with counseling. Adherence to an MD was evaluated with a validated food-frequency questionnaire (MEDI-LITE score). Results: The cross-sectional analysis showed that higher consumption of dairy products correlated independently with higher levels of total cholesterol (TC), high-density lipoprotein cholesterol (HDL-C), and low-density lipoprotein cholesterol (LDL-C) and with lower triglycerides (TG) levels. Instead, lower HDL-C and TG levels and higher TC levels were independently associated with higher consumption of meat products. Adherence to an MD significantly improved after the follow-up period, from a mean value of 10 ± 3 (median 10, IQR 8–12) to 13 ± 2 (median 14, IQR 12–15), $p < 0.0001$. Conclusions: Dyslipidemic patients benefit from counseling for improving their adherence to an MD. The high intake of dairy products was associated with less atherogenic hyperlipidemia, which was characterized by higher levels of TC and HDL-C as compared withs the intake of an excessive amount of meat products, which was associated with higher levels of TC and TG and lower levels of HDL-C.

Keywords: Mediterranean diet; saturated fatty acids; ASCVD prevention

Citation: Formisano, E.; Pasta, A.; Cremonini, A.L.; Di Lorenzo, I.; Sukkar, S.G.; Pisciotta, L. Effects of a Mediterranean Diet, Dairy, and Meat Products on Different Phenotypes of Dyslipidemia: A Preliminary Retrospective Analysis. *Nutrients* **2021**, *13*, 1161. https://doi.org/10.3390/nu13041161

Academic Editors: Michael Chourdakis and Emmanuella Magriplis

Received: 21 February 2021
Accepted: 30 March 2021
Published: 1 April 2021

1. Introduction

Dyslipidemia is a major cause of atherosclerotic cardiovascular disease (ASCVD) [1–3]. In particular, the most atherogenic form of dyslipidemia is associated with diabetes, insulin resistance conditions, and familial combined hypercholesterolemia, and it is characterized by elevated levels of low-density lipoprotein cholesterol (LDL-C) and triglycerides (TG), and low levels of high-density lipoprotein cholesterol (HDL-C) [4,5]. Considering the different risk factors for ASCVD, diet plays a key role [6]. A Mediterranean diet (MD) is the main dietary model recommended for the prevention of ASCVD [7] and is the reference diet model of the 2019 European Society of Cardiology/European Atherosclerosis Society (ESC/EAS) guidelines for the management of dyslipidemia [8]. In patients affected by hyperlipidemia, the MD recommends low intake of saturated fatty acids (SFAs), at least less than 10% of total energy intake (i.e., <7% in patients with hypercholesterolemia). Consequently, moderate restriction of milk and dairy product consumption should be balanced by a limited intake of meat and meat products [9], in particular, the preferred consumption of milk and dairy products should not exceed 180 g/day, while no more than 80 g/day of meat and meat products should be consumed [10]. Low-fat cheeses and semi-skimmed milk should be preferred for patients with dyslipidemia [11], and processed meats should not be recommended [12]. A high prevalence of plant-based food, such as whole grains, vegetables, and fruits are highly advisable according to the MD in order to reach a total amount of carbohydrates between 45 and 55% of total energy intake, and 25–40 g per day of total dietary fiber [8]. Furthermore, the MD encourages a moderate amount of seafood, regular consumption of olive oil, and increased physical activity [13,14]. A reduction in sugar intake and elimination of alcohol consumption is recommended for patients with hypertriglyceridemia [15].

In recent years, several studies have investigated the relationship between diet and ASCVD risk. Different studies have mostly recommended that consumption of SFAs is not recommended for prevention of ASCVD and increased LDL-C levels [16,17], while recent epidemiological studies in the literature support the fact that SFAs do not increase the risk of ASCVD [18]. The Prospective Urban and Rural Epidemiology study (PURE) was a large observational study that clarified the relationship between macronutrient intake and mortality, concluding that SFA intake did not influence mortality rate, while high carbohydrate intake was associated with higher mortality risk [19]. In the European Prospective Investigation into Cancer and Nutrition (EPIC) study, a significantly lower mortality was observed among subjects with the highest intake of saturated fatty acids as compared with those with minimum intake [20]. In a recent meta-analysis, de Souza et al. checked the relationship between SFAs intake and cardiovascular mortality and did not observe an increased risk of ASCVD events in subjects with a high consumption of SFAs as compared with those with low consumption [21]. Therefore, ASCVD risk may be influenced by the dietary source of SFAs, mainly represented by dairy and meat products. Meat consumption is considered to be a dietary risk factor for atherogenic dyslipidemia [12]. De Oliveira et al. reported, on the one hand, that a higher intake of SFAs from meat products is related to the development of ASCVD; on the other hand, a lower ASCVD risk is correlated to a higher intake of SFAs from dairy products [22]. However, the literature is still controversial regarding the relationship between meat and dairy products intake and alterations in lipid profile. Therefore, this study aims to evaluate adherence to an MD at baseline and at follow-up in a cohort of dyslipidemic patients and to evaluate how different food intakes can influence the lipid profile, especially how different sources of saturated fatty acids act on the lipid phenotype.

2. Materials and Methods

2.1. Study Design and Subjects

In the current study, a retrospective analysis was performed on the medical charts of 106 patients, 53 women and 53 men, suffering from different forms of hyperlipidemias. All subjects had been referred to the outpatient section of the Lipid Clinic, IRCCS Policlinic San Martino Hospital, University of Genoa, Italy, from February to July 2019. The exclusion criteria were age <18 years, active neoplasm, malignant hematological disease, endocrinopathy, inflammatory bowel disease, connective tissue disease, chronic and acute liver disease, congestive heart failure (NYHA class III–IV), acute and chronic nephropathy (GRF < 45 mL/min according to the Chronic Kidney Disease—Epidemiology Collaboration equation), acute and chronic infection, and therapy with hormones (including insulin) or with recombinant cytokines.

At baseline, height and weight, blood pressure, and smoking habits were recorded during a medical evaluation and body mass index (BMI) and the risk score (RS) were calculated. Blood test results provided a complete lipid profile (total cholesterol, high-density lipoprotein cholesterol, and triglycerides), tested without lipid lowering treatment and analyzed by an experienced physician who specialized in the management of hyperlipidemias. The LDL-C level calculation was performed using the Friedewald formula. Patients' food habits at the time of the first evaluation (baseline) were assessed using a validated food frequency questionnaire, i.e., the MEDI-LITE score [10,23]. At the follow-up visit, i.e., after three months, weight and blood pressure were reported, as well as BMI and the blood lipid profile were recalculated; food habits were re-assessed using the same food frequency questionnaire, however, participants responded referring to the period between the baseline and the follow-up.

Informed written consent for the use of personal data was obtained from patients. The study was conducted in accordance with the Declaration of Helsinki and was approved by the Ethics Committee of IRCCS Policlinic Hospital San Martino in Genoa (Italy) (project number 44/2021).

2.2. *Dietary Assessment*

Food intake and adherence to an MD were assessed in common clinical practice through the MEDI-LITE score, which is a food frequency questionnaire that had been previously proposed and validated [10,24]. Daily and weekly food intake were evaluated by nine questions regarding foods recommended by the MD. The highest consumption of fruits, vegetables, cereals, legumes, fish, and olive oil corresponds to a score of 2, a score of 1 represents average consumption, and a score of 0 indicates the lowest consumption. Conversely, a score of 2 corresponds to the lowest consumption of meat and meat products, dairy products, and alcohol; a score of 1 indicates average intake; and a score of 0 represents the highest intake. The final score obtained ranged from 0 (low adherence to the MD) to 18 (high adherence to the MD) points.

Lifestyle Intervention

A lipid lowering diet based on the ESC/EAS guidelines for the management of dyslipidemias [8], was proposed to all patients. Lipid intake ranged between 25 and 35% of the daily kcal, with cholesterol lower than 300 mg/day and saturated fats <7% of the total kcal. The protein and carbohydrate intakes were 15–25% and 45–55% of the total daily kcal, respectively. Normal weight and overweight patients were advised to perform moderate-intense exercise at least 30 min per day. The following four different types of diets were administered, in an outpatient setting, after anthropometric and biochemical parameter evaluation:

- General advice with weekly counseling on food frequency for patients with primary hypercholesterolemia and normal weight patients.
- General advice with counseling on food frequency for non-overweight patients with mixed hyperlipemia or hypertriglyceridemia or with a reduction in alcohol and carbohydrates.
- General advice based on the frequency of food and control of food with an overall energy intake of 1700 kcal/day for overweight women.
- General advice based on the frequency of food and control of food portions with a total energy intake of 2100 kcal/day for overweight men.

The compositions of the diets are reported in Supplementary Table S1.

2.3. *Statistical Analysis*

Statistical analysis was performed using SPSS Statistics 25, Version 25.0 (SPSS Inc., Chicago, IL, USA) (https://www.ibm.com/it-it/analytics/spss-statistics-software, accessed on 31 March 2021). Detailed statistical analysis is reported in the Supplementary Materials.

3. Results

3.1. Characteristics of the Population and Adherence to an MD

The general characteristics of the study population at baseline are shown in Table 1. The median age was 55 (IQR 45–64) and the 106 patients were equally male and female. Most of them (n = 98, 92.5%) were natives of Liguria, a region in the North-West of Italy, while six patients were born in South America (5.7%) and one subject came from each of UK and Romania. Most of the enrolled patients (except two subjects) did not practice moderate physical activity for more than 15 min every day. The comedications used by patients are reported in Supplementary Table S2.

Table 1. Characteristics of all 106 dyslipidemic patients.

VARIABLE	VALUE
Sex [F/M: n; %]	53 (50.0%)/53 (50.0%)
Age [years: mean ± SD; median; IQR]	54 ± 14; 55 (45–64)
Weight [kg: mean ± SD; median; IQR]	73.9 ± 17.3; 72.5 (60.0–84.0)
BMI [kg/m^2: mean ± SD; median; IQR]	26.1 ± 4.7; 25.8 (22.6–29.2)
SBP [mm/Hg: mean ± SD; median; IQR]	137 ± 17; 135 (128–146)
DBP [mm/Hg: mean ± SD; median; IQR]	82 ± 9; 80 (77–88)
Smoking habits [Never + Past/Current: n; %]	84 (79.2%)/22 (20.8%)
Risk SCORE [%: mean(SD; median; IQR] Low-Risk: <1% [n; %] Moderate-Risk: ≥1% and <5% [n; %] High-Risk: ≥5% and <10% [n; %] Very-High-Risk: ≥10% [n; %]	4.0 ± 6.3; 1.4 (0.6–4.2) 41 (38.7%) 41 (38.7%) 10 (9.4%) 14 (13.2%)
TC [mg/dl: mean ± SD; median, IQR]	245 ± 55; 248 (210–278)
HDL-C [mg/dl: mean ± SD; median, IQR]	57 ± 19; 53 (42–66)
LDL-C [mg/dl: mean ± SD; median, IQR]	159 ± 51; 154 (130–189)
TG [mg/dl: mean ± SD; median, IQR]	186 ± 156; 127 (97–208)

Abbreviations: M = male, F = female, BMI = body mass index, SBP = systolic blood pressure, DBP = diastolic blood pressure, IQR= Interquartile range, TC = total cholesterol, HDL-C = high-density lipoprotein cholesterol, LDL-C = low-density lipoprotein cholesterol, TG = triglycerides.

The mean MEDI-LITE score for the patients was 10 ± 3 (median 10, IQR 8–12) points. A regression analysis of the lipid profile adjusted for sex, age, BMI, and smoking habits showed that the presence of a higher MEDI-LITE score was independently correlated with higher levels of HDL-C levels ($\beta \pm$ SE 1.099 ± 0.413, r = 0.253, p = 0.009) and TC ($\beta \pm$ SE 1.353 ± 0.449, r = 0.283, p = 0.003) and lower levels of TG ($\beta \pm$ SE 3.712 ± 2.272, r = 159, p = 0.105). LDL-C levels did not correlate with the MEDI-LITE score.

3.2. Cross-Sectional Analysis: Relationship between Lipid Profile and Different Food Categories

Table 2 shows the number of patients based on the MEDI-LITE scores obtained for specific food categories. Lipid levels normalized by sex, age, BMI, and smoking habits were divided according to food categories and the score assigned (Table 2). Independent sample comparison tests were preliminarily performed. Patients with fruit intake >300 g/day had significantly higher levels of TC and HDL-C than those who ate <150 g/day or between 150 and 300 g/day. The levels of TC and HDL-C were significantly lower in subjects who ate fewer vegetables (<150 g/day) than in moderate and higher consumers of vegetables (150–300 and >300 g/day, respectively). No statistically significant differences were observed in the serum levels of LDL-C. Patients who consumed more meat and meat products (>120 g/day) had significantly lower levels of TC and HDL-C than moderate (80–120 g/day) and low (<80 g/day) meat consumers, while levels of TG were significantly higher in the latter (<80 g/day) than subjects who ate >120 g/day. LDL-C levels did not vary significantly. Patients who consumed the most (270 g/day) dairy products had significantly higher levels of TC, HDL-C, and LDL-C and lower levels of TG than patients with the lowest intake of dairy products (<180 g/day). No alcohol consumption was significantly associated with higher levels of TC and HDL-C and significantly lower levels of TG than alcohol consumption by patients. None differences in LDL-C levels have been observed in different alcohol consumer groups.

Table 2. Lipid profile and patient distribution according to food categories and the score assigned.

	Patients [*n*, %]	TC [Median, IQR]	HDL-C [Median, IQR]	LDL-C [Median, IQR]	TG [Median, IQR]
Fruit					
<150 g/day	26 (24.5%)	238 (229–250)	52 (42–58)	156 (148–164)	220 (142–270)
150–300 g/day	20 (18.9%)	238 (232–247)	54 (48–66)	161 (147–164)	209 (132–227)
>300 g/day	60 (56.6%)	251 (239–259)	59 (51–68)	163 (150–165)	149 (134–225)
p-value †		$p = 0.003$ <150 vs. >300 g/day $p = 0.01$ ($p = 0.003$) 150–300 vs. >300 g/day $p = 0.04$ ($p = 0.01$)	$p = 0.03$ <150 vs. >300 g/day $p = 0.04$ ($p = 0.01$)	NS	NS
Vegetables					
<100 g/day	36 (34.0%)	237 (230–249)	51 (45–60)	155 (149–164)	217 (145–235)
100–250 g/day	32 (30.2%)	249 (238–257)	57 (51–70)	163 (155–164)	145 (126–222)
>250 g/day	38 (35.8%)	249 (238–259)	57 (52–68)	164 (149–166)	149 (137–217)
p-value †		$p = 0.01$ <100 vs. >250 g/day $p = 0.02$ ($p = 0.008$) <100 vs. 100–250 g/day $p = 0.06$ ($p = 0.02$)	$p = 0.04$ <100 vs. >250 g/day $p = 0.10$ ($p = 0.03$) <100 vs. 100–250 g/day $p = 0.06$ ($p = 0.02$)	NS	NS
Legumes					
<70 g/week	50 (47.2%)	245 (233–255)	55 (49–67)	162 (149–164)	157 (134–229)
70–140 g/week	46 (43.4%)	246 (236–259)	56 (50–68)	164 (150–165)	149 (148–163)
>140 g/week	10 (9.4%)	239 (237–254)	56 (49–61)	157 (128–227)	216 (153–231)
p-value †		NS	NS	NS	NS
Cereals					
<130 g/day	40 (37.7%)	247 (233–259)	57 (50–68)	162 (149–165)	150 (130–230)
130–200 g/day	20 (18.9%)	244 (237–256)	58 (50–64)	163 (155–165)	180 (137–230)
>200 g/day	46 (43.4%)	243 (235–253)	55 (49–62)	163 (149–165)	198 (139–227)
p-value †		NS	NS	NS	NS
Fish					
<100 g/week	32 (30.2%)	240 (232–252)	55 (45–64)	161 (149–164)	212 (125–252)
100–250 g/week	58 (54.7%)	248 (236–258)	59 (50–67)	164 (149–165)	150 (133–220)
>250 g/week	16 (15.1%)	241 (237–254)	54 (50–63)	150 (149–165)	209 (150–231)
p-value †		NS	NS	NS	NS
Meat Products					
>120 g/day	21 (19.8%)	236 (228–249)	48 (40–56)	158 (148–165)	228 (169–270)
80–120 g/day	31 (29.2%)	240 (233–249)	53 (49–61)	155 (148–164)	214 (139–230)
<80 g/day	54 (50.9%)	253 (240–259)	60 (52–69)	164 (156–165)	147 (127–212)
p-value †		$p = 0.001$ <80 vs. >120 g/day $p = 0.001$ ($p < 0.0001$) <80 vs. 80–120 g/day $p = 0.06$ ($p = 0.02$)	$p < 0.0001$ <80 vs. 80–120 g/day $p = 0.06$ ($p = 0.02$) <80 vs. >120 g/day $p < 0.0001$ ($p < 0.0001$)	NS	$p = 0.008$ <80 vs. >120 g/day $p = 0.009$ ($p = 0.003$)
Dairy Products					
>270 g/day	51 (48.1%)	249 (240–259)	58 (52–68)	164 (150–166)	145 (127–216)
180–270 g/day	11 (10.4%)	237 (231–255)	53 (42–61)	161 (152–165)	219 (149–240)
<180 g/day	44 (41.5%)	240 (233–253)	53 (47–66)	156 (148–164)	211 (138–258)
p-value †		$p = 0.01$ <180 vs. >270 g/day $p = 0.02$ ($p = 0.005$)	$p = 0.074$ <180 vs. >270 g/day $p = 0.04$	$p = 0.02$ <180 vs. >270 g/day $p = 0.02$ ($p = 0.006$)	$p = 0.02$ <180 vs. >270 g/day $p = 0.04$ ($p = 0.01$)

Table 2. *Cont.*

	Patients [*n*, %]	TC [Median, IQR]	HDL-C [Median, IQR]	LDL-C [Median, IQR]	TG [Median, IQR]
Alcohol					
>2 AU/day	35 (33.0%)	239 (233–254)	54 (47–67)	157 (149–164)	213 (147–234)
1–2 AU/day	34 (32.1%)	241 (234–252)	53 (48–60)	161 (149–164)	180 (124–236)
<1 AU/day	37 (34.9%)	253 (242–260)	59 (54–68)	164 (150–165)	146 (134–213)
p-value †		$p = 0.009$ 1–2 vs. <1 AU $p = 0.02$ ($p = 0.006$) >2 vs. <1 AU $p = 0.04$ ($p = 0.01$)	$p = 0.01$ 1–2 vs. <1 AU $p = 0.05$ ($p = 0.02$) >2 vs. <1 AU $p = 0.12$ ($p = 0.04$)	NS	>2 vs. <1 AU $p = 0.01$
Olive Oil					
Occasional	3 (2.8%)	255 (233–259)	60 (43–63)	166 (166–166)	150 (149–234)
Frequent	5 (4.7%)	247 (245–248)	59 (51–71)	163 (155–169)	135 (106–230)
Regular	98 (92.5%)	243 (235–256)	56 (49–67)	162 (149–165)	191 (134–228)
p-value †		NS	NS	NS	NS

Abbreviations: AU = Alcoholic Unit; NS = Non-statistically significant. † Independent samples Kruskal–Wallis tests. Significance values have been adjusted by the Bonferroni correction for multiple tests. Unadjusted *p*-values have been also reported.

Finally, the relationships among the lipid profile (TC, HDL-C, LDL-C, and TG adjusted for sex, age, BMI, and smoking habits) and all food categories considered in the baseline analysis was investigated through a cross-sectional multivariate analysis (details of the statistical analysis are reported in Table 3. Higher consumption of dairy products correlated independently with higher levels of TC, HDL-C, and LDL-C and with a lower level of TG. Instead, lower levels of HDL-C and TG and higher levels of TC were independently associated with higher consumption of meat and meat products. Finally, a lower level of TC also correlated independently with the frequent use of olive oil. No other statistically significant differences were observed in LDL-C levels.

Table 3. Multivariate analysis on baseline lipid profile in all 106 patients.

VARIABLE and PREDICTORS	β	SE	*p*-Value	r^2	F (*p*-Value) †
TC				0.317	4.952 (<0.0001)
Fruit (high intake: >300 g/day)	2.373	1.434	0.101		
Vegetables (high intake: >250 g/day)	2.628	1.429	0.069		
Legumes (high intake: >140 g/day)	1.292	1.726	0.456		
Cereals (high intake: >200 g/day)	−0.387	1.186	0.745		
Fish (high intake: >250 g/day)	0.594	1.830	0.746		
Meat products (low intake: <80 g/day)	4.784	1.408	0.001		
Dairy Products (low intake: <180 g/day)	−2.596	1.160	0.028		
Olive Oil (Frequent use)	−5.495	2.868	0.058		
Alcohol (low intake: < 1 AU/day)	2.082	1.340	0.124		
HDL-C				0.268	3.904 (<0.0001)
Fruit (high intake: >300 g/day)	1.791	1.353	0.189		
Vegetables (high intake: >250 g/day)	1.626	1.347	0.230		
Legumes (high intake: >140 g/day)	1.53	1.627	0.350		
Cereals (high intake: >200 g/day)	−0.328	1.118	0.770		
Fish (high intake: >250 g/day)	−0.766	1.726	0.658		
Meat products (low intake: <80 g/day)	5.359	1.328	<0.0001		
Dairy Products (low intake: <180 g/day)	−2.433	1.094	0.048		
Olive Oil (Frequent use)	−2.643	2.704	0.331		
Alcohol (low intake: < 1 AU/day)	1.034	1.264	0.416		

Table 3. *Cont.*

VARIABLE and PREDICTORS	β	SE	p-Value	r²	F (p-Value) †
LDL-C				0.149	1.540 (0.149)
Fruit (high intake: >300 g/day)	0.406	1.187	0.733		
Vegetables (high intake: >250 g/day)	1.700	1.229	0.171		
Legumes (high intake: >140 g/day)	0.301	1.515	0.843		
Cereals (high intake: >200 g/day)	0.038	1.013	0.970		
Fish (high intake: >250 g/day)	−0.602	1.589	0.706		
Meat products (low intake: <80 g/day)	1.186	1.246	0.344		
Dairy Products (low intake: <180 g/day)	−2.190	0.976	0.028		
Olive Oil (Frequent use)	−4.877	2.663	0.071		
Alcohol (low intake: < 1 AU/day)	0.840	1.185	0.481		
TG				0.233	3.202 (0.002)
Fruit (high intake: >300 g/day)	−6.806	7.468	0.364		
Vegetables (high intake: >250 g/day)	−9.251	7.474	0.219		
Legumes (high intake: >140 g/day)	−0.479	9.005	0.958		
Cereals (high intake: >200 g/day)	3.714	6.225	0.552		
Fish (high intake: >250 g/day)	0.955	9.530	0.920		
Meat products (low intake: <80 g/day)	−19.321	7.358	0.010		
Dairy Products (low intake: <180 g/day)	15.326	6.065	0.013		
Alcohol (low intake: < 1 AU/day)	−9.931	7.080	0.164		
Olive Oil (Frequent use)	17.823	14.928	0.235		

Abbreviations: TC = total cholesterol, HDL-C = high-density lipoprotein cholesterol, LDL-C = low-density lipoprotein cholesterol, TG = triglycerides. Dependent variable were TC, HDL-C, LDL-C and TG (bold text) and were adjusted for sex, age, BMI and smoking habits. Predictors were fruit intake (<150 g/day = 0, 150–300 g/day = 1 and >300 g/day = 2), vegetables intake (<100 g/day = 0, 100–250 g/day =1 and >250 g/day = 2), legumes intake (<70 g/week = 0, 70–140 g/week = 1 and >140 g/week = 2), cereals intake (<130 g/day = 0, 130–200 g/day = 1 and >200 g/day = 2), fish intake (<100 g/week = 0, 100–250 g/week = 1 and >250 g/week = 2), meat products intake (>120 g/day = 0, 80–120 g/day = 1 and <80 g/day = 2), dairy products intake (>270 g/day = 0, 180–270 g/day = 1 and <180 g/day = 2), alcohol consume (>2 AU/day = 0, 1–2 AU/day = 1 and <1 AU/day = 2) and olive oil use (Occasional = 0, Frequent = 1 and Regular = 2). Abbreviation: β = angular coefficient, SE = standard error, r^2 = square correlation coefficient, F = F-value, *p*-values for predictors, † *p*-value for model fitting significance.

3.3. Follow-Up Analysis

Thirty-four patients (32.1%) did not attend the follow-up visit, and therefore were excluded from the follow-up analysis. Thus, demographical and clinical characteristics of the remaining 72 patients are reported in Table 4. The median follow-up period was 12 weeks (10–13 weeks).

Adherence to an MD significantly improved after the follow-up period, from a mean value of 10 ± 3 (median 10, IQR 8–12) to 13 ± 2 (median 14, IQR 12–15) with $p < 0.0001$ (Table 4). Overall, the number of patients with higher scores in the specific food categories considered in the MEDI-LITE score increased significantly, with the exception of olive oil and cereal consumption which did not statistically differ from baseline (Supplementary Table S3).

Nutritional counseling was effective for improving weight, BMI, and lipid profile excluding HDL-C levels. The addition of a nutraceutical or lipid-lowering drug was further effective in reducing TC, LDL-C, and TG levels (Table 5).

Table 4. Characteristics of the 72 dyslipidemic patients included in follow-up analysis.

VARIABLE	VALUE
Sex [F/M: *n*; %]	34 (47.2%)/38 (52.8%)
Age [years: mean ± SD; median; IQR]	55 ± 13; 55 (48–64)
SBP [mm/Hg: mean ± SD; median; IQR]	138 ± 17; 136 (130–150)
DBP [mm/Hg: mean ± SD; median; IQR]	83 ± 10; 81 (78–89)
Smoking habits [Never + Past/Current: *n*; %]	55 (76.4%)/17 (23.6%)
Risk SCORE [%: mean(SD; median; IQR] Low-Risk: <1% [*n*; %] Moderate-Risk: ≥1% and <5% [*n*; %] High-Risk: ≥5% and <10% [*n*; %] Very-High-Risk: ≥10% [*n*; %]	4.3 ± 7.0; 1.5 (0.7–4.1) 25 (34.7%) 31 (43.1%) 6 (8.3%) 10 (13.9%)
Lipid Lowering Intervention	
Diet alone [*n*; %]	31 (43.1%)
Lipid-lowering Nutraceuticals [*n*; %]	13 (18.1%)
Lipid-lowering Drugs [*n*; %]	28 (38.9%)

Abbreviations: M = male, F = female, IQR = Interquartile range, SBP = systolic blood pressure, DBP = diastolic blood pressure.

Table 5. Variation in anthropometric measures, MEDI-LITE score, and lipid profile after the nutritional counseling.

VARIABLES	Baseline [Mean ± SD; Median; IQR]	Follow-up [Mean ± SD; Median; IQR]	Absolute Variation [Mean ± SD; Median; IQR]	Percentage Variation [%]	*p*-Value †
Weight [kg: mean ± SD; median; IQR]	75.7 ± 17.5; 74.3 (62.5, 84.0)	72.8 ± 15.8; 71.0 (60.0, 83.5)	−2.5 ± 3.5; −2.0 (−3.3, 0)	−3.2%	<0.0001
BMI [kg/m^2: mean ± SD; median; IQR]	26.3 ± 4.7; 26.0 (22.9, 28.8)	25.2 ± 4.0; 25.5 (22.1, 27.4)	−9 ± 1.2; −0.6 (−1.2, 0)	−3.3%	<0.0001
MEDI-LITE [Points: mean ± SD; median; IQ range]	10 ± 3; 10 (8, 12)	13 ± 2; 14 (12, 15)	3 ± 3; 3 (1, 5)	+43.4%	<0.0001
TC [mg/dl: mean ± SD; median, IQR]					
Diet alone	249 ± 36; 255 (222, 267)	207 ± 54; 204 (158, 248)	−42 ± 54; −23 (−87, −1)	−16.2%	0.002
Lipid-lowering Nutraceuticals	257 ± 39; 261 (232, 270)	211 ± 39; 204 (190, 213)	−38 ± 34; −42 (−67, 0)	−15.1%	0.046
Lipid-lowering Drugs	238 ± 67; 234 (179, 294)	170 ± 30; 173 (140, 196)	−83 ± 61; −73 (−119, −33)	−29.3%	<0.0001
HDL-C [mg/dl: mean ± SD; median, IQR]					
Diet alone	58 ± 21; 53 (42, 67)	60 ± 20; 54 (47, 68)	0 ± 7; 0 (−3, 4)	2.5%	0.641
Lipid-lowering Nutraceuticals	58 ± 26; 46 (40, 63)	55 ± 17; 50 (40, 72)	0 ± 9; 0 (−2, 7)	3.4%	0.753
Lipid-lowering Drugs	54 ± 15; 52 (42, 66)	50 ± 12; 48 (40, 61)	−2 ± 8; −3 (−5, 4)	−2.5%	0.383
LDL-C [mg/dl: mean ± SD; median, IQR]					
Diet alone	161 ± 35; 150 (138, 187)	123 ± 47; 129 (83, 170)	−32 ± 49; −22 (−78, 0)	−18.6%	0.026
Lipid-lowering Nutraceuticals	180 ± 33; 179 (154, 196)	132 ± 34; 131 (102, 145)	−39 ± 37; −39 (−52, −9)	−22.6%	0.068
Lipid-lowering Drugs	146 ± 60; 147 (95, 185)	90 ± 29; 100 (70, 112)	−71 ± 50; −66 (−111, −22)	−38.3%	0.001
TG [mg/dl: mean ± SD; median, IQR]					
Diet alone	184 ± 123; 130 (103, 254)	129 ± 66; 111 (85, 167)	−39 ± 83; −17 (−44, 0)	−15.2%	0.025
Lipid-lowering Nutraceuticals	192 ± 149; 119 (102, 208)	125 ± 56; 102 (90, 177)	−54 ± 104; −10 (−81, 0)	−16.8%	0.173
Lipid-lowering Drugs	218 ± 228; 138 (104, 206)	152 ± 105; 123 (90, 158)	−80 ± 200; −45 (−63, 0)	−16.7%	0.013

Abbreviations: BMI = body mass index, IQR= Interquartile range. † *p*-values for dependent samples nonparametric Wilcoxon Signed Ranks Test between baseline and follow-up values.

4. Discussion

The main purpose of this study was to evaluate the influence of different eating habits on the lipid profile of patients suffering from dyslipidemia.

A preliminary result is that greater adherence to an MD based on MEDI-LITE scores correlated with a better lipid profile characterized by higher levels of HDL-C and lower levels of TG, which is a finding that is strongly supported by the scientific literature [24]. Moreover, a recent study highlighted that high MEDI-LITE total scores were associated with low prevalence of dyslipidemia [25]. The results for fruits and vegetables intake showed an association with higher total cholesterol and HDL, but these data also indicate adherence to an MD and the effect on lipid profile may be mediated by dairy and olive oil consumption.

One of the main results of this study is the different impacts on the lipid profiles of patients with excessive consumption of meat and dairy products according to the MEDI-LITE scores. In fact, subjects with higher meat consumption had atherogenic dyslipidemia with significantly lower levels of HDL-C and higher levels of TG, while higher levels of TC and LDL-C were balanced by higher levels of HDL-C and lower levels of TG in patients with higher consumption of dairy products. These findings are questionable with respect to the dietary recommendations of the 2019 ESC/EAS guidelines for the management of dyslipidemia [8] which recommend an SFA intake less than 10% of the total caloric intake (i.e., about 22 g of SFAs considering a daily total caloric intake of 2000 kcal), and less than 7% in dyslipidemic patients, without distinguishing the food sources (i.e., meat or dairy products). In the literature, the effect of SFAs on ASCVD risk has been extensively studied but is not yet fully understood. Two large prospective analysis, the Nurses' Health Study (NHS) [26] and the Health Professionals Follow-Up Study (HPFS) [27], on the one hand, reported that an increase in consumption of SFAs was related to increased risk of an ASCVD event [28]. On the other hand, a recent prospective study (PURE) clearly highlighted that the higher the consumption of SFAs, the lower the cardiovascular mortality, even in large consumers [19]. A similar correlation emerged in the EPIC study's cohort of subjects, i.e., a minimum intake of SFAs was associated with significantly higher total mortality as compared with a maximum intake of SFAs [20]. A possible match point was proposed by the MESA study which prospectively observed a higher incidence of ASCVD events in patients who consumed more SFAs from meat, while SFAs from dairy products were associated with a decrease in ASCVD occurrence [22].

Furthermore, the correlation between ASCVD risk and higher meat consumption could also be due to the pro-atherogenic effect of some biomolecules in meat, such as choline, carnitine, and lecithin. Conversely, dairy products provide micronutrients and vitamins with a proven protective effect on the risk of ASCVD. In addition, Lordan et al. [29] highlighted the anti-inflammatory properties of dairy products because of their content in inhibitors of the platelet activating factor (PAF). The latter biomolecule is a lipoid factor of thrombosis and inflammation and plays a pivotal role in atherogenesis and atherosclerosis progression. To date, the protective effect of PAF inhibitors present in dairy products has been confirmed in vitro [30] and in vivo in both animals and humans [31]. Furthermore, beneficial anti-inflammatory properties for fermented dairy products have been hypothesized due to the presence of specific bacteria such as lactic acid bacteria and bifidobacteria, as well as the presence of specific fermentation products [32].

In brief, the source of SFAs could have different impacts on the ASCVD risk, in fact, most of the correlation studies between ASCVD and SFAs conducted in the USA, of a population consuming large quantities of meat products [33,34], have shown an increase in ASCVD risk proportional to the consumption of SFAs [26,27]. Conversely, the latter correlation between SFA consumption and ASCVD risk is negative in European patients [20] whose prevalent source of SFAs is represented by dairy products [35].

Moreover, the cross-sectional analysis highlights that frequent use of olive oil correlates with lower levels of TC; a meta-analysis by George, E. S. et al. reported that TC levels decreased linearly with high consumption of polyphenols olive oil [36].

The follow-up analysis showed that adherence to an MD and lipid profile levels improved with dietary counseling. In fact, it is known that nutritional counseling improves adherence to an MD, as highlighted in a recent study by Sialvera, T.E. et al., in which a positive change in lipid profile levels was also observed [37]. Overall, we observed a statistically significant shift from the categories with the lowest MEDI-LITE scores to those with the highest scores, except for olive oil and cereals, whose consumption was already high at the baseline. The reduction in dietary intake of SFAs has mostly been encouraged in accordance with current ESC/EAS guideline recommendations [8]. However, the reduction in meat products was preferred, and the categories of both high and medium consumption were reduced. Conversely, moderate consumption of dairy products was encouraged despite the high and low consumption categories. Further research and scientific debate will be needed to adapt the correct dietary recommendations to the results of the recent scientific literature [38].

Furthermore, dietary counseling was effective in reducing BMI, and the efficacy of dietary intervention in the treatment of weight is well known in the literature [39]. The use of lipid-lowering nutraceuticals had a valuable impact on the lipid profile as compared with diet alone and their effects have been previously highlighted in the literature [14,40,41].

The main limitation of the present study was the relatively small sample size analyzed; thus, the findings should be considered as preliminary. Other limitations are the lack of information about physical activity, employment, and family income; however, these indicators could be homogeneous as most patients live in the same local geographic area. Finally, the use of a food frequency questionnaire may be subject to recall bias.

5. Conclusions

In conclusion, high intake of dairy products was associated with a balanced hyperlipidemia, characterized by higher levels of TC and HDL-C, while a diet with an excessive amount of meat products caused a form of mixed atherogenic dyslipidemia with higher TC and TG levels and lower HDL-C levels. In the light of these findings and according to the recent literature, dietary recommendations should distinguish between SFA sources (i.e., meat products or dairy products) rather than suggesting a general reduction in SFA intake. In addition, dietary counseling is effective in improving adherence to MD in dyslipidemic patients.

Supplementary Materials: The following are available online at https://www.mdpi.com/article/10.3390/nu13041161/s1: Supplementary Table S1, Composition of diets for overweight patients; 1.1 General advice with counselling on weekly food frequency for patients with primary hypercholesterolemia and normal weight patients; 1.2 General advice with advising on food frequency in non-overweight patients with mixed hyperlipemia or hypertriglyceridemia or with reduction in alcohol and carbohydrates; 1.3 General advice based on frequency of food and control of food with an overall energy intake of 1700 kcal/day for overweight women; 1.4 General advice based on frequency of food and control of food portions with a total energy intake of 2100 kcal/day for overweight men; 1.5 Statistical Analysis; Supplementary Table S2, Comedications used by the 106 patients; Supplementary Table S3, Variation of patient distribution according to food categories and the score assigned.

Author Contributions: Conceptualization, L.P.; methodology, L.P. and E.F.; formal analysis, A.P.; investigation, L.P., I.D.L., E.F., A.L.C. and A.P.; data curation, I.D.L., E.F. and A.P.; writing—original draft preparation, E.F. and A.P.; writing—review and editing, L.P. and A.L.C.; supervision, L.P. and S.G.S.; project administration, L.P. All authors have read and agreed to the published version of the manuscript.

Funding: This research received no external funding.

Institutional Review Board Statement: The study was conducted according to the guidelines of the Declaration of Helsinki, and approved by the Ethics Committee of Liguria Region (N. CER Liguria: 44/2021).

Informed Consent Statement: Informed consent was obtained from all subjects involved in the study.

Data Availability Statement: The data presented in this study are available on request from the corresponding author. The data are not publicly available due to privacy policy.

Conflicts of Interest: The authors declare no conflict of interest.

References

1. Pol, T.; Held, C.; Westerbergh, J.; Lindbäck, J.; Alexander, J.H.; Alings, M.; Erol, C.; Goto, S.; Halvorsen, S.; Huber, K.; et al. Dyslipidemia and Risk of Cardiovascular Events in Patients With Atrial Fibrillation Treated With Oral Anticoagulation Therapy: Insights From the ARISTOTLE (Apixaban for Reduction in Stroke and Other Thromboembolic Events in Atrial Fibrillation) Trial. *J. Am. Heart Assoc.* **2018**, *7*. [CrossRef] [PubMed]
2. Nelson, R.H. Hyperlipidemia as a Risk Factor for Cardiovascular Disease. *Prim. Care* **2013**, *40*, 195–211. [CrossRef] [PubMed]
3. Yu, J.N.; Cunningham, J.A.; Thouin, S.R.; Gurvich, T.; Liu, D. Hyperlipidemia. *Prim. Care* **2000**, *27*, 541–587. [CrossRef]
4. Musunuru, K. Atherogenic dyslipidemia: Cardiovascular risk and dietary intervention. *Lipids* **2010**, *45*, 907–914. [CrossRef]
5. Manjunath, C.N.; Rawal, J.R.; Irani, P.M.; Madhu, K. Atherogenic dyslipidemia. *Indian J. Endocrinol. Metab.* **2013**, *17*, 969–976. [CrossRef] [PubMed]
6. Pan, A.; Lin, X.; Hemler, E.; Hu, F.B. Diet and Cardiovascular Disease: Advances and Challenges in Population-Based Studies. *Cell Metab.* **2018**, *27*, 489–496. [CrossRef] [PubMed]
7. Mattioli, A.V.; Palmiero, P.; Manfrini, O.; Puddu, P.E.; Nodari, S.; Dei Cas, A.; Mercuro, G.; Scrutinio, D.; Palermo, P.; Sciomer, S.; et al. Mediterranean diet impact on cardiovascular diseases: A narrative review. *J. Cardiovasc. Med. Hagerstown Md* **2017**, *18*, 925–935. [CrossRef]
8. Mach, F.; Baigent, C.; Catapano, A.L.; Koskinas, K.C.; Casula, M.; Badimon, L.; Chapman, M.J.; De Backer, G.G.; Delgado, V.; Ference, B.A.; et al. 2019 ESC/EAS Guidelines for the management of dyslipidaemias: Lipid modification to reduce cardiovascular risk. *Eur. Heart J.* **2020**, *41*, 111–188. [CrossRef]
9. Lăcătușu, C.-M.; Grigorescu, E.-D.; Floria, M.; Onofriescu, A.; Mihai, B.-M. The Mediterranean Diet: From an Environment-Driven Food Culture to an Emerging Medical Prescription. *Int. J. Environ. Res. Public Health* **2019**, *16*, 942. [CrossRef]
10. Sofi, F.; Dinu, M.; Pagliai, G.; Marcucci, R.; Casini, A. Validation of a literature-based adherence score to Mediterranean diet: The MEDI-LITE score. *Int. J. Food Sci. Nutr.* **2017**, *68*, 757–762. [CrossRef]
11. Drouin-Chartier, J.-P.; Côté, J.A.; Labonté, M.-È.; Brassard, D.; Tessier-Grenier, M.; Desroches, S.; Couture, P.; Lamarche, B. Comprehensive Review of the Impact of Dairy Foods and Dairy Fat on Cardiometabolic Risk123. *Adv. Nutr.* **2016**, *7*, 1041–1051. [CrossRef] [PubMed]
12. Simpson, E.J.; Clark, M.; Razak, A.A.; Salter, A. The impact of reduced red and processed meat consumption on cardiovascular risk factors; an intervention trial in healthy volunteers. *Food Funct.* **2019**, *10*, 6690–6698. [CrossRef] [PubMed]
13. Rees, K.; Takeda, A.; Martin, N.; Ellis, L.; Wijesekara, D.; Vepa, A.; Das, A.; Hartley, L.; Stranges, S. Mediterranean-style diet for the primary and secondary prevention of cardiovascular disease. *Cochrane Database Syst. Rev.* **2019**, *3*, CD009825. [CrossRef] [PubMed]
14. Pasta, A.; Formisano, E.; Cremonini, A.L.; Maganza, E.; Parodi, E.; Piras, S.; Pisciotta, L. Diet and Nutraceutical Supplementation in Dyslipidemic Patients: First Results of an Italian Single Center Real-World Retrospective Analysis. *Nutrients* **2020**, *12*, 2056. [CrossRef]
15. Brinton, E.A. Management of hypertriglyceridemia for prevention of atherosclerotic cardiovascular disease. *Cardiol. Clin.* **2015**, *33*, 309–323. [CrossRef]
16. Briggs, M.A.; Petersen, K.S.; Kris-Etherton, P.M. Saturated Fatty Acids and Cardiovascular Disease: Replacements for Saturated Fat to Reduce Cardiovascular Risk. *Healthcare* **2017**, *5*, 29. [CrossRef]
17. Siri-Tarino, P.W.; Sun, Q.; Hu, F.B.; Krauss, R.M. Saturated fatty acids and risk of coronary heart disease: Modulation by replacement nutrients. *Curr. Atheroscler. Rep.* **2010**, *12*, 384–390. [CrossRef]
18. Astrup, A.; Magkos, F.; Bier, D.M.; Brenna, J.T.; de Oliveira Otto, M.C.; Hill, J.O.; King, J.C.; Mente, A.; Ordovas, J.M.; Volek, J.S.; et al. Saturated Fats and Health: A Reassessment and Proposal for Food-Based Recommendations: JACC State-of-the-Art Review. *J. Am. Coll. Cardiol.* **2020**, *76*, 844–857. [CrossRef]
19. Dehghan, M.; Mente, A.; Zhang, X.; Swaminathan, S.; Li, W.; Mohan, V.; Iqbal, R.; Kumar, R.; Wentzel-Viljoen, E.; Rosengren, A.; et al. Associations of fats and carbohydrate intake with cardiovascular disease and mortality in 18 countries from five continents (PURE): A prospective cohort study. *Lancet Lond. Engl.* **2017**, *390*, 2050–2062. [CrossRef]
20. Praagman, J.; Beulens, J.W.; Alssema, M.; Zock, P.L.; Wanders, A.J.; Sluijs, I.; van der Schouw, Y.T. The association between dietary saturated fatty acids and ischemic heart disease depends on the type and source of fatty acid in the European Prospective Investigation into Cancer and Nutrition-Netherlands cohort. *Am. J. Clin. Nutr.* **2016**, *103*, 356–365. [CrossRef]
21. de Souza, R.J.; Mente, A.; Maroleanu, A.; Cozma, A.I.; Ha, V.; Kishibe, T.; Uleryk, E.; Budylowski, P.; Schünemann, H.; Beyene, J.; et al. Intake of saturated and trans unsaturated fatty acids and risk of all cause mortality, cardiovascular disease, and type 2 diabetes: Systematic review and meta-analysis of observational studies. *BMJ* **2015**, *351*, h3978. [CrossRef]
22. de Oliveira Otto, M.C.; Mozaffarian, D.; Kromhout, D.; Bertoni, A.G.; Sibley, C.T.; Jacobs, D.R.; Nettleton, J.A. Dietary intake of saturated fat by food source and incident cardiovascular disease: The Multi-Ethnic Study of Atherosclerosis. *Am. J. Clin. Nutr.* **2012**, *96*, 397–404. [CrossRef]

23. Sofi, F.; Macchi, C.; Abbate, R.; Gensini, G.F.; Casini, A. Mediterranean diet and health status: An updated meta-analysis and a proposal for a literature-based adherence score. *Public Health Nutr.* **2014**, *17*, 2769–2782. [CrossRef] [PubMed]
24. Kastorini, C.-M.; Milionis, H.J.; Esposito, K.; Giugliano, D.; Goudevenos, J.A.; Panagiotakos, D.B. The effect of Mediterranean diet on metabolic syndrome and its components: A meta-analysis of 50 studies and 534,906 individuals. *J. Am. Coll. Cardiol.* **2011**, *57*, 1299–1313. [CrossRef] [PubMed]
25. Platania, A.; Zappala, G.; Mirabella, M.U.; Gullo, C.; Mellini, G.; Beneventano, G.; Maugeri, G.; Marranzano, M. Association between Mediterranean diet adherence and dyslipidaemia in a cohort of adults living in the Mediterranean area. *Int. J. Food Sci. Nutr.* **2018**, *69*, 608–618. [CrossRef] [PubMed]
26. Hu, F.B.; Stampfer, M.J.; Manson, J.E.; Ascherio, A.; Colditz, G.A.; Speizer, F.E.; Hennekens, C.H.; Willett, W.C. Dietary saturated fats and their food sources in relation to the risk of coronary heart disease in women. *Am. J. Clin. Nutr.* **1999**, *70*, 1001–1008. [CrossRef]
27. Zong, G.; Li, Y.; Wanders, A.J.; Alssema, M.; Zock, P.L.; Willett, W.C.; Hu, F.B.; Sun, Q. Intake of individual saturated fatty acids and risk of coronary heart disease in US men and women: Two prospective longitudinal cohort studies. *BMJ* **2016**, *355*, i5796. [CrossRef] [PubMed]
28. Li, Y.; Hruby, A.; Bernstein, A.M.; Ley, S.H.; Wang, D.D.; Chiuve, S.E.; Sampson, L.; Rexrode, K.M.; Rimm, E.B.; Willett, W.C.; et al. Saturated Fats Compared With Unsaturated Fats and Sources of Carbohydrates in Relation to Risk of Coronary Heart Disease: A Prospective Cohort Study. *J. Am. Coll. Cardiol.* **2015**, *66*, 1538–1548. [CrossRef] [PubMed]
29. Lordan, R.; Zabetakis, I. Invited review: The anti-inflammatory properties of dairy lipids. *J. Dairy Sci.* **2017**, *100*, 4197–4212. [CrossRef]
30. Lordan, R.; Vidal, N.P.; Huong Pham, T.; Tsoupras, A.; Thomas, R.H.; Zabetakis, I. Yoghurt fermentation alters the composition and antiplatelet properties of milk polar lipids. *Food Chem.* **2020**, *332*, 127384. [CrossRef]
31. Lordan, R.; Tsoupras, A.; Zabetakis, I.; Demopoulos, C.A. Forty Years Since the Structural Elucidation of Platelet-Activating Factor (PAF): Historical, Current, and Future Research Perspectives. *Molecules* **2019**, *24*, 4414. [CrossRef]
32. Linares, D.M.; Gómez, C.; Renes, E.; Fresno, J.M.; Tornadijo, M.E.; Ross, R.P.; Stanton, C. Lactic Acid Bacteria and Bifidobacteria with Potential to Design Natural Biofunctional Health-Promoting Dairy Foods. *Front. Microbiol.* **2017**, *8*. [CrossRef] [PubMed]
33. United Nations Food and Agricultural Organization (FAO). Average Supply of Meat across the Population, Measured in Kilograms Per Person Per Year. Available online: http://www.fao.org/faostat/en/#home (accessed on 18 January 2021).
34. Meat Food Supply Quantity (Kg/Capita/Yr) (Fao, 2020). Available online: https://ourworldindata.org/grapher/meat-supply-per-person (accessed on 18 January 2021).
35. Per Capita Consumption of Processed and Fresh Dairy Products in Milk Solids. OECD/FAO (2020), "OECD-FAO Agricultural Outlook", OECD Agriculture Statistics (Database). Available online: http://dx.doi.org/10.1787/agr-outl-data-en (accessed on 18 January 2021).
36. George, E.S.; Marshall, S.; Mayr, H.L.; Trakman, G.L.; Tatucu-Babet, O.A.; Lassemillante, A.-C.M.; Bramley, A.; Reddy, A.J.; Forsyth, A.; Tierney, A.C.; et al. The effect of high-polyphenol extra virgin olive oil on cardiovascular risk factors: A systematic review and meta-analysis. *Crit. Rev. Food Sci. Nutr.* **2019**, *59*, 2772–2795. [CrossRef] [PubMed]
37. Sialvera, T.E.; Papadopoulou, A.; Efstathiou, S.P.; Trautwein, E.A.; Ras, R.T.; Kollia, N.; Farajian, P.; Goumas, G.; Dimakopoulos, I.; Papavasiliou, K.; et al. Structured advice provided by a dietitian increases adherence of consumers to diet and lifestyle changes and lowers blood low-density lipoprotein (LDL)-cholesterol: The Increasing Adherence of Consumers to Diet & Lifestyle Changes to Lower (LDL) Cholesterol (ACT) randomised controlled trial. *J. Hum. Nutr. Diet. Off. J. Br. Diet. Assoc.* **2018**, *31*, 197–208. [CrossRef]
38. Poli, A. The PURE study and the enigmatic aspects of the diet: Is it possible that an high saturated fat consumption would not be harmful? *Eur. Heart J. Suppl. J. Eur. Soc. Cardiol.* **2020**, *22*, E113–E115. [CrossRef] [PubMed]
39. Williams, L.T.; Barnes, K.; Ball, L.; Ross, L.J.; Sladdin, I.; Mitchell, L.J. How Effective Are Dietitians in Weight Management? A Systematic Review and Meta-Analysis of Randomized Controlled Trials. *Healthcare* **2019**, *7*, 20. [CrossRef] [PubMed]
40. Cicero, A.F.G.; Colletti, A.; Bajraktari, G.; Descamps, O.; Djuric, D.M.; Ezhov, M.; Fras, Z.; Katsiki, N.; Langlois, M.; Latkovskis, G.; et al. Lipid-lowering nutraceuticals in clinical practice: Position paper from an International Lipid Expert Panel. *Nutr. Rev.* **2017**, *75*, 731–767. [CrossRef]
41. Formisano, E.; Pasta, A.; Cremonini, A.L.; Favari, E.; Ronca, A.; Carbone, F.; Semino, T.; Di Pierro, F.; Sukkar, S.G.; Pisciotta, L. Efficacy of Nutraceutical Combination of Monacolin K, Berberine, and Silymarin on Lipid Profile and PCSK9 Plasma Level in a Cohort of Hypercholesterolemic Patients. *J. Med. Food* **2020**, *23*, 658–666. [CrossRef]

nutrients

MDPI

Article

Assessment of Sodium Knowledge and Urinary Sodium Excretion among Regions of the United Arab Emirates: A Cross-Sectional Study

Amjad H. Jarrar [1], Lily Stojanovska [1,2], Vasso Apostolopoulos [2], Leila Cheikh Ismail [3,4], Jack Feehan [2,5], Eric O. Ohuma [6,7], Ala Z. Ahmad [1], Asma A. Alnoaimi [1], Latifa S. Al Khaili [1], Najah H. Allowch [1], Fatima T. Al Meqbaali [1], Usama Souka [1] and Ayesha S. Al Dhaheri [1,*]

1 Food, Nutrition and Health Department, College of Food and Agriculture, United Arab Emirates University, Al Ain 15551, UAE; AmjadJ@uaeu.ac.ae (A.H.J.); lily.stojanovska@uaeu.ac.ae (L.S.); 201050547@uaeu.ac.ae (A.Z.A.); 201050511@uaeu.ac.ae (A.A.A.); 201005105@uaeu.ac.ae (L.S.A.K.); 201050006@uaeu.ac.ae (N.H.A.); fatmadiab@uaeu.ac.ae (F.T.A.M.); usamasouka@uaeu.ac.ae (U.S.)

2 Institute for Health and Sport, Victoria University, Melbourne 14428, Australia; vasso.apostolopoulos@vu.edu.au (V.A.); jfeehan@student.unimelb.edu.au (J.F.)

3 Clinical Nutrition and Dietetics Department, College of Health Sciences, University of Sharjah, Sharjah 27272, UAE; lcheikhismail@sharjah.ac.ae

4 Nuffield Department of Women's & Reproductive Health, University of Oxford, Oxford OX1 2JD, UK

5 Department of Medicine—Western Health, The University of Melbourne, Melbourne 3021, Australia

6 Maternal, Adolescent, Reproductive & Child Health (MARCH) Centre, London School of Hygiene &Tropical Medicine (LSHTM), London WC1E 7HT, UK; eric.ohuma@ndm.ox.ac.uk

7 Centre for Tropical Medicine and Global Health, Nuffield Department of Medicine, University of Oxford, Oxford OX3 7LG, UK

* Correspondence: ayesha_aldhaheri@uaeu.ac.ae; Tel.: +971-50-6167671; Fax: +971-37-134593

Received: 15 August 2020; Accepted: 7 September 2020; Published: 9 September 2020

Abstract: Non-communicable diseases (NCDs) such as cardiovascular disease, cancer and diabetes, are increasing worldwide and cause 65% to 78% of deaths in the Gulf Cooperation Council (GCC). A random sample of 477 healthy adults were recruited in the United Arab Emirates (UAE) in the period March–June 2015. Demographic, lifestyle, medical, anthropometric and sodium excretion data were collected. A questionnaire was used to measure knowledge, attitude and practice regarding salt. Mean sodium and potassium excretion were 2713.4 ± 713 mg/day and 1803 ± 618 mg/day, respectively, significantly higher than the World Health Organization (WHO) recommendations for sodium (2300 mg/day) and lower for potassium (3150 mg/day). Two-thirds (67.4%) exceeded sodium guidelines, with males 2.6 times more likely to consume excessively. The majority of the participants add salt during cooking (82.5%) and whilst eating (66%), and 75% identified processed food as high source of salt. Most (69.1%) were aware that excessive salt could cause disease. Most of the UAE population consumes excess sodium and insufficient potassium, likely increasing the risk of NCDs. Despite most participants being aware that high salt intake is associated with adverse health outcomes, this did not translate into salt reduction action. Low-sodium, high-potassium dietary interventions such as the Mediterranean diet are vital in reducing the impact of NCDs in the UAE.

Keywords: urinary sodium excretion; urinary potassium excretion; salt; sodium; non-communicable diseases; United Arab Emirates

1. Introduction

Chronic diseases are long-lasting conditions with continuous effects, and include cardiovascular disease (CVD), chronic respiratory disease (CRD), cancer and type 2 diabetes (T2D). Globally, their incidence is increasing becoming a growing burden to global economies and people's quality of life. Collectively, these non-communicable diseases (NCDs) are the leading cause of death globally [1], making it a significant priority in healthcare systems. In some countries, up to 40% of those dying from NCDs are younger than 60 years of age [1].

The rapid improvement in the socio-economic status of the countries making up the Gulf Cooperation Council (GCC) (Bahrain, Kuwait, Oman, Qatar, Saudi Arabia and the United Arab Emirates (UAE) has contributed to changing food consumption patterns, lifestyle habits and health status over the last four decades, with diet quality decreasing through the addition of more processed Westernized food. These changes have resulted in an increasingly sedentary lifestyle, high blood pressure and obesity, known to be major risk factors of NCDs [2,3]. Thus, it is not surprising that CVD is the major cause of morbidity and mortality in the Gulf region [4]. It is estimated that NCDs cause between 65% and 78% of deaths in the GCC member countries [5].

In particular, the lifestyle of the Emirati population has changed considerably in the last 40 years due to rapid improvement in socio-economic indicators in the UAE. This transition has led to less physical activity and altered eating habits, including increased intake of processed foods. These changes, in addition to the adoption of a Western lifestyle and diet, have led to the rise in prevalence of overweight, obesity and the risk of metabolic syndrome in the UAE. In the UAE, CVD accounts for more than 25% of all deaths countrywide, however, this has increased in the major metropolitan center, accounting for 29% of all deaths in the Emirate of Abu Dhabi [6].

Diet, environmental factors, lifestyle, physical inactivity and genetics have been shown to contribute to the risk of NCDs [1]. Control of these primary risk factors could reduce the incidence of some NCDs by up to 80% and cancers by 40% [1]. As such, in recent years, there has been a significant effort to improve diet and increase physical activity to control the prevalence of NCDs. Hypertension is the most common outcome of excessive sodium intake independent of age and is a key risk factor for many NCDs [7]. Globally, over 7.5 million people die from hypertension-related complications per year, which surpasses deaths from tobacco smoking (5 million), obesity (2.8 million) and cholesterol (2.6 million) [8]. Hypertension, secondary to excessive salt consumption, is a major risk factor for CVD, responsible for 62% of strokes and 49% of coronary heart disease (CHD) [7]. In the UAE, approximately 30% of the population is hypertensive, [9] and the disease is thought to be widely underdiagnosed [10]. High salt intake is considered one of the major contributors to premature adult death in developed and developing countries [11]. A systematic review and meta-analysis of 5508 participants across 61 studies showed that higher salt intake was associated with significantly increased risk of stroke, stroke mortality and coronary heart disease [11]. Unfavorably high sodium intake remains prevalent worldwide and varies widely, ranging from 4–17 g/day, with mainland China having the greatest intake, and some less developed island nations the lowest [12], but for many countries it remains well above the World Health Organization (WHO) recommendation of less than 5 g of salt intake per day [13]. The UK Food Standards Agency highlighted in 2012 that 75% of salt intake comes from processed foods and proposed that a reduction in the sodium content of processed food and drink would be required to achieve the recommended daily intake in the community [14,15].

Alongside appropriate sodium consumption, ensuring adequate intake of potassium is vital to ensuring normal mineral homeostasis and healthy blood pressure. Potassium is the paired ion for sodium in a range of different physiologies—from nerve transmission to renal function. Having adequate potassium in the diet ensures that the kidney is able to remove sodium from the plasma, and hence allows more effective regulation of blood pressure. While frank potassium deficiency (hypokalemia) is well understood and monitored, chronic, insufficient dietary intake is not, despite being associated with an increase in systolic blood pressure, and in the face of declining diet quality, insufficient intake is becoming more common [16]. Despite its important role in health, potassium intake has not been investigated in the UAE, however, globally, it has been reported that there is widespread dietary insufficiency, and this is likely to be mirrored in the Gulf region.

The impact of diet on NCDs is critical, and dietary approaches such as the Mediterranean diet have been suggested to have a role in improving health outcomes globally. The Mediterranean diet, with its high fruit and vegetable and low meat and processed food content, is an effective way to reduce salt and sodium intake, leading to a subsequent improvement in health outcomes [17]. Its high vegetable content also lends itself to improving potassium intake—making it an effective intervention to reduce hypertension [17].

There are numerous methods used for assessing salt intake, including estimation by weighing ingested food, dietary recall questionnaires, estimating the salt content of food before ingestion and taking measurements of 24-h (hr) sodium excretion [18]. Measurement of 24-h urinary sodium excretion is considered to be the golden standard for estimating daily sodium intake on the premise that the majority (90–95%) of sodium ingested is excreted via the urine [18].

The aim of this study was to assess sodium intake using 24-h urinary sodium excretion from a sample of the healthy UAE population and to assess their knowledge, attitudes and practices (KAP) surrounding salt intake.

2. Materials and Methods

2.1. Study Design and Participants

A cross-sectional study with an anonymized self-reported questionnaire and the collection of 24-h urine for the assessment of sodium, potassium and creatinine excretion was conducted between March 2015 and June 2015 in the UAE. The questionnaire consisted of items to assess participants' attitudes, behavior and knowledge (KAP) regarding salt consumption and knowledge. The sample size was calculated based on the following formula to be representative of the UAE, with a confidence interval level of 95%.

Sample size of an unknown population was calculated by Cochrane's formula ($n = z^2 \times p \times (1 - p)/e2$), with z = level of confidence (for a level of confidence of 95%, z = 1.96); p = the estimated proportion of the population that presents the characteristic of having high knowledge $p = 0.5$; e = margin of error accepted, e = 0.05; N (sample size) = 385 participants, plus 20% estimated dropouts = approximately 461 participants. Hence, a sample of 530 healthy individuals were recruited to participate in the study from the seven Emirates (Abu Dhabi, Dubai, Sharjah, Ajman, Ras Al Khaimah, Fujairah and Umm Al Quwain) aged between 20 and 65 years. Two methods were used for recruitment: face to face recruitment at community, school or university events and posters displayed in shopping malls, health centers, schools and university hostels. The WHO/PAHO (2010) protocol for 24-h urine collection and analysis was used. Four age groups were considered for recruitment in the current study; 20–30, 31–40, 41–50 and 51–65 years old with a ratio of 1:1 male to female. This demographic was used to ensure a sample of the 'healthy' population—participants older than 65 are likely to have comorbid disease which may have affected the urine analysis. All participants provided written informed consent to participate in the study.

A screening questionnaire was designed to collect data regarding demographic information, lifestyle habits, past medical history, medication and current health status. Questionnaires were administered by the research team. Exclusion criteria at screening were those with self-reported chronic diseases (i.e., heart disease, using medication for hypertension, renal failure, liver disease), pregnant and lactating women, those on diuretics and women who had their menstrual period during the time of urine collection. Inclusion and exclusion criteria are summarized in Table 1. Inclusion criteria at screening were participants aged 20 to 65 years for both genders, non-pregnant and non-lactating, no known chronic kidney disease, renal failure, hypertension with medications and liver diseases, no medical condition(s) or medication(s) known to affect urination and able to collect 24-h (hr) urine. Exclusion criteria following urine collection included those that were unable to collect adequate urine within the 24-h time period (i.e., volume < 500 mL), and creatinine levels below 500 or above 2000 mg/day, which is equivalent to <9 or >26 mg/kg of body mass for female participants and <13 or >29 mg/kg of body mass for male participants [19]. Forty-one participants were excluded due to limited urine sample collection (<500 mL urine) or being unable to effectively urinate into the collection bottle, and 12 participants due to creatinine levels below 500 mg. The creatinine cutoffs were used to screen for renal abnormalities that may have skewed the results [19]. One urine sample was also excluded during testing due to abnormalities, leaving 476 urine samples for the final urine analysis, alongside 477 questionnaire responses. The enrolment process of the study participants is shown in Figure 1.

Table 1. Summary of inclusion and exclusion criteria.

Inclusion	Exclusion
Age 20–65	Renal or urinary pathology
Non-pregnant	Chronic disease
Non-lactating	Current menstrual period
No chronic kidney disease	24-h urine volume <500 mL
No medical conditions	Urine creatinine <500 mg or >2000 mg
Not currently taking prescribed medications known to affect urine	

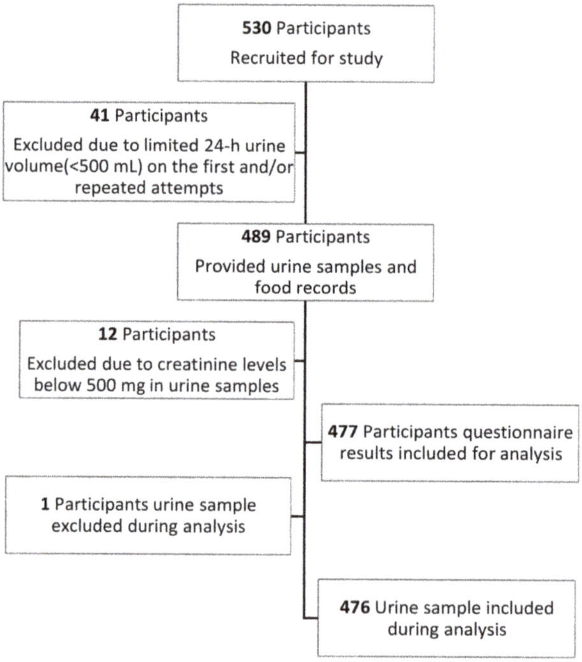

Figure 1. Flow diagram of the study design.

Participants were given full details of the study protocol with the opportunity to ask questions after which written informed consent to participate was sought. Each participant was allocated a personal identification number to provide anonymity and data confidentiality. Ethical approval for the study protocol was obtained from the UAE University (UAEU) Scientific Research Ethics Committee (Reference number: DVCRGS/36/2015).

2.2. *Anthropometric Measurements*

Body weight and height were measured for each participant and their body mass index (BMI) was calculated as weight (kg) divided by height (m) squared (kg/m^2). Height was recorded to the nearest 1 cm using a stadiometer (Seca Stadiometer, Seca Ltd., Birmingham, UK) and weight was recorded using a balance (Biospace Co., Seoul, Korea) to the nearest 0.1 kg having removed their shoes and heaviest clothing. An appropriately trained member of the research team took all the measurements [20].

2.3. *Knowledge, Attitude and Practice (KAP) Questionnaire*

Participants were asked to complete a self-reported questionnaire. The questionnaire assessed knowledge relating to salt and health outcomes, frequency of consumption and their perceived salt consumption, and was developed according to the WHO/PAHO recommendations for the assessment of population sodium intake and behaviors. The development and performance of the specific questionnaire has been described elsewhere [21].

2.4. *24-h Urine Collections and Analysis*

A single timed 24-h urine collection was obtained for the estimation of sodium excretion. Participants were given written and verbal instructions for the 24-h urine collection procedure. A 3-L coded plastic bottle was given to each participant for urine collection. Participants were asked to discard the first urine of the day and to collect all urine in the plastic bottle provided over the following 24-h. Participants were also asked to write on a separate sheet the time and date at the start and end of the urine collection, indicating occasions they missed urination. Urine samples with less than 500 mL or those who missed urine collection were rejected and participants were asked to repeat the process on another day.

Urine analysis for sodium, potassium and creatinine were conducted in the College of Food and Agriculture laboratories at UAEU. For the measurement of sodium and potassium levels in the urine, 50 mL of the urine sample was mixed with 200 µL of 1% nitric acid. Analytical solutions were introduced to a Varian ICP-OES model 710-ES spectrometer for sodium and potassium measurements [18]. Urinary creatinine was measured using a Cary 50 MPR Micro plate Reader-Varian and the concentration determined using a standard curve [22].

2.5. *Statistical Analysis*

Continuous variables were summarized by means and standard deviations or medians and inter-quartile ranges (25th–75th percentile) as appropriate. Continuous variables were checked visually for any departure from normality using histograms and quantile-quantile plots (Q–Q plots). All continuous data were reasonably normally distributed and therefore no transformations were applied. Categorical variables from the KAP questionnaire were reported as the percentage of responses per category. The Student's *t*-test was used to compare the mean difference in sodium and potassium excretion in urine against the recommended dietary allowance. Measures of association for categorical variables were evaluated using a chi-square or Fisher's exact test as appropriate. All analyses were conducted using the Statistical Package for the Social Sciences (SPSS) version 21. All statistical significance was determined at 5%.

3. Results

3.1. *Characteristics of the Study Population*

A total of 530 participants provided urine specimens, out of which 41 participants were excluded due to limited urine sample collection (<500 mL urine), and 12 participants due to creatinine levels below 500 mg in the urine, to give a final sample size of 477. One urine sample was excluded from the sample during analysis, due to excessive creatinine levels, leading to one less participant in the urine analysis (n = 476). The mean age was 37.31 years (standard deviation (SD) = 12.5 years, range 20–65 years), of which 55% were female (Table 2). The mean weight, height and BMI for participants were 73.37 ± 15.4 kg, 165.8 ± 8.95 cm and 26.7 ± 5.15 kg/m^2, respectively (Table 2). The prevalence of underweight, normal weight, overweight and obese individuals was 3.14%, 37.11%, 36.06% and 23.69%, respectively.

Table 2. Summary of study population demographics (N = 477).

Variable	Mean ± SD
Age (years)	37.31 ± 12.5
Weight (kg)	73.37 ± 15.4
Height (cm)	165.8 ± 8.95
Body Mass Index (BMI)	26.7 ± 5.15
	N (%)
Emirates [1]	
Abu Dhabi (West)	137 (28.72)
Al-Ain (East)	150 (31.45)
Northern Emirates [2]	190 (39.83)
Age Category (years)	
20–30	156 (32.70)
31–40	113 (23.69)
41–50	123 (25.78)
51–65	85 (17.82)
BMI Classifications (WHO definition)	
Underweight (<18.5 kg/m^2)	15 (3.14)
Normal-weight (18.5–24.9 kg/m^2)	177 (37.11)
Overweight (25.0–29.9 kg/m^2)	172 (36.06)
Obese (30.0–34.9 kg/m^2)	113 (23.69)
Gender Distribution, N (%)	
Males	214 (44.86)
Females	263 (55.14)

[1] Geographic divisions of United Arab Emirates; [2] Dubai, Sharjah, Ajman, Umm Al Quwain and Fujairah.

3.2. *Major Findings of the Knowledge, Attitude and Practice (KAP) Questionnaire*

The knowledge, attitude and practice (KAP) questionnaire (Table 3) indicated that the majority of the participants added salt during cooking (N = 393; 82.4%) and while eating (N = 315; 66%). Most participants reported that they always or sometimes use stock cubes during cooking (N = 346; 72.6%), and 69.1% reported that they were aware that high salt intake could cause serious health problems. However, a large proportion (62.1%) thought that their salt consumption was within the recommended amounts, with 60% claiming to have tried to control their salt or sodium intake. Most of the participants (45.2%) reported that high salt intake was associated with high blood pressure, followed by kidney stones (18.7%) and obesity (17.8%), but only 11.7% associated it with heart disease, and 6.5% with T2D. More than 75% of the participants reported that they considered processed foods as a high source of salt.

Table 3. Knowledge, attitude and practice (KAP) of salt intake and participants' knowledge on health consequences (N = 477). * This question is multiple choice with more than one selection allowed.

	Gender				Age Category (Year)				
Do you Add Salt during Cooking (Missing Answers = 0)	**Male** N = 214 (%)	**Female** N = 263 (%)	**Total** N = 477 (%)	**Chi-Square (*p*-Value)**	**20–30** N = 156 (%)	**31–40** N = 113 (%)	**41–50** N = 123 (%)	**51–65** N = 85 (%)	**Chi-Square (*p*-Value)**
Never	46 (21.6)	38 (14.1)	84 (17.5)		28 (18.0)	26 (23.0)	13 (10.6)	17 (19.0)	
Sometimes	80 (37.6)	96 (36.6)	176 (37.1)	5.60 (0.061)	65 (41.7)	42 (37.2)	46 (37.4)	23 (27.4)	20.01 (0.01)
Always	88 (40.8)	129 (49.2)	217 (45.5)		63 (40.4)	45 (39.8)	64 (52.0)	45 (54.2)	
Do you Add Salt to Food at the Table (Missing Answers = 1)	**Male** N (%)	**Female** N (%)	**Total** N = 476 N (%)	**Chi-Square (*p*-Value)**	**20–30** N (%)	**31–40** N (%)	**41–50** N (%)	**51–65** N (%)	**Chi-Square (*p*-Value)**
Never	71 (33.3)	90 (34.4)	161 (33.8)		54 (34.6)	31 (27.4)	40 (32.8)	36 (42.8)	
Sometimes	93 (43.7)	122 (46.60	215 (45.2)	2.12 (0.548)	75 (48.1)	53 (46.9)	51 (41.8)	36 (42.8)	12.71 (0.391)
Always	49 (23.0)	51 (19.0)	100 (21.0)		27 (17.3)	29 (25.7)	31 (25.4)	13 (14.3)	
Do you Use Stock Cubes during Cooking (Missing Answers = 0)	**Male** N (%)	**Female** N (%)	**Total** N = 477 N (%)	**Chi-Square (*p*-Value)**	**20–30** N (%)	**31–40** N (%)	**41–50** N (%)	**51–65** N (%)	**Chi-Square (*p*-Value)**
Never	55 (25.8)	76 (28.6)	131 (27.4)		39 (25.0)	30 (26.6)	33 (26.8)	29 (34.1)	
Sometimes	61 (28.6)	74 (28.2)	135 (28.4)	0.50 (0.779)	42 (26.9)	35 (31.0)	36 (29.2)	22 (25.9)	4.65 (0.794)
Always	98 (45.5)	113 (43.1)	211 (44.2)		75 (48.1)	48 (42.5)	54 (44.0)	34 (40.0)	
How Much Salt do you Think you Consume (Missing Answers = 0)	**Male** N (%)	**Female** N (%)	**Total** N = 477 N (%)	**Chi-Square (*p*-Value)**	**20–30** N (%)	**31–40** N (%)	**41–50** N (%)	**51–65** N (%)	**Chi-Square (*p*-Value)**
Too much	49 (23.0)	47 (17.6)	96 (20.0)		32 (20.5)	26 (23.0)	22 (18.0)	16 (19.1)	
Just the right amount	125 (58.2)	171 (65.3)	296 (62.1)	2.85 (0.240)	96 (61.5)	70 (62.0)	80 (65.0)	50 (59.5)	3.101 (0.928)
Far too little	40 (18.8)	45 (17.2)	85 (17.9)		28 (17.9)	17 (15.0)	21 (17.0)	19 (21.4)	
Do you Think that High Salt Diet could Cause Serious Health Problems? (Missing Answers = 0)	**Male** N (%)	**Female** N (%)	**Total** N = 477 N (%)	**Chi-Square (*p*-Value)**	**20–30** N (%)	**31–40** N (%)	**41–50** N (%)	**51–65** N (%)	**Chi-Square (*p*-Value)**
Yes	149 (69.6)	181 (68.8)	330 (69.1)		113 (72.4)	73 (64.6)	84 (68.4)	60 (70.0)	
No	45 (21.0)	68 (25.8)	113 (23.7)	3.682 (0.158)	32 (20.6)	32 (28.3)	31 (25.2)	18 (23.7)	4.782 (0.780)
Don't know	20 (9.3)	14 (5.4)	34 (7.2)		11 (7.1)	8 (7.1)	8 (6.56)	7 (8.4)	
What are the Health Problems Associated with High Salt Intake *	**Male** N (%)	**Female** N (%)	**Total** N = 477N (%)	**Chi-Square (*p*-Value)**	**20–30** N (%)	**31–40** N (%)	**41–50** N (%)	**51–65** N (%)	**Chi-Square (*p*-Value)**
High blood pressure	90 (42.1)	126 (47.9)	216 (45.2)		73 (46.8)	47 (41.6)	59 (48.0)	37 (43.5)	
Kidney stones	43 (20.1)	46 (17.5)	89 (18.7)		31 (19.9)	22 (19.5)	21 (17.1)	15 (17.6)	
Obesity	38 (17.8)	47 (17.9)	85 (17.8)	3.43 (0.414)	25 (16.0)	23 (20.3)	18 (14.6)	19 (22.3)	4.23 (0.624)
Diabetes	18 (8.4)	13 (4.9)	31 (6.5)		8 (5.1)	9 (8.0)	8 (6.5)	6 (7.1)	
Heart disease	25 (11.7)	31 (11.8)	56 (11.7)		19 (12.2)	12 (10.6)	17 (13.8)	8 (9.4)	
Do you Think Processed Foods are High in Sodium? (Missing Answers = 0)	**Male** N (%)	**Female** N (%)	**Total** N = 477 (%)	**Chi-Square (*p*-Value)**	**20–30** N (%)	**31–40** N (%)	**41–50** N (%)	**51–65** N (%)	**Chi-Square (*p*-Value)**
Yes	159 (74.2)	207 (78.6)	366 (76.7)	1.620 (0.444)	123 (78.9)	88 (77.9)	88 (71.5)	68 (80.0)	6.578 (0.574)
No	55 (25.8)	56 (21.4)	111 (23.3)		33 (21.1)	25 (22.1)	35 (28.5)	17 (20.0)	
Do you do Anything on a Regular Basis to Control your Salt or Sodium Intake? (Missing Answers = 0)	**Male** N (%)	**Female** N (%)	**Total** N = 477 (%)	**Chi-Square (*p*-Value)**	**20–30** N (%)	**31–40** N (%)	**41–50** N (%)	**51–65** N (%)	**Chi-Square (*p*-Value)**
Yes	131 (61.2)	158 (60.1)	289 (60.6)	0.935 (0.626)	88 (56.4)	69 (61.1)	76 (61.8)	56 (65.9)	4.823 (0.764)
No	83 (38.8)	105 (39.9)	188 (39.4)		68 (43.6)	44 (38.9)	47 (38.2)	29 (34.1)	

3.3. High Levels of Sodium Secretion in the UAE Population within 24-h Urine Collection

The mean 24-h urine volume was 1338.3 ± 553 mL, with a range of 550–4000 mL. The mean sodium excretion in urine was 2713.4 ± 713 mg. The average values for sodium excretion in urine exceeded the WHO recommendations of sodium intake of less than 2300 mg (Table 4) [23]. Of the 476 participants, 320 (67.4%) had a sodium excretion above the WHO recommended level of 2300 mg. Males were more likely (51.6%) to exceed the WHO recommendation compared to females (odds ratio (OR): 2.60; 95% confidence interval (CI): 1.71 to 3.96; $p < 0.001$). However, there were no significant differences by age of those surpassing the recommendation (OR: 0.99; 95% CI: 0.98 to 1.02; $p = 0.98$).

Table 4. Mean sodium, potassium and creatinine urinary excretion and ratio of sodium to potassium (n = 476).

Nutrients	Mean ± SD	Recommendation	*p*-Value
Mean 24-h sodium excretion in urine (mg)	2713.40 ± 713	<2300 mg	<0.001
Mean 24-h potassium excretion in urine (mg)	1803.30 ± 618.03	>3510 mg	<0.001
Mean 24-h creatinine excretion in urine (mg)	1284.81 ± 607.0		
Mean 24-h creatinine (mg/kg body mass)	16.83 ± 4.84		
Mean 24-h creatinine (mg/kg body mass)—female	13.42 ± 1.95		
Mean 24-h creatinine (mg/kg body mass)—male	21.81 ± 3.80		
Mean 24-h urinary Na/K ratio	1.64 ± 0.55		

Mean urinary excretion for potassium and creatinine and the sodium to potassium ratio were 1803.30 ± 618.03 mg, 1284.81 ± 607.0 mg and 1.64 ± 0.55 mg, respectively (Table 4). While it is challenging to use potassium excretion to estimate intake, it is likely that it is well below the WHO recommendations of 3500 mg/day [24]. Moreover, mean urinary excretion for creatinine for female participants was 13.42 ± 1.95 mg/kg body mass, with a minimum to maximum reading of 10.23 to 19.87 mg/kg body mass, while for male participants it was 21.81 ± 3.80 mg/kg body mass, with a minimum to maximum reading of 13.60 to 28.63 mg/kg body mass (Table 4). Mean urinary excretions for sodium, potassium and creatinine for male and female participants according to the different age groups are shown in Figure 2.

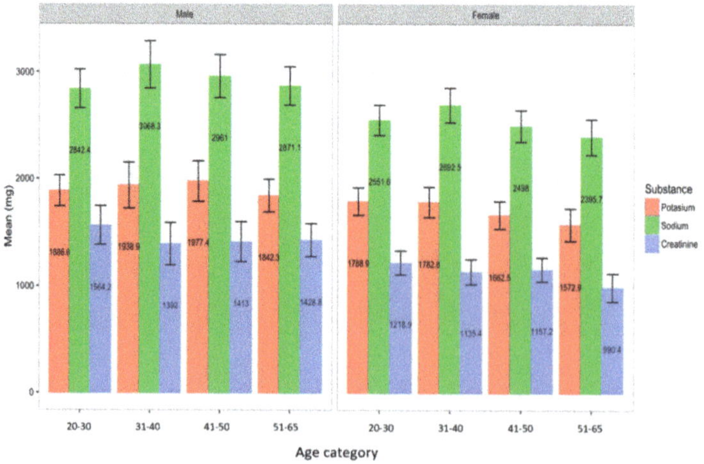

Figure 2. Mean creatinine, sodium and potassium levels for male (left panel) and female (right panel) participants according to age groups. The capped bars represent the 95% confidence intervals of the means.

4. Discussion

This study showed that sodium intake of the participants exceeds WHO recommendations with concurrent low intakes of potassium. Moreover, most of the participants were unaware that their consumption was beyond the recommended levels of the WHO, however, most were able to identify some common sources of sodium, such as stock cubes and processed foods, as well as its deleterious effect on health. To our knowledge, this is the first study in the UAE reporting 24-h urinary sodium excretion. A 24-h collection period is necessary to capture the marked diurnal variation in sodium, chloride and water excretion. Electrolyte excretion in healthy individuals normally reaches the maximum at or before midday, and the minimum at night towards the end of sleep [25]. This study is also the first to report on potassium excretion in the UAE, another critical indicator of dietary hypertension risk.

The results from the current study were similar to the results in a study conducted in Eastern Saudi Arabia that showed the mean intake of sodium assessed by 24-h sodium excretion to be 3200 ± 1100 mg/day and 2700 ± 850 mg/day for men and women, respectively [26]. Similar findings were noted in a Jordan study using 24-h urinary sodium excretion, which showed that the average sodium intake was 4100 mg/day (10.4 g/day salt) and sodium intake was higher in males, 4300 mg, compared with 4000 mg by females. It was clear that the Jordanian participants consumed at least double the current WHO recommended daily sodium amount of 2000 mg (5 g salt) [27]. Likewise, a study conducted in Oman using the National Nutrition Survey based on a 24-h dietary recall noted the average intake of salt to be 11–12 g/day [28], again significantly higher than the WHO recommendation. Two further studies analyzing food consumption in Kuwait [29,30] reported the average salt intake to be within 8–10 g/day. These results, and our own, are strong indicators that consumption of sodium exceeds the WHO recommendations in the GCC countries. It is well known high sodium intake is associated with hypertension and stroke, as well as contributes to myocardial infarction and heart and kidney failure [31,32]. Consequently, this prevalent increase in sodium consumption is likely to contribute to the incidence of NCDs in the UAE. Globally, the mean intake of sodium is high in East Asia, Central Asia, Eastern Europe, Central Europe and the Middle East/North Africa, in the range of 3900–4200 mg/day, which is equivalent to 9.75–10.5 g/day of salt [33], far exceeding the WHO recommendations, and is similar to our findings. While higher than the recommendations, the results of our study would suggest that the UAE was at the lower end of the scale of sodium intake in these geographic areas, however, comparisons between urinary excretion and sodium intake must be drawn with care. This may reflect the relatively high levels of education and other key socio-economic indicators when compared to these countries, which may manifest in more health-promoting behaviors. Urinary excretion of sodium as a function of intake has also been assessed in other nations, with generally higher socio-economic and health indicators. For example, in Japan and the United Kingdom (UK), sodium intake was 4470 ± 1600 mg/day and 3289 mg/day, respectively, and was attributed to a high intake of canned and processed foods [34,35].

High dietary sodium and low dietary potassium intakes are associated with hypertension and increased risk of cardiovascular disease (CVD) [36]. In the current study, the sodium to potassium ratio was 1.64 ± 0.55, suggesting that not only did sodium intake exceed WHO recommendations but insufficient dietary potassium was also prevalent. The amount of potassium excreted in 24-h urine is well correlated with dietary potassium intake [37]. A high urinary sodium–potassium ratio is an indicator of a need to reduce sodium and increase potassium intake [1,3]. The WHO has suggested that achieving guidelines for sodium and potassium intake would yield a sodium–potassium ratio close to 1.00 [23,24].

In our study, 67.4% of the participants exceeded the WHO recommendations for salt intake, with more males (51.6%) than females exceeding the recommendations. This finding is consistent with previous studies conducted in Kuwait, where males (74.7%) and females (50.9%) exceeded recommendations [29]. Similarly, a study conducted in Eastern Saudi Arabia also found that males tend to consume more sodium compared to females [26]. This finding is also consistent outside the GCC countries. In Brazil, 90% of the of study population exceeded WHO recommendations for salt intake with excess consumption again more common in males [38]. Another study aimed to estimate sodium intake in New York City, noting the mean sodium intake to be 3239 mg/day, with 81% of participants exceeding recommendations [39]. Brown et al. (2013), reported that sodium intake tends to be higher in men than women, based on 5693 participants recruited in 1984–1987 aged 20–59 years from 29 North American and European samples [31]; the findings again echoed those in our study. The sex differences in sodium excretion could have a number of causes, however, it is likely that increased appetite and calorie consumption is a major driver behind the variance. It is also possible that socio-cultural norms lead men to make more salt-heavy diet choices in both social and home situations, both in the UAE and globally. This is particularly relevant when viewed against the increased risk profile of a number of NCDs in men, and also makes it more challenging for males to meet sodium guidelines, as they are required to reduce their intake considerably compared to women.

The data on urinary potassium excretion is also of significant importance to the health of the population of the UAE. It is well known that potassium is a key part of effective blood pressure regulation, because of its role in effective sodium clearance. The mean potassium intake shown in this study was well below the WHO guidelines, providing opportunities for improvement of the health of the UAE. Encouraging a varied diet, high in fruit and leafy vegetables, would provide a ready means of improving health outcomes. Potassium is not amenable to fortification, due to the negative consequences of excessive intake and a flavor-masking effect of common chemical formats of the mineral, which means improving diet quality is the major means of increasing intake in the community.

It was also found that 82.5% of the participants in this study added salt sometimes or always during cooking, which is similar to that noted in Lebanon, where 100% of the participants have been found to add salt during cooking [40]. In the current study, the majority of participants reported that they added stock cubes and additional table salt while eating, sometimes or always. These findings are similar to the Lebanon study which showed that 60% of the participants used table salt [40]. Likewise, 61% of university students in the UAE reported adding salt while cooking, and 14% of the participants often added salt to food even before tasting it [21].

Despite the fact that 67.4% of the participants exceeded the WHO recommended salt intake in the current study, only 20.0% reported that their consumption was beyond the recommended threshold (Table 3). In light of our data showing widespread sodium excess, this suggests that many people are unaware of how much they are consuming. In this regard, education and public awareness programs are required so that the general population is more aware of salt portion sizes and the sodium content of processed foods, drinks and other foods in general.

Interestingly, about 60% of the participants claimed to be taking measures to control their salt intake, again similar to reports from Lebanon (65.8%) [40]. These findings are also similar to a study conducted in five sentinel countries of the Americas (Argentina, Canada, Chile, Costa Rica and Ecuador), where almost 90% of the participants reported excess intake of salt is associated with adverse health conditions, and over 60% of the participants indicated they were conscious of their salt intake and taking measures to reduce it. They also found that more than 30% of their participants believed that reducing dietary salt intake was highly important [41]. Most of these studies reported that the majority of the participants were aware that high salt intake was associated with adverse health outcomes, however, this awareness does not translate into effective behavioral change in salt reduction. These interesting findings have some important implications for strategies to reduce sodium intake. One of the mainstays of sodium reduction is public education, however, these results would indicate that the general knowledge is adequate. However, education campaigns on effective ways to reduce intake, while increasing potassium and hydration, would play a role in the general reduction in sodium across the UAE, alongside effective regulations and sodium targets.

The results of the current study indicate that there is prevalent high sodium and low potassium intake within the general population of the UAE, which consequently may increase the risk of hypertension, CVD and other NCDs. This emphasizes the need for coordinated salt reduction programs to aid in the reduction of NCDs in the UAE. Strategies such as educational campaigns, regulation of sodium content of widely consumed food items and setting targets for sodium intake will allow for a more cohesive approach to improving the health of the UAE in this regard. In the last two decades, a number of countries have put sodium reduction strategies in place, and they have generally been somewhat successful, however, there are still significant strides to be made [42]. The most effective population interventions are likely to be salt reduction targets in common food stuffs, specific to the geographical areas and the local cuisines. In the metropolitan centers of the UAE, this will likely need to target processed and fast foods, which are becoming more of a staple in the Emirati diet, however, future research to identify significant sources of sodium in the UAE is needed to guide policy makers. Other nations with successful sodium reduction strategies have used salt targets, typically between 5–8 g/day [42], to help guide these regulations and interventions. Decreasing the sodium consumption of the UAE will also require regulation of industry to offer more low-salt options, as well as improve standards on labeling and nutritional declaration on packaged foodstuffs.

The Mediterranean diet could play a role in combatting the widespread salt imbalance in the UAE. The Mediterranean diet is inherently low in sodium and high in potassium due to its high vegetable and low meat and processed food content. The Mediterranean diet is also accessible to the local region, as it contains a number of similarities to traditional food practices in the Arab nations, such as an emphasis on vegetables, dairy, grains and spices, however, the Emirati cuisine traditionally features meat products more strongly [43]. The Mediterranean diet has been shown to reduce hypertension [44], however, there is some debate surrounding the role of sodium in this. Some authors have found that the Mediterranean diet does not readily offer reductions in sodium [45], however, this may be due to variations in adherence and specific components of the diet, as well as the amount of other minerals, such as potassium, which are abundant in plant-rich diets.

Despite the significant findings, a limitation of this study was that urinary sodium was assessed by a single 24-h urine collection and this may not represent the average sodium intake in a person due to daily individual variability. However, a single urine measurement is considered a more accurate measure of sodium intake at a population level [18], though it may possibly be less accurate for individuals. There is also a potential that the recruited population may have been broadly healthier, as they were likely more health conscious, better educated and possibly of a higher socio-economic status. Future studies should account for key socio-economic indicators, such as years of education and household income in both their recruitment and analysis to ensure a representative sample of the population. This may have led to an underestimation of the UAE's sodium intake found in this study. Additionally, while the KAP questionnaire used in this study captures some important facets of the participants' knowledge and behavior surrounding salt, there is further room for additional information, particularly surrounding important sources of sodium in the modern diet. An expanded questionnaire, and other measures such as food diaries, would provide more reliable information on the true intake of sodium, and how that compares to the participants' knowledge. Despite these limitations, the study described was statistically sound and powered to reliably identify the sodium practices in the UAE. The large sample, with demographically representative participants, and the validated analytical methods, are also strengths of the research presented here.

5. Conclusions

In this cross-sectional sample of the UAE population, the majority consumed salt well above the international WHO recommendations with a concurrent low intake of potassium, suggesting significant room for improvement in the intake of these minerals. There are significant differences by gender, with males more likely to exceed the WHO recommendations for salt and sodium intake.

It is imperative for communities, as well as local and national governments, to play a leading role in the development and implementation of salt reduction strategies, such as increasing adherence to the Mediterranean diet, as well as setting standards for industry. Future research should aim to validate these findings with larger studies, as well as to identify important sources of sodium in the diet of the UAE. Awareness programs should be established to educate the population about the risk factors for excess salt consumption. A nationwide assessment should be conducted to evaluate the level of the problem, and to enable identification of appropriate priorities for the implementation of population-based diet-related interventions to reduce the prevalence of NCDs and their associated rates of morbidity and mortality.

Author Contributions: Conceptualization, A.S.A.D.; Formal analysis, E.O.O., F.T.A.M. and U.S.; Investigation, A.H.J., A.Z.A., A.A.A., L.S.A.K. and N.H.A.; Methodology, A.S.A.D.; Resources, A.S.A.D.; Supervision, A.H.J. and A.S.A.D.; Writing—original draft, A.H.J. and A.S.A.D.; Writing—review and editing, A.H.J., L.S., V.A., L.C.I., J.F., E.O.O. and A.S.A.D. All authors have read and agreed to the published version of the manuscript.

Funding: This research received no external funding.

Acknowledgments: Authors would like to express their sincere gratitude to everyone who participated in the study.

Conflicts of Interest: The authors declare no conflict of interest.

References

1. World Health Organization. *Plan of Action for the Prevention and Control of Noncommunicable Diseases in the Eastern Mediterranean Region*; World Health Organization: Geneva, Switzerland, 2011.
2. Stamler, J.; Rose, G.; Stamler, R.; Elliott, P.; Dyer, A.; Marmot, M. Intersalt study findings. Public health and medical care implications. *Hypertension* **1989**, *14*, 570–577. [CrossRef] [PubMed]
3. He, F.J.; MacGregor, G.A. Effect of modest salt reduction on blood pressure: A meta-analysis of randomized trials. Implications for public health. *J. Hum. Hypertens.* **2002**, *16*, 761–770. [CrossRef] [PubMed]
4. Morrison, A.C.; Ness, R.B. Sodium intake and cardiovascular disease. *Ann. Rev. Public Health* **2011**, *32*, 71–90. [CrossRef]
5. World Health Organization. *Noncommunicable Diseases Country Profiles 2018*; World Health Organization: Geneva, Switzerland, 2018.
6. Loney, T.; Aw, T.-C.; Handysides, D.G.; Ali, R.; Blair, I.; Grivna, M.; Shah, S.M.; Sheek-Hussein, M.; El-Sadig, M.; Sharif, A.A. An analysis of the health status of the United Arab Emirates: The 'Big 4'public health issues. *Glob. Health Action* **2013**, *6*, 20100. [CrossRef] [PubMed]
7. He, F.J.; Burnier, M.; MacGregor, G.A. Nutrition in cardiovascular disease: Salt in hypertension and heart failure. *Eur. Heart J.* **2011**, *32*, 3073–3080. [CrossRef]
8. World Health Organization. Global Status Report on Noncommunicable Diseases 2010, Geneva. 2011. Available online: http://www.who.int/nmh/publications/ncd_report_full_en.pdf (accessed on 28 August 2020).
9. Shah, S.M.; Loney, T.; Sheek-Hussein, M.; El Sadig, M.; Al Dhaheri, S.; El Barazi, I.; Al Marzouqi, L.; Aw, T.-C.; Ali, R. Hypertension prevalence, awareness, treatment, and control, in male South Asian immigrants in the United Arab Emirates: A cross-sectional study. *BMC Cardiovasc. Disord.* **2015**, *15*, 30. [CrossRef]
10. Abdulle, A.M.; Nagelkerke, N.J.; Abouchacra, S.; Pathan, J.Y.; Adem, A.; Obineche, E.N. Under-treatment and under diagnosis of hypertension: A serious problem in the United Arab Emirates. *BMC Cardiovasc. Disorders* **2006**, *6*, 24. [CrossRef]
11. Aburto, N.J.; Ziolkovska, A.; Hooper, L.; Elliott, P.; Cappuccio, F.P.; Meerpohl, J.J. Effect of lower sodium intake on health: Systematic review and meta-analyses. *BMJ* **2013**, *346*, f1326. [CrossRef]
12. Brown, I.J.; Tzoulaki, I.; Candeias, V.; Elliott, P. Salt intakes around the world: Implications for public health. *Int. J. Epidemiol.* **2009**, *38*, 791–813. [CrossRef]
13. World Health Organization. *Diet, Nutrition, and the Prevention of Chronic Diseases: Report of a Joint WHO/FAO Expert Consultation*; World Health Organization: Geneva, Switzerland, 2003; Volume 916, p. 5.
14. Chobanian, A.V.; Bakris, G.L.; Black, H.R.; Cushman, W.C.; Green, L.A.; Izzo, J.L., Jr.; Jones, D.W.; Materson, B.J.; Oparil, S.; Wright, J.T., Jr. The seventh report of the joint national committee on prevention, detection, evaluation, and treatment of high blood pressure: The JNC 7 report. *JAMA* **2003**, *289*, 2560–2571. [CrossRef]
15. Wyness, L.A.; Butriss, J.L.; Stanner, S.A. Reducing the population's sodium intake: The UK Food Standards Agency's salt reduction programme. *Public Health Nutr.* **2012**, *15*, 254–261. [CrossRef] [PubMed]

16. Newberry, S.J.; Chung, M.; Anderson, C.A.; Chen, C.; Fu, Z.; Tang, A.; Zhao, N.; Booth, M.; Marks, J.; Hollands, S.; et al. *Sodium and Potassium Intake: Effects on Chronic Disease Outcomes and Risks*; Agency for Healthcare Research and Quality: Rockville, MD, USA, 2018.
17. Kokkinos, P.; Panagiotakos, D.B.; Polychronopoulos, E. Dietary influences on blood pressure: The effect of the Mediterranean diet on the prevalence of hypertension. *J. Clin. Hypertens.* **2005**, *7*, 165–172. [CrossRef] [PubMed]
18. Wielgosz, A.; Robinson, C.; Mao, Y.; Jiang, Y.; Campbell, N.R.; Muthuri, S.; Morrison, H. The impact of using different methods to assess completeness of 24-hour urine collection on estimating dietary sodium. *J. Clin. Hypertens.* **2016**, *18*, 581–584. [CrossRef] [PubMed]
19. Johnson, R.J.; Feehally, J.; Floege, J. *Comprehensive Clinical Nephrology E-Book*; Elsevier Health Sciences: Amsterdam, The Netherlands, 2014.
20. Lee, R.; Nieman, D. *Nutritional Assessment*; McGraw-Hill Education: New York, NY, USA, 2012.
21. Ismail, L.C.; Hashim, M.; Jarrar, A.H.; Mohamad, M.N.; Saleh, S.T.; Jawish, N.; Bekdache, M.; Albaghli, H.; Kdsi, D.; Aldarweesh, D. Knowledge, Attitude, and Practice on Salt and Assessment of Dietary Salt and Fat Intake among University of Sharjah Students. *Nutrients* **2019**, *11*, 941. [CrossRef] [PubMed]
22. Bowers, L.D.; Wong, E.T. Kinetic serum creatinine assays. II. A critical evaluation and review. *Clin. Chem.* **1980**, *26*, 555–561. [CrossRef]
23. World Health Organization. *Guideline: Sodium Intake for Adults and Children*; 9241504838; World Health Organization (WHO): Geneva, Switzerland, 2012.
24. World Health Organization. *Guideline: Potassium Intake for Adults and Children*; World Health Organization: Geneva, Switzerland, 2012.
25. Wesson, L.G. Electrolyte excretion in relation to diurnal cycles of renal function: Plasma electrolyte concentrations and aldosterone secretion before and during salt and water balance changes in normotensive subjects. *Medicine* **1964**, *43*, 547–592. [CrossRef]
26. Alkhunaizi, A.; Al Jishi, H.; Al Sadah, Z. Salt intake in Eastern Saudi Arabia. *East Mediterr. Health J.* **2013**, *19*, 915–918. [CrossRef]
27. Alawwa, I.; Dagash, R.; Saleh, A.; Ahmad, A. Dietary salt consumption and the knowledge, attitudes and behavior of healthy adults: A cross-sectional study from Jordan. *Libyan J. Med.* **2018**, *13*, 1479602. [CrossRef]
28. Al-Ghannami, S.; Library of Ministry of Health; Ministry of Health; Sultanate of Oman. National Nutrition Survey. 2004. Available online: https://www.moh.gov.om/en/web/statistics/ (accessed on 1 August 2020).
29. Zaghloul, S.; Al-Hooti, S.N.; Al-Hamad, N.; Al-Zenki, S.; Alomirah, H.; Alayan, I.; Al-Attar, H.; Al-Othman, A.; Al-Shami, E.; Al-Somaie, M. Evidence for nutrition transition in Kuwait: Over-consumption of macronutrients and obesity. *Public Health Nutr.* **2013**, *16*, 596–607. [CrossRef]
30. Alomirah, H.; Al-Zenki, S.; Husain, A. *Assessment of Acrylamide Levels in Heat-Processed Foodstuffs Consumed by Kuwaitis*; KISR No. 9316; Library of the Kuwait Institute of Scientific Research: Safat, Kuwait, 2008.
31. Brown, I.J.; Dyer, A.R.; Chan, Q.; Cogswell, M.E.; Ueshima, H.; Stamler, J.; Elliott, P.; Group ICOR. Estimating 24-hour urinary sodium excretion from casual urinary sodium concentrations in Western populations: The INTERSALT study. *Am. J. Epidemiol.* **2013**, *177*, 1180–1192. [CrossRef]
32. Lichtenstein, A.H.; Appel, L.J.; Brands, M.; Carnethon, M.; Daniels, S.; Franch, H.A.; Franklin, B.; Kris-Etherton, P.; Harris, W.S.; Howard, B. Diet and lifestyle recommendations revision 2006: A scientific statement from the American Heart Association Nutrition Committee. *Circulation* **2006**, *114*, 82–96. [CrossRef] [PubMed]
33. Micha, R.; Khatibzadeh, S.; Shi, P.; Fahimi, S.; Lim, S.; Andrews, K.G.; Engell, R.E.; Powles, J.; Ezzati, M.; Mozaffarian, D. Global, regional, and national consumption levels of dietary fats and oils in 1990 and 2010: A systematic analysis including 266 country-specific nutrition surveys. *BMJ* **2014**, *348*, g2272. [CrossRef] [PubMed]
34. Anderson, C.A.; Appel, L.J.; Okuda, N.; Brown, I.J.; Chan, Q.; Zhao, L.; Ueshima, H.; Kesteloot, H.; Miura, K.; Curb, J.D. Dietary sources of sodium in China, Japan, the United Kingdom, and the United States, women and men aged 40 to 59 years: The INTERMAP study. *J. Am. Diet. Assoc.* **2010**, *110*, 736–745. [CrossRef]
35. Ashford, R.; Jones, K.; Collins, D.; Earl, K.; Moore, S.; Koulman, A.; Yarde, J.; Polly, B.; Swan, G. *Assessment of Salt Intake from Urinary Sodium in Adults (Aged 19 to 64 Years) in England, 2018 to 2019. National Diet and Nutrition Survey*; Public Health England: London, UK, 2020.

36. Geleijnse, J.M.; Witteman, J.C.; Stijnen, T.; Kloos, M.W.; Hofman, A.; Grobbee, D.E. Sodium and potassium intake and risk of cardiovascular events and all-cause mortality: The Rotterdam Study. *Eur. J. Epidemiol.* **2007**, *22*, 763–770. [CrossRef] [PubMed]
37. Taylor, E.N.; Stampfer, M.J.; Mount, D.B.; Curhan, G.C. DASH-style diet and 24-hour urine composition. *Clin. J. Am. Soc. Nephrol.* **2010**, *5*, 2315–2322. [CrossRef]
38. Nilson, E.A. The strides to reduce salt intake in Brazil: Have we done enough? *Cardiovasc. Diagn. Ther.* **2015**, *5*, 243.
39. Angell, S.Y.; Yi, S.; Eisenhower, D.; Kerker, B.D.; Curtis, C.J.; Bartley, K.; Silver, L.D.; Farley, T.A. Sodium intake in a cross-sectional, representative sample of New York City adults. *Am. J. Public Health* **2014**, *104*, 2409–2416. [CrossRef]
40. Nasreddine, L.; Akl, C.; Al-Shaar, L.; Almedawar, M.M.; Isma'eel, H. Consumer knowledge, attitudes and salt-related behavior in the Middle-East: The case of Lebanon. *Nutrients* **2014**, *6*, 5079–5102. [CrossRef]
41. Claro, R.M.; Linders, H.; Ricardo, C.Z.; Legetic, B.; Campbell, N.R. Consumer attitudes, knowledge, and behavior related to salt consumption in sentinel countries of the Americas. *Rev. Panam. Salud. Publica* **2012**, *32*, 265–273. [CrossRef]
42. World Health Organization. *Mapping Salt Reduction Initiatives in the WHO European Region*; WHO Regional Office for Europe: Copenhagen, Denmark, 2013.
43. Berry, E.M.; Arnoni, Y.; Aviram, M. The Middle Eastern and biblical origins of the Mediterranean diet. *Public Health Nutr.* **2011**, *14*, 2288–2295. [CrossRef]
44. La Verde, M.; Mulè, S.; Zappalà, G.; Privitera, G.; Maugeri, G.; Pecora, F.; Marranzano, M. Higher adherence to the Mediterranean diet is inversely associated with having hypertension: Is low salt intake a mediating factor? *Int. J. Food Sci. Nutr.* **2018**, *69*, 235–244. [CrossRef] [PubMed]
45. Magriplis, E.; Farajian, P.; Pounis, G.D.; Risvas, G.; Panagiotakos, D.B.; Zampelas, A. High sodium intake of children through 'hidden' food sources and its association with the Mediterranean diet: The GRECO study. *J. Hypertens.* **2011**, *29*, 1069–1076. [CrossRef] [PubMed]

nutrients

MDPI

Article

Eating Habits and Lifestyle during COVID-19 Lockdown in the United Arab Emirates: A Cross-Sectional Study

Leila Cheikh Ismail [1,2,3,*], Tareq M. Osaili [1,3,4], Maysm N. Mohamad [5], Amina Al Marzouqi [6], Amjad H. Jarrar [5], Dima O. Abu Jamous [3], Emmanuella Magriplis [7], Habiba I. Ali [5], Haleama Al Sabbah [8], Hayder Hasan [1,3], Latifa M. R. AlMarzooqi [9], Lily Stojanovska [5,10], Mona Hashim [1,3], Reyad R. Shaker Obaid [1,3], Sheima T. Saleh [1] and Ayesha S. Al Dhaheri [5]

1 Department of Clinical Nutrition and Dietetics, College of Health Sciences, University of Sharjah, Sharjah 27272, UAE; tosaili@sharjah.ac.ae (T.M.O.); haidarah@sharjah.ac.ae (H.H.); mhashim@sharjah.ac.ae (M.H.); robaid@sharjah.ac.ae (R.R.S.O.); U14120207@sharjah.ac.ae (S.T.S.)
2 Nuffield Department of Women's & Reproductive Health, University of Oxford, Oxford OX1 2JD, UK
3 Research Institute of Medical and Health Sciences (RIMHS), University of Sharjah, Sharjah 27272, UAE; d_abujamous@yahoo.com
4 Department of Nutrition and Food Technology, Faculty of Agriculture, Jordan University of Science and Technology, Irbid 22110, Jordan
5 Department of Nutrition and Health, College of Medicine and Health Sciences, United Arab Emirates University, Al Ain 15551, UAE; drmaysm@gmail.com (M.N.M.); amjadj@uaeu.ac.ae (A.H.J.); habAli@uaeu.ac.ae (H.I.A.); lily.stojanovska@uaeu.ac.ae (L.S.); ayesha_aldhaheri@uaeu.ac.ae (A.S.A.D.)
6 Department of Health Services Administration, College of Health Sciences, University of Sharjah, Sharjah 27272, UAE; amalmarzouqi@sharjah.ac.ae
7 Department of Food Science and Human Nutrition, Agricultural University of Athens, Iera Odos 75, 11855 Athens, Greece; emagriplis@aua.gr
8 College of Natural and Health Sciences, Zayed University, Dubai 19282, UAE; haleemah.alsabah@zu.ac.ae
9 Nutrition Section, Ministry of Health and Prevention, Dubai 1853, UAE; latefa.rashed@moh.gov.ae
10 Institute for Health and Sport, Victoria University, Melbourne 14428, Australia
* Correspondence: lcheikhismail@sharjah.ac.ae; Tel.: +971-56-191-4363 or +971-6-505-7508

Received: 5 October 2020; Accepted: 27 October 2020; Published: 29 October 2020

Abstract: The coronavirus disease is still spreading in the United Arab Emirates (UAE) with subsequent lockdowns and social distancing measures being enforced by the government. The purpose of this study was to assess the effect of the lockdown on eating habits and lifestyle behaviors among residents of the UAE. A cross-sectional study among adults in the UAE was conducted using an online questionnaire between April and May 2020. A total of 1012 subjects participated in the study. During the pandemic, 31% reported weight gain and 72.2% had less than eight cups of water per day. Furthermore, the dietary habits of the participants were distanced from the Mediterranean diet principles and closer to "unhealthy" dietary patterns. Moreover, 38.5% did not engage in physical activity and 36.2% spent over five hours per day on screens for entertainment. A significantly higher percentage of participants reported physical exhaustion, emotional exhaustion, irritability, and tension "all the time" during the pandemic compared to before the pandemic ($p < 0.001$). Sleep disturbances were prevalent among 60.8% of the participants during the pandemic. Although lockdowns are an important safety measure to protect public health, results indicate that they might cause a variety of lifestyle changes, physical inactivity, and psychological problems among adults in the UAE.

Keywords: United Arab Emirates; COVID-19; eating habits; lifestyle behaviors

1. Introduction

The novel coronavirus disease (COVID-19) pandemic has added various challenges and changes to human life worldwide, causing an unprecedented impact on human health, lifestyle, and social life, and has affected the local and international economy [1]. Following its first emergence in December 2019, in the city of Wuhan in China and its subsequent outbreak throughout the world in the following months it was characterized as a global pandemic by the World Health Organization (WHO) on 11 March 2020 [2]. On 28 September 2020, over 32.7 million confirmed cases of novel coronavirus and around 991,000 deaths worldwide were reported by the WHO [3]. In the United Arab Emirates (UAE) a total of 90,618 confirmed cases were reported in the same period [3]. In response to the rapid spread of the disease governments all around the world had to implement strict measures such as complete or partial lockdowns, isolation, quarantine and social distancing [4,5].

In the UAE, as a response to this outbreak, the government had to act quickly to contain the spread of the virus. Parallel with measures taken by most countries worldwide, complete and partial lockdowns were implemented, non-essential public places were closed, telework and distance learning was initiated, delivery services like delivering drugs to chronically ill patients were provided and sanitizing cities during night as part of the National Disinfection Program was implemented [6]. According to the World Bank, the total population of the UAE in 2019 was about 9.8 million [7]. However, nearly 75% of the population is concentrated in Abu Dhabi and Dubai as they have more than 3 million residents each. Moreover, the UAE is a multicultural country with expatriates and immigrants accounting for about 88% of the population [8]. Thus, this study provides unique opportunities to examine the impact of COVID-19 on lifestyle behaviors in the UAE.

There is no doubt that during times of confinement, food accessibility and availability may be affected, which in turn affects diet quality [9]. The imposed possibility of reduced income, job losses and anxiety about an uncertain future might lead the population to cut down expenditure including their expenses for food, making them go for more palatable, affordable and possibly unhealthy options [10]. Diet can affect many areas, but most importantly it can affect immune status [11] in the short term, a time during which heightened activity should be at its best. Available literature, however, has shown trends toward unfavorable dietary behaviors during the lockdown such as increased caloric intake, more frequent snacking, reduced consumption of fresh fruits and vegetable, and weight gain [10,12]. Traditionally, the diet in the UAE consists of fruits (such as dates), vegetables and fish and it is characterized by a high-fiber content and low fat and cholesterol content [13]; foods that characterize the Mediterranean diet and that are rich in vitamins A, D, C, folate, E and B-complex, required for an optimal immune response. Moreover, a large portion of UAE residents are from Arab countries in which fruits, vegetables and olive oils constitute key components of their diets. Therefore, it would be of interest to assess any shift in dietary habits during the COVID-19 situation.

Levels of physical activity were also negatively affected during quarantine [10,14,15]. Factors like complete lockdowns, closure of sport facilities and parks, and overall movement restrictions have reduced the ability to engage in physical activity. This was accompanied with an increase in sedentary behaviors related to quarantine, including distance learning and telework [16]. A meta-analysis on physical activity prior to COVID-19 pandemic revealed that a quarter of the population residing in the UAE had a sedentary lifestyle and were not engaged in any type of physical activity [17].

The emergence of infectious diseases reaching pandemic levels induces a huge psychological impact and distressed mental health symptoms in the population with anxiety being the most common as was shown following the Middle East respiratory syndrome coronavirus (MERS-CoV), severe acute respiratory syndrome coronavirus (SARS-CoV), and severe acute respiratory syndrome coronavirus 2 (SARS-CoV-2) [18,19]. Anxiety and uncertainty along with food insecurity and restricted healthcare access might also impact individuals with eating disorders and obesity [20,21]. Multiple factors influence the extent of psychological impact of outbreaks including unknown means of virus transmission, future unpredictability, media misinformation, and quarantine [19,22]. Consequently, such stressful events strongly aggravate disturbed sleep patterns and insomnia, poor eating habits along with decreased levels of physical activity and increased sedentary behaviors [23,24].

This study aimed to investigate the effect of quarantine on eating habits, physical activity, stress and sleep behaviors among adult UAE residents using a formulated online survey. A comparison of lifestyle and dietary behaviors before and during the lockdown was also conducted to allow better understanding of the effects of Covid-19-induced confinement policies on lifestyle changes among the UAE residents. Dietary intake was examined during the lockdown to evaluate potential risks of nutritional inadequacies.

2. Materials and Methods

2.1. Study Design and Participants

To assess the effect of the coronavirus pandemic and the effect of lockdown on eating habits and lifestyle of residents of the UAE, a population-based (cross-sectional) study was conducted in the UAE between April and May 2020. Although cross-sectional studies are rarely used to compare before and after, since there is no temporal sequence, it is the best design to use when previous information is not available, in order to draw inferences. Considering the sudden outbreak of COVID-19, this study aimed to evaluate the effect of the pandemic by examining highly modifiable factors including lifestyle and dietary.

The target population included all adults ≥18 years and from all seven emirates, residing in UAE. These were invited to participate in an online survey using snowball sampling methods in order to guarantee a large-scale distribution and recruitment of participants. A total of 1012 participants (24.1% males) were included in this study.

A web link was retrieved for the survey and was distributed using e-mail invitations and social media platforms, e.g., LinkedIn™ (Mountain View, CA, USA), Facebook™ (Cambridge, MA, USA), and WhatsApp™ (Menlo Park, CA, USA). The first page of the survey included an information sheet and consent form indicating the participants' right to withdraw at any time. Consenting participants then chose their desired language and proceeded to complete and submit their responses. All data were collected anonymously with no indication of any personal information and participants were not rewarded. The study protocol was approved by the Research Ethics Committee at the University of Sharjah (REC-20-04-25-02) and the Social Sciences Research Ethics Committee at United Arab of Emirates University (ERS_2020_6106).

2.2. Survey Questionnaire

A multicomponent, self-administrated online survey was designed using Google document forms in English, Arabic, and French. This survey contained questions on dietary and lifestyle habits prior to and during the COVID-19 confinement. A researcher from the College of Health Sciences at the University of Sharjah (UAE) and a researcher from the College of Food and Agriculture at United Arab Emirates University (UAE) developed the draft of the survey in English. Questions were developed based on a previous national nutrition survey [25], the International Physical Activity Questionnaire Short Form (IPAQ-SF) [26] and the Copenhagen Psychosocial Questionnaire (COPSOQ-II) [27]. It was then translated and culturally adapted following an internationally accepted methodology [28,29]. The survey was later reviewed by the research team and was pilot tested with 25 people from the UAE. Following the pilot-testing, slight modifications were made to the survey. The online survey included 37 questions and was divided into seven sections: (1) socio-demographic background (10 questions): gender, age, marital status, number of children the participant has, education level, employment status, whether they were working or studying from home during the lockdown, weight change, perceived health status, and emirate of residence; (2) sources of information (2 questions): where do they obtain health and nutrition related information; (3) eating habits (8 questions): meal type, meal frequency, eating breakfast, skipping meals, reasons for skipping meals, water intake, and food frequency of specific foods; (4) shopping habits (5 questions): preparing a grocery list, stocking up on foods, using online shopping, reading food labels, and cleaning/sanitizing groceries; (5) physical activity (4 questions): exercising frequency, household chores frequency, computer time for work or study, and screen time for entertainment; (6) stress and irritability (4 questions): physical exhaustion, emotional exhaustion, irritability, and tension; (7) sleep (4 questions) sleep duration, sleep quality, sleep disturbances, and energy level. The full version of the questionnaire is available as a Supplementary File.

Questions on eating habits, physical activity, stress and irritability, and sleep were asked twice, once regarding the period before the pandemic (pre-COVID-19) and the other regarding the period during lockdown (during COVID-19).

2.2.1. Dietary Assessment

A total of 10 specific dietary questions were included in the questionnaire to assess frequency of specific food groups only during COVID-19 pandemic [30]. Food groups were included based on usual intakes of the population residing in the United Arab Emirates [31,32]. These characterize the basic Mediterranean type diet but also include food high in sugar and fat, observed to be recently trending in the UAE [25]. Specifically, the questionnaire included the following food groups: fruit, vegetables, milk and milk products, meat and meat products (red meat, chicken and fish), grains (bread, rice pasta), sweets, sugar sweetened beverages (ssbs), coffee and tea, and energy drinks. Response options included never; 1–4 times per week; once a day; 2–3 times a day; 4 or more times a day. Internal consistency of the food added in the food frequency questionnaire was evaluated using Cronbach's alpha for this section of the questionnaire specifically, to decrease false high internal consistency, since this test is affected by the length of the test [33]. A value of 0.81 was derived showing strong inter-relatedness of the food items, ensuring validity (Cronbach's alpha = 0.81, from a scale of 0 to 1.0; small cohort error variance of 0.34).

2.2.2. Physical Activity Assessment

A modified version of the International Physical Activity Questionnaire Short Form (IPAQ-SF) was used to assess frequency of physical activity pre-COVID-19 and during COVID-19 among surveyed participants [26]. Participants were asked to indicate "how many days per week did they engage in moderate to vigorous physical activity", and "how many days per week did they engage in household chores". They were also asked to indicate "how many hours per day did they spend on the computer for work or study", and "how many hours per day did they spend on screens for fun and entertainment".

2.2.3. Stress, Irritability and Sleep Assessment

Questions on stress and sleep were adopted from the second version of the Copenhagen Psychosocial Questionnaire (COPSOQ-II) with modifications [27]. Regarding stress and irritability, participants were asked to provide the frequency of experiencing physical exhaustion; emotional exhaustion; irritability; and tension. The same questions were asked once regarding the period before the pandemic (pre-COVID-19) and once during the pandemic. The response options included all the time; a small part of the time; part of the time; a large part of the time; all the time.

With regard to sleep, participants were asked if they experienced sleep disturbances including sleeping badly and restlessly; having difficulty to go to sleep; waking up too early and not being able to get back to sleep; waking up several times and found it difficult to get back to sleep; or none of the options. The questionnaire also included the following questions: "number of sleeping hours per night", "rating sleep quality", and "describing energy level during the day". The repose options for rating sleep quality were very good; good; poor. The repose options for describing energy level were energized; neutral; lazy. Questions were repeated twice, once about the period pre-COVID-19 and the second regarding the period during COVID-19.

2.3. Statistical Analysis

Categorical variables are presented as counts and percentages. The chi square test was used to determine the association between categorical variables, and the McNemar test was used to investigate the difference between categorical variables before and during the COVID-19 pandemic. A sub-analysis was also performed for weight and specific behavioral variables' differences between groups. Specifically, data were stratified (i) by sex, (ii) by age group (18–35 and ≥36 years), and (iii) level of education. Principal component analysis (PCA) was used to group related dietary practice into components [34]. The correlation of each food group with the underlying component was calculated with component loadings. In this analysis, values >0.3 were considered as having an effect in the component construction. Each participant was given a score based on the sum of the component loadings of each food group. The identified components were rotated (varimax rotation) to retrieve orthogonal, uncorrelated factors, decreasing variance errors. The Kaiser–Meyer–Olkin (KMO) measure of sample adequacy was used to assess PCA adequacy. Results were significant for p value < 0.05. Statistical analysis was performed using Statistical Package for the Social Sciences (SPSS) version 26.0 (IBM, Chicago, IL, USA).

3. Results

3.1. Demographic Characteristics

The survey was completed by 1012 participants. The sample distribution from different emirates was representative of the population distribution in the UAE. With the highest number of participants residing in Abu Dhabi and Dubai. More specifically, local coverage spreads over all regions in the UAE: 33.9% of participants live in the capital Abu Dhabi, 32.5% in Dubai, and 33.6% in Sharjah and northern Emirates. The majority of the participants completed the survey in Arabic (60.4%), followed by English (39.3%), and only 0.3% chose the French language. Comprehensive information relating to demographic characteristics of the study population is presented in Table 1. The majority of participants were females (75.9%), aged 26–35 years (29.1%), were married (56.4%), had no children (50%), completed a bachelor's degree (54.1%), worked full-time (53.3%), and were working or studying from home during quarantine (61.6%). Almost one third of the participants reported weight gain since the start of the lockdown (31%). However, 20.9% reported weight loss, 40.1% maintained their weight, and 7.9% did not know if there was a change in their weight. The majority of participants described their health status during the outbreak as very good (39.7%) and only 0.7% indicated poor health status.

Table 1. Demographic characteristics of study participants (n = 1012).

Characteristics	n	%
Gender		
Male	244	24.1
Female	768	75.9
Age (years)		
18–25	280	27.7
26–35	294	29.1
36–45	240	23.7
46–55	154	15.2
>55	44	4.3
Marital status		
Married	571	56.4
Single	403	39.8
Divorced	30	3.0
Widowed	8	0.8

Table 1. *Cont.*

Characteristics	*n*	%
Number of children		
None	506	50.0
1–2	230	22.7
≥ 3	276	27.3
Education level		
Less than high school	8	0.8
High school	111	11.0
College/Diploma	102	10.1
Bachelor's degree	547	54.1
Higher than bachelor's degree	244	24.1
Employment status		
Full-time	539	53.3
Part-time	44	4.3
Self-employed	31	3.1
Student	156	15.4
Unemployed	230	22.7
Retired	12	1.2
Working/studying from home		
Yes	623	61.6
No	309	30.5
Not applicable	80	7.9
Weight change during pandemic		
Lost weight	212	20.9
Gained weight	314	31.0
Maintained weight	406	40.1
Do not know	80	7.9
Perceived health state during pandemic		
Excellent	217	21.4
Very good	402	39.7
Good	284	28.1
Fair	102	10.1
Poor	7	0.7
Emirate of residence		
Abu Dhabi	343	33.9
Dubai	329	32.5
Sharjah	244	24.1
Ajman	52	5.1
Ras al Khaimah	20	2.0
Fujairah	16	1.6
Umm al Quwain	8	0.8

3.2. *Source of Information*

When asked about the most common source of information for health and nutrition updates, 69.1% and 67.8% of participants reported relying on social media applications, respectively (Table 2). Local and international health authorities were selected as the second source of information for both health and nutrition updates (65.4% and 48.7%, respectively).

Table 2. Source of health and nutrition information during COVID-19 pandemic ($n = 1012$).

Source of Information *	Health-Related Information, n (%)	Nutrition-Related Information, n (%)
Local and international health authorities	662 (65.4)	493 (48.7)
Social media	699 (69.1)	686 (67.8)
Healthcare professionals	409 (40.4)	462 (45.7)
Television	231 (22.8)	172 (17.0)
Newspapers	75 (7.4)	51 (5.0)
Friends and family	339 (33.5)	386 (38.1)

* As multiple responses were allowed, the total number of responses is greater than the number of surveyed participants and the percent of cases is displayed.

3.3. Eating Habits

Table 3 presents the eating habits of the study participants pre- and during the COVID-19 pandemic. Results showed a significant increase in the percentage of participants consuming mostly homemade meals during the pandemic and a significant reduction in those mainly consuming fast-food ($p < 0.001$). Moreover, the percentage of participants consuming five or more meals per day increased from 2.1% before the pandemic to 7% during the pandemic ($p < 0.001$). Also, the percentage of participants consuming breakfast increased from 66% to 74.2%, and the percentage of those skipping meals decreased from 64.5% to 46.2% during the pandemic ($p < 0.001$). Participants reported skipping meals mainly due to lack of time before the pandemic (62.3%), however, the main reason behind that was lack of appetite (36%). With regards to water intake, only 24.1% of participants consumed eight or more cups per day before the pandemic, and the percentage increased to 27.8% during the pandemic ($p = 0.003$).

Table 3. Eating habits pre- and during COVID-19 pandemic ($n = 1012$).

Variables	Pre-COVID-19 n (%)	During COVID-19 n (%)	p-Value (2-Sided)
Most consumed meals during the week *			
Homemade	838 (82.8)	974 (96.2)	<0.001
Frozen ready-to-eat meals	119 (11.8)	97 (9.6)	0.032
Fast food	270 (26.7)	80 (7.9)	<0.001
Restaurants [1]	289 (28.6)	58 (5.7)	<0.001
Healthy restaurants [2]	98 (9.7)	46 (4.5)	<0.001
Number of meals per day			
1–2 meals	470 (46.4)	369 (36.5)	<0.001
3–4 meals	521 (51.5)	572 (56.5)	0.009
≥5 meals	21 (2.1)	71 (7.0)	<0.001
Eating breakfast on most days			
Yes	668 (66.0)	751 (74.2)	<0.001
No	344 (34.0)	261 (25.8)	
Skipping meals			
Yes	663 (65.5)	468 (46.2)	<0.001
No	349 (34.5)	544 (53.8)	
Reasons for skipping meals (If the answer was yes) *			
To reduce food intake	143 (21.7)	136 (29.1)	0.011
Lack of time	410 (62.3)	143 (30.6)	<0.001
To lose weight	122 (18.5)	110 (23.6)	0.001
Lack of appetite	182 (27.7)	168 (36.0)	0.016
Fasting	68 (10.3)	120 (25.7)	<0.001

Table 3. *Cont.*

Variables	Pre-COVID-19 *n* (%)	During COVID-19 *n* (%)	*p*-Value (2-Sided)
Amount of water consumed per day			
1–4 cups	410 (40.5)	337 (33.3)	<0.001
5–7 cups	358 (35.4)	394 (38.9)	0.036
≥8 cups	244 (24.1)	281 (27.8)	0.003

* As multiple responses were allowed, the total number of responses is greater than the number of surveyed participants and the percent of cases is displayed. [1] Restaurants: included all ethnic restaurants (Asian, Middle Eastern, International, etc.), casual dining and family style restaurants; [2] healthy restaurants: included food outlets with the "Weqaya logo", restaurants categorized as "healthy" on food mobile apps (such as Zomato, Talabat, and Uber Eats) or catering services providing meal plan services based on nutritional needs (such as Kcal, right bite, Eat Clean ME, etc.).

The frequency of consumption for particular food products during the COVID-19 pandemic among residents of the UAE are presented in Table 4. Over half of the participants (51.2%) did not consume fruits daily, 37% did not consume vegetables daily, and 46.2% did not consume milk and dairy products on daily basis. However, 46.1% of the participants consumed sweets and desserts at least once per day, and 37.1% reported consuming salty snacks (chips, crackers, and nuts) every day.

Table 4. The frequency of consumption of particular foods during COVID-19 pandemic (*n* = 1012).

Food Items	≥4 Times/Day	2–3 Times/Day	Once/Day	1–4 Times/Week	Never
			n (%)		
Fruits	20 (2.0)	133 (13.1)	341 (33.7)	462 (45.7)	56 (5.5)
Vegetables	32 (3.2)	244 (24.1)	362 (35.8)	356 (35.2)	18 (1.8)
Milk and milk products	17 (1.7)	167 (16.5)	361 (35.7)	374 (37.0)	93 (9.2)
Meat/fish/chicken	32 (3.2)	133 (13.1)	440 (43.5)	383 (37.8)	24 (2.4)
Bread/rice/pasta	43 (4.2)	263 (26.0)	350 (34.6)	311 (30.7)	45 (4.4)
Sweets/desserts	29 (2.9)	106 (10.5)	331 (32.7)	437 (43.2)	109 (10.8)
Salty snacks	14 (1.4)	85 (8.4)	276 (27.3)	500 (49.4)	137 (13.5)
Coffee/tea	80 (7.9)	321 (31.7)	300 (29.6)	222 (21.9)	89 (8.8)
Sweetened drinks	18 (1.8)	51 (5.0)	156 (15.4)	340 (33.6)	447 (44.2)
Energy drinks	4 (0.4)	11 (1.1)	35 (3.5)	87 (8.6)	875 (86.5)

Additionally, 69.2% had tea or coffee at least once per day. Sweet drinks such as fruit juices and beverages were less popular among the study participants, as 44.2% reported never consuming them and an even higher percentage (86.5%) reported never consuming energy drinks during the pandemic.

A total of two components from the PCA output were derived, based on eigenvalue (at least 1) and scree plots obtained (Table 5). These two components explained 47% of the variance in eating behavior and were named based on the interpretation of the component loadings. The first pattern explained 31% of eating variation and was named "Western-type diet" since it was characterized by significantly positive loadings in dairy, meat, sweets, salted foods and vegetables. The second pattern explained 16% of the variance and loaded positively with ssbs and energy drinks and negatively on fruits and vegetables. Therefore, it was named "Free Sugars diet". A KMO of 0.78 was obtained, which is considered substantial.

Table 5. Component loading for the two major dietary patterns of the participants during COVID-19.

Food Groups	Western	Free Sugars
Fruits	0.2839	**−0.3807**
Vegetable	**0.3302**	**−0.4219**
Milk	**0.3247**	−0.1932
Meat	**0.3599**	−0.0732
Carbs	**0.3975**	−0.0764
Sweets	**0.3845**	0.2917
Salted Foods	**0.3356**	0.2776
Coffee/Tea	0.2457	−0.1641
Sweet Drinks	0.2678	**0.4929**
Energy Drinks	0.1575	**0.4433**
KMO	**0.78**	

KMO: Kaiser–Meyer–Olkin (KMO) test. The unique characteristics of each component (dietary pattern) are presented in bold. Marginally unique dietary characteristic for each component. Loadings ≥0.30 and ≤−0.30.

3.4. *Shopping*

The results revealed that the majority of participants prepared a shopping list beforehand (80.3%), started stocking up on foods during the pandemic (43.9%), did not order their groceries online (58.0%), read the food label before purchasing products (52.4%), and sanitized or cleaned groceries before storing them (71.9%) (Table 6).

Table 6. Shopping practices during COVID-19 pandemic (n = 1012).

Variables	n	%
Prepare shopping list		
Yes	813	80.3
No	199	19.7
Start stocking up on foods		
Yes	444	43.9
No	412	40.7
Already stocking up	156	15.4
Online grocery shopping		
Yes	425	42.0
No	587	58.0
Reading food labels		
Yes	530	52.4
No	113	11.2
Sometimes	369	36.5
Sanitizing/cleaning groceries		
Yes	728	71.9
No	113	11.2
Sometimes	171	16.9

3.5. *Physical Activity*

Figure 1a shows that 32.1% of the participants reported not engaging in any physical activity before the coronavirus pandemic, and the percentage increased to 38.5% during the pandemic ($p < 0.001$). Moreover, Figure 1b shows that there was a significant association between the frequency of performing physical activity during the pandemic and the reported change in weight among participants ($p < 0.001$). Of those who reported performing physical activity more than three times per week, 29.9% lost weight and 49.5% maintained their weight ($p < 0.001$). Furthermore, 40.3% of people who did not perform physical activity reported weight gain.

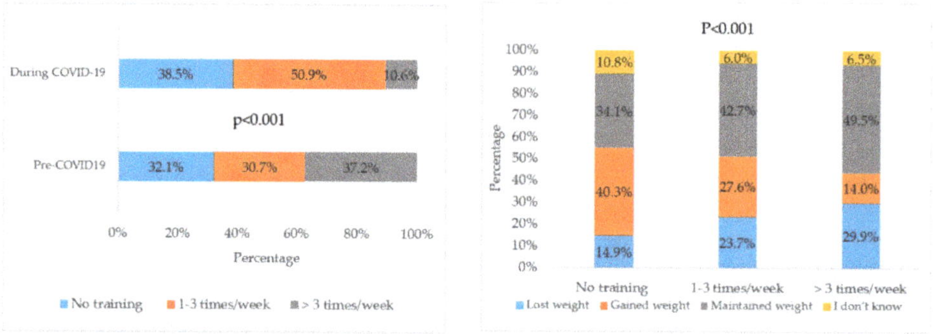

(**a**) (**b**)

Figure 1. Physical activity pre- and during COVID-19 pandemic (**a**) Frequency; (**b**) Change in weight. The p values indicate the statistical significance of McNemar test. The p values indicate the statistical significance of chi-square test.

A significantly higher percentage of participants spent more than five hours per day on the computer for study or work purposes during the pandemic (47.6%) compared to before the pandemic (32%) ($p < 0.001$). Similarly, the percentage of participants spending more than five hours per day on screens for fun increased from 12.9% before the lockdown to 36.2% during the lockdown ($p < 0.001$) (Table 7).

Table 7. Daily activities pre- and during COVID-19 pandemic (n = 1012).

Variables	**Pre-COVID-19** *n* **(%)**	**During COVID-19** *n* **(%)**	***p*-Value (2-Sided)**
Doing household chores			
Never	302 (29.8)	207 (20.5)	<0.001
1–3 times/week	404 (39.8)	333 (32.9)	<0.001
4–5 times/week	62 (6.1)	114 (11.3)	<0.001
Everyday	244 (24.1)	358 (35.4)	<0.001
Screen time for study or work			
None	188 (18.6)	160 (15.8)	0.004
1–2 h/day	282 (27.9)	136 (13.4)	<0.001
3–5 h/day	218 (21.5)	234 (23.1)	0.375
>5 h/day	324 (32.0)	482 (47.6)	<0.001
Screen time for entertainment			
Less than 30 min/day	113 (11.2)	62 (6.1)	<0.001
1–2 h/day	456 (45.1)	231 (22.8)	<0.001
3–5 h/day	312 (30.8)	353 (34.9)	0.053
>5 h/day	131 (12.9)	366 (36.2)	<0.001

3.6. Stress

Participants were asked to indicate the frequency of experiencing physical exhaustion; emotional exhaustion; irritability; and tension before and during the pandemic. Figure 2 presented the response distribution in percentages for each of the four stress parameters.

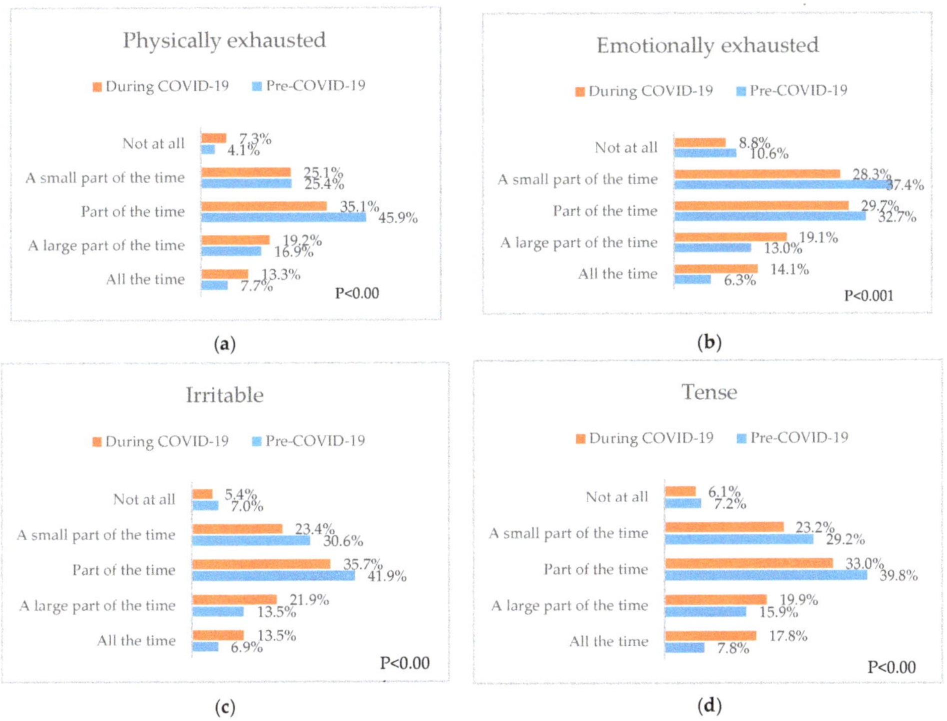

Figure 2. Stress and irritability pre- and during COVID-19 pandemic (**a**) Physical exhaustion; (**b**) Emotional exhaustion; (**c**) Irritability; (**d**) Tension. The p values indicate the statistical significance of McNemar test.

The results indicate a significant increase in the percentage of participants reporting all four stress parameters "all the time" during the coronavirus pandemic compared to before the pandemic (13.3% vs. 7.7% for physical exhaustion; 14.1% vs. 6.3% for emotional exhaustion; 13.5% vs. 6.9% for irritability; and 17.8% vs. 6.3% for tension) (all $p < 0.001$).

3.7. Sleep

Results showed a significant decrease in the percentage of participants who reported sleeping less than seven hours per night from 51.7% before the pandemic to 39% during the pandemic ($p < 0.001$) (Table 8). However, a higher percentage of participants reported poor sleep quality during the pandemic (28.1%) compared to before the pandemic (17.3) ($p < 0.001$), and sleep disturbances were also more common during the pandemic (60.8%) compared to before (52.9%). Consequently, 30.9% of the surveyed participants reported feeling lazy and less energized during the pandemic, compared to only 4.7% before the pandemic ($p < 0.001$) (Table 8).

An analysis of weight and behavioral factors by sex and age groups is depicted in Table 9. Significantly more males reported decreased engagement in physical activity (50% vs. 39.3%; $p = 0.013$) and increased screen time (54.5% vs. 51%; $p = 0.002$). Sleep disturbances increase was, however, significantly higher in females ($p = 0.011$). Moreover, those aged over 36 years reported a higher weight gain as well as an increase in the number of meals consumed per day ($p = 0.042$ and $p = 0.024$, respectively). Sleep duration and quality was most affected among participants aged 18–35 ($p < 0.001$). There was no significant association between different education levels and lifestyle changes (Table 9).

Table 8. Sleep pre- and during COVID-19 pandemic (n = 1012).

Variables	Pre-COVID-19 n (%)	During COVID-19 n (%)	p-Value (2-Sided)
Hours of sleep per night			
<7 h	523 (51.7)	395 (39.0)	<0.001
7–9 h	459 (45.4)	499 (49.3)	0.057
>9 h	30 (3.0)	118 (11.7)	<0.001
How would you rate your sleep quality			
Very good	308 (30.4)	282 (27.9)	0.134
Good	529 (52.3)	446 (44.1)	<0.001
Poor	175 (17.3)	284 (28.1)	<0.001
Did you experience any of the following *			
Slept badly and restlessly	251 (24.8)	285 (28.2)	0.057
Hard to go to sleep	199 (19.7)	358 (35.4)	<0.001
Woken up too early and not been able to get back to sleep	232 (22.9)	147 (14.5)	<0.001
Woken up several times and found it difficult to get back to sleep	187 (18.5)	334 (33.0)	<0.001
None	477 (47.1)	397 (39.2)	<0.001
Describe your energy level			
Energized	369 (36.5)	189 (18.7)	<0.001
Neutral	596 (58.9)	510 (50.4)	<0.001
Lazy	47 (4.7)	313 (30.9)	<0.001

* As multiple responses were allowed, the total number of responses is greater than the number of surveyed participants and the percent of cases is displayed.

Table 9. Lifestyle changes during COVID-19 pandemic by demographic factors (n = 1012).

Variables	All n = 1012	Gender			Age Group (Year)			Education Level		
		Female n = 768	Male n = 244	p Value	18–35 n = 574	≥36 n = 438	p Value	High School n = 119	Higher Degree n = 893	p Value
Weight, n, (%)										
Decreased	212 (20.9)	166 (21.6)	46 (18.9)	0.143	131 (22.8)	81 (18.5)	0.042	19 (16.0)	193 (21.6)	0.350
Same as before	486 (48.0)	376 (49.0)	110 (45.1)		273 (47.6)	213 (48.6)		62 (52.1)	424 (47.5)	
Increased	314 (31.0)	226 (29.4)	88 (36.1)		170 (29.6)	144 (32.9)		38 (31.9)	276 (30.9)	
Meals per day, n (%)										
Decreased	124 (12.3)	96 (12.5)	28 (11.5)	0.140	84 (14.6)	40 (9.1)	0.024	13 (10.9)	111 (12.4)	0.352
Same as before	628 (62.1)	464 (60.4)	164 (67.2)		342 (59.6)	272 (61.9)		69 (58.0)	559 (62.6)	
Increased	260 (25.7)	208 (27.1)	52 (21.3)		148 (25.8)	127 (29.0)		37 (31.1)	223 (25.0)	
Physical activity, n (%)										
Decreased	424 (41.9)	302 (39.3)	122 (50.0)	0.013	226 (39.4)	198 (45.2)	0.171	42 (35.3)	382 (42.8)	0.169
Same as before	438 (43.3)	346 (45.1)	92 (37.7)		258 (44.9)	180 (41.1)		61 (51.3)	377 (42.2)	
Increased	150 (14.8)	120 (15.6)	30 (12.3)		90 (15.7)	60 (13.7)		16 (13.4)	134 (15.0)	

Table 9. *Cont.*

Variables	All $n = 1012$	Gender			Age Group (Year)			Education Level		
		Female $n = 768$	Male $n = 244$	*p* Value	18–35 $n = 574$	≥36 $n = 438$	*p* Value	High School $n = 119$	Higher Degree $n = 893$	*p* Value
Screen time (entertainment), n (%)										
Decreased	72 (7.1)	67 (8.7)	5 (2.0)	0.002	46 (8.0)	26 (5.9)	0.150	8 (6.7)	64 (7.2)	0.984
Same as before	415 (41.0)	309 (40.2)	106 (43.4)		222 (38.7)	193 (44.1)		49 (41.2)	366 (41.0)	
Increased	525 (51.9)	392 (51.0)	133 (54.5)		306 (53.3)	219 (50.0)		62 (52.1)	463 (51.8)	
Sleep (h), n (%)										
Decreased	148 (14.6)	124 (16.1)	24 (9.8)	0.051	100 (17.4)	48 (11.0)	<0.001	23 (19.3)	125 (14.0)	0.302
Same as before	534 (52.8)	397 (51.7)	137 (56.1)		270 (47.0)	264 (60.3)		59 (49.6)	475 (53.2)	
Increased	330 (32.6)	247 (32.2)	83 (34.0)		204 (35.5)	126 (28.8)		37 (31.1)	293 (32.8)	
Sleep disturbances, n (%)										
Decreased	157 (15.5)	119 (15.5)	38 (15.6)	0.011	90 (15.7)	67 (15.3)	<0.001	16 (13.4)	141 (15.8)	0.135
Same as before	552 (54.5)	401 (52.2)	151 (61.9)		285 (49.7)	267 (61.0)		58 (48.7)	494 (55.3)	
Increased	303 (29.9)	248 (32.3)	55 (22.5)		199 (34.7)	104 (23.7)		45 (37.8)	258 (28.9)	

p value was based on chi-square test at 5% level.

4. Discussion

This population-based, cross-sectional study assessed eating habits and lifestyle behaviors among residences of the UAE, via an online survey during the COVID-19 pandemic between April and May 2020. The results indicate that the COVID-19 pandemic and the subsequent lockdown resulted in weight gain in about one-third of the respondents with changes in important and highly modifiable dietary and lifestyle behaviors that are considered essential for optimal somatic and psychological health. Specifically, participants also reported an increase in the number of meals consumed per day and a reduction in the percentage of skipping meals particularly breakfast during the pandemic. The present study also indicated that dietary habits were distanced from the Mediterranean diet principles and closer to "unhealthy" dietary patterns, characterized as high in energy but with low nutrient density; viewed as a detrimental combination for immune status. Although more homemade meals were prepared, a factor associated with healthy weight status, at the same time more non-nutritious foods were chosen, as well as being more frequently consumed (since an increase was also seen among frequency of meals per day). These data, therefore, are informative on the potential alterations of food prepared and consumed although at home.

In agreement with our study, the results from Kuwait, United States, Italy and France revealed an increase in caloric intake and indicated weight gain during the current COVID-19 home confinement [10,35–37]. Data from Kuwait, a close Gulf country to UAE, showed a significant increase in weight of respondents during the quarantine and the weight gain was 4.5 times higher among those consuming unhealthy diets [38]. The actual weight increase was not assessed in this study considering the short time interval of COVID-19 lockdown, however, the large percentage of the population that reported an increase in weight can be used as a proxy pertaining to changes in eating behavior and activity level. It has been suggested that the negative alterations in eating behaviors could be due to anxiety or boredom [39], lack of motivation to maintain healthy habits [40], or reduced availability of goods and limited access to food due to restricted store opening hours [41]. The prevalence of overweight and obesity in the UAE even before COVID-19 was high and has increased over time [42]. It is estimated that over one third of the population in the UAE is living with obesity with higher rates among females [43]. Thus, extra efforts are needed to reduce the burden of obesity and its risk factors especially during the COVID-19 pandemic.

Over half of the surveyed participants in this study did not consume fruits daily and about one third did not consume vegetables and dairy products on daily basis. Instead, almost half of the same population reported consuming sweets and desserts at least once per day and over one third consumed salty snacks daily. This transition towards a Westernized diet in the UAE was reported in 1998, where the consumption of fresh fruit and vegetables and of milk and dairy products was found low [32]. Moreover, in 2003, 77.5% of males and 75.7% of females in the UAE had less than five servings of fruit and vegetables per day [44]. Likewise, a recent study among Emirati adolescents revealed that only 28% of them met the recommended daily fruit and vegetable intake [45]. This is concerning especially as fruits and vegetables are an important source of fiber, vitamins, minerals, and antioxidants. Diets rich in antioxidants (such as the Mediterranean diet and Dietary Approaches to Stop Hypertension (DASH) diet) are vascular protective. The Mediterranean diet is recognized as an anti-inflammatory dietary pattern, focusing on high consumption of plant foods, low red meat and dairy and moderate consumption of monounsaturated fat sources such as olive oil [46]. Evidence suggests that the Mediterranean diet is associated with better health status, lower risk of chronic disease and inflammation as well as increased immunity [47–49]. The Mediterranean diet is not only a healthy dietary pattern, but is also a sustainable diet that has a lower environmental impact than the typical Western diet [50]. Moreover, mounting evidence indicates that the Mediterranean diet has a favorable effect on diseases related to chronic inflammation, including visceral obesity, type 2 diabetes mellitus and the metabolic syndrome [51–55]. Knowing that the prevalence of cardiovascular disease incidence is high in the UAE (40%) [56] and rates of dyslipidemia are strikingly elevated (72.5%) [57] makes it imperative that diets such as the Mediterranean diet should be encouraged to prevent the potentially negative effect of quarantine on dietary habits and overall health [41].

Due to the increase in obesogenic behaviors related to the COVID-19 pandemic, two dietary patterns were revealed among the studied population, named the "Western-type diet" and the "Free Sugars diet". These patterns indicate unhealthy eating behaviors during the period of the pandemic. This is in agreement with previous studies reporting a transformation of the diet in Eastern Mediterranean countries from a traditional Mediterranean diet to a more Westernized diet which is high in energy, saturated fat, cholesterol, salt, and refined carbohydrates, and low in fruits, vegetables, fiber, and polyunsaturated fats [25,58–60]. Therefore, current dietary behaviors in the UAE may not be effective against the COVID-19 virus since it can adversely affect the immune system response among other health factors. Furthermore, it is unclear whether these dietary patterns were due to the lockdown that followed the COVID-19 outbreak; however, the implications can be detrimental considering an adequate supply of macro- and micro-nutrients are essential for optimal immune function and response [11,61].

Amidst these passive changes in food behavior, some beneficial aspects emerged from this study, such as a significant increase in home-made food preparations, regular breakfast consumption and lower intakes of fast foods. Similarly, a consumer online based survey conducted by Ipsos across the Middle East and North Africa (MENA) region revealed that 57% out of the 5000 consumers who took part in the survey were preparing their own meals, and 79% were eating less often at restaurants [62].

Among the surveyed participants, more than one third reported a non-engagement in any physical activity during coronavirus pandemic lockdown. This was mostly observed among males in this study, with a simultaneously greater likelihood of increased sedentary time, compared to females. The findings of this questionnaire are in accordance with other studies indicating that the current COVID-19 pandemic had a dramatic impact on lifestyle behaviors globally, including diminished engagement in sports and physical activity in general [63–65]. Moreover, the "Effects of home Confinement on multiple Lifestyle Behaviours during the COVID-19 outbreak (ECLB-COVID-19)" international survey revealed that the COVID-19 pandemic had a negative effect on all levels of physical activity (vigorous, moderate, walking and overall) and increased daily sedentary time by more than 28% [14]. Similarly, in the current study the proportion of participants who spent more than five hours per day on screens for entertainment increased by 23.3%. Together with the unhealthy diet, the reduction of physical activity would not only contribute to weight gain, but also to an increase in cardiovascular risk during quarantine. Thus, awareness about the importance of regular physical activity and its benefits on overall health is necessary during such times [66,67]. It is also important to identify groups at a higher risk of unhealthy lifestyle behaviors during the COVID-19 pandemic to design interventions targeted towards these groups.

During the COVID-19 pandemic higher levels of anxiety, stress and depression have been observed among individuals [68–70]. In this study, the percentage of participants experiencing exhaustion, irritability, and tension more often during the coronavirus pandemic increased significantly. Sleep was mostly affected in females and needs to be further evaluated since it is linked with multiple endocrine functions, as well risk for obesity and depression. The risk of obesity is underlined by the significant increase in daily meal frequency among participants over 36 years with the majority being female. Also, despite WHO recommendations to minimize listening to unreliable news that could cause anxiety or distress and to seek information only from trusted sources [71], over two thirds of participants in this survey used social media as a main source for health updates. Studies have shown the negative and harmful effect of misinformation overload "infodemic" on the mental health of individuals [72,73]. Moreover, stress and anxiety could disrupt sleep quality during the night and energy levels during the day. Results of the current survey indicated a 10.8% increase in participants reporting poor sleep quality and 26.2% increase in those feeling lazy during the pandemic. Xiao and his co-workers found a significant negative correlation between anxiety levels and sleep quality and suggested the use of telepsychiatry consultation as an important therapeutic strategy [74]. The use of telehealth has been shown to be useful in providing support to patients and is appropriate for the delivery of mental health services [75]. Additionally, the Mediterranean diet does not only have a protective effect on the risk of cardiovascular diseases and certain types of cancer [54,76], but also an increased compliance with it could be associated with lesser mental distress, better sleep quality, and higher scoring for self-perceived health status [77–79].

It is acknowledged that this study has limitations related to the use of self-reported questionnaire, snowball sampling method and the cross-sectional study design. The study information was acquired after lockdown, and although comparisons are critical to be made in order to draw inferences, no conclusive remarks can be drawn. Results stratified by sex should be interpreted with caution, since the majority of the participants were females. Furthermore, in order to minimize selection bias that may arise with snowball sampling (including interrelated-similar individuals), each individual could refer a maximum of three people who were not family members, and only one individual per age group (young adults, older adults, elderly) was enrolled from a household. Moreover, the change in dietary pattern was not assessed in this study, since data on food frequency were only obtained during COVID-19 pandemic, although these can be used as a reference for further studies performed, in these uncertain times. This was done to reduce the probability of including recall bias, since the participants had to respond to multiple questions on food frequency and quantity during COVID-19 lockdown and for a prolonged period prior to that. Also, the presence of obesity and eating disorders were not determined in the study, nor was information on infection with COVID-19 reported. Such analysis would require a longer questionnaire, hence may have decreased the compliance and response rate, but also would have required a larger sample size based on the prevalence of all factors to acquire adequate study power. Another potential limitation of the study was that respondents were mostly females. Although this is usual in online questionnaires [80], it should be considered when generalizing the results. However, using an online survey facilitated data collection during COVID-19 pandemic from all seven emirates. It also guaranteed the anonymity of the participants, thus reducing the social desirability bias. The strengths of this research include data collection timing one month after lockdown which minimizes memory failure for previous habits. In addition, the survey provided was in multiple languages in a multilingual environment like UAE.

The results of the study indicate that individuals in the UAE experienced negative lifestyle changes, unbalanced food choices, a reduction in physical activity, and psychological problems during the COVID-19 pandemic. Although quarantine is an essential measure to protect public health and control the transmission of the virus, these findings should be taken into consideration for future regulations in the UAE.

Supplementary Materials: The following are available online at http://www.mdpi.com/2072-6643/12/11/3314/s1, Eating Habits and Lifestyle during COVID-19 Lockdown in the United Arab Emirates: A Cross-Sectional Study.

Author Contributions: Conceptualization, L.C.I., T.M.O. and A.S.A.D.; methodology, L.C.I., T.M.O., A.S.A.D., M.N.M., M.H., and S.T.S.; validation, L.C.I., T.M.O., A.S.A.D., M.N.M. and E.M.; formal analysis, L.C.I., M.N.M., S.T.S., E.M. and H.H.; investigation, L.C.I., T.M.O., M.N.M., A.S.A.D., A.A.M., A.H.J., D.O.A.J., H.I.A., H.A.S., H.H., L.M.R.A., L.S., M.H., R.R.S.O., and S.T.S.; writing—original draft preparation, L.C.I., M.N.M., A.S.A.D. and S.T.S.; writing—review and editing, L.C.I., T.M.O., M.N.M., A.S.A.D., A.A.M., A.H.J., D.O.A.J., E.M.,H.I.A., H.A.S., H.H., L.M.R.A., L.S., M.H., R.R.S.O., and S.T.S. All authors have read and agreed to the published version of the manuscript.

Funding: This research received no external funding.

Conflicts of Interest: The authors declare no conflict of interest.

References

1. Barro, R.J.; Ursúa, J.F.; Weng, J. *The Coronavirus and the Great Influenza Pandemic: Lessons from the "Spanish flu" for the Coronavirus's Potential Effects on Mortality and Economic Activity*; 0898-2937; National Bureau of Economic Research: Cambridge, MA, USA, 2020.
2. WHO. WHO Director-General's Opening Remarks at the Media Briefing on COVID-19—11 March 2020. Available online: https://www.who.int/dg/speeches/detail/who-director-general-s-opening-remarks-at-the-media-briefing-on-covid-19---11-march-2020 (accessed on 16 August 2020).
3. WHO. Coronavirus Disease (COVID-19) Weekly Epidemiological and Operational Updates September 2020. Available online: https://www.who.int/docs/default-source/coronaviruse/situation-reports/20200928-weekly-epi-update.pdf?sfvrsn=9e354665_6 (accessed on 29 September 2020).
4. Wilder-Smith, A.; Freedman, D. Isolation, quarantine, social distancing and community containment: Pivotal role for old-style public health measures in the novel coronavirus (2019-nCoV) outbreak. *J. Travel Med.* **2020**, *27*, taaa020. [CrossRef] [PubMed]
5. Koh, D. COVID-19 lockdowns throughout the world. *Occup. Med.* **2020**. [CrossRef]
6. Bloukh, S.H.; Shaikh, A.; Pathan, H.M.; Edis, Z. Prevalence of COVID-19: A Look behind the Scenes from the UAE and India. *Preprints* **2020**. [CrossRef]
7. Bank, T.W. United Arab Emirates: Data Source: United Nations World Population Prospects. Available online: https://data.worldbank.org/country/AE (accessed on 16 August 2020).
8. De Bel-Air, F. *Demography, Migration, and the Labour Market in the UAE*; Migration Policy Center, Gulf Labour Markets and Migration (GLMM): Firenze, Italy, 2015.
9. Scarmozzino, F.; Visioli, F. Covid-19 and the Subsequent Lockdown Modified Dietary Habits of Almost Half the Population in an Italian Sample. *Foods* **2020**, *9*, 675. [CrossRef] [PubMed]
10. Deschasaux-Tanguy, M.; Druesne-Pecollo, N.; Esseddik, Y.; Szabo de Edelenyi, F.; Alles, B.; Andreeva, V.A.; Baudry, J.; Charreire, H.; Deschamps, V.; Egnell, M.; et al. Diet and physical activity during the COVID-19 lockdown period (March-May 2020): Results from the French NutriNet-Sante cohort study. *medRxiv* **2020**. [CrossRef]
11. Calder, P.C. Nutrition, immunity and COVID-19. *BMJ Nutr. Prev. Health* **2020**, *3*, 74. [CrossRef]
12. Zachary, Z.; Brianna, F.; Brianna, L.; Garrett, P.; Jade, W.; Alyssa, D.; Mikayla, K. Self-quarantine and Weight Gain Related Risk Factors During the COVID-19 Pandemic. *Obes. Res. Clin. Pract.* **2020**. [CrossRef]
13. Musaiger, A.O. Diet and Prevention of Coronary Heart Disease in the Arab Middle East Countries. *Med. Princ. Pract.* **2002**, *11*, 9–16. [CrossRef]
14. Ammar, A.; Brach, M.; Trabelsi, K.; Chtourou, H.; Boukhris, O.; Masmoudi, L.; Bouaziz, B.; Bentlage, E.; How, D.; Ahmed, M. Effects of COVID-19 Home Confinement on Eating Behaviour and Physical Activity: Results of the ECLB-COVID19 International Online Survey. *Nutrients* **2020**, *12*, 1583. [CrossRef]

15. Lippi, G.; Henry, B.M.; Sanchis-Gomar, F. Physical inactivity and cardiovascular disease at the time of coronavirus disease 2019 (COVID-19). *Eur. J. Prev. Cardiol.* **2020**. [CrossRef]
16. Hall, G.; Laddu, D.R.; Phillips, S.A.; Lavie, C.J.; Arena, R. A tale of two pandemics: How will COVID-19 and global trends in physical inactivity and sedentary behavior affect one another? *Prog. Cardiovasc. Dis.* **2020**. [CrossRef] [PubMed]
17. Yammine, K. The prevalence of physical activity among the young population of UAE: A meta-analysis. *Perspect. Public Health* **2017**, *137*, 275–280. [CrossRef] [PubMed]
18. Wu, P.; Fang, Y.; Guan, Z.; Fan, B.; Kong, J.; Yao, Z.; Liu, X.; Fuller, C.J.; Susser, E.; Lu, J. The psychological impact of the SARS epidemic on hospital employees in China: Exposure, risk perception, and altruistic acceptance of risk. *Can. J. Psychiatry* **2009**, *54*, 302–311. [CrossRef]
19. Pfefferbaum, B.; North, C.S. Mental health and the Covid-19 pandemic. *N. Engl. J. Med.* **2020**. [CrossRef] [PubMed]
20. Todisco, P.; Donini, L.M. Eating disorders and obesity (ED&O) in the COVID-19 storm. *Eat. Weight Disord.* **2020**, *1*. [CrossRef]
21. Touyz, S.; Lacey, H.; Hay, P. Eating disorders in the time of COVID-19. *J. Eat. Disord.* **2020**, *8*, 19. [CrossRef] [PubMed]
22. Rajkumar, R.P. COVID-19 and mental health: A review of the existing literature. *Asian J. Psychiatry* **2020**, *52*, 102066. [CrossRef]
23. Holmes, E.A.; O'Connor, R.C.; Perry, V.H.; Tracey, I.; Wessely, S.; Arseneault, L.; Ballard, C.; Christensen, H.; Silver, R.C.; Everall, I. Multidisciplinary research priorities for the COVID-19 pandemic: A call for action for mental health science. *Lancet Psychiatry* **2020**. [CrossRef]
24. Torales, J.; O'Higgins, M.; Castaldelli-Maia, J.M.; Ventriglio, A. The outbreak of COVID-19 coronavirus and its impact on global mental health. *Int. J. Soc. Psychiatry* **2020**. [CrossRef]
25. Ng, S.W.; Zaghloul, S.; Ali, H.; Harrison, G.; Yeatts, K.; El Sadig, M.; Popkin, B.M. Nutrition transition in the United Arab Emirates. *Eur. J. Clin. Nutr.* **2011**, *65*, 1328–1337. [CrossRef]
26. Lee, P.H.; Macfarlane, D.J.; Lam, T.H.; Stewart, S.M. Validity of the international physical activity questionnaire short form (IPAQ-SF): A systematic review. *Int. J. Behav. Nutr. Phys. Act.* **2011**, *8*, 115. [CrossRef] [PubMed]
27. Pejtersen, J.H.; Kristensen, T.S.; Borg, V.; Bjorner, J.B. The second version of the Copenhagen Psychosocial Questionnaire. *Scand. J. Public Health* **2010**, *38*, 8–24. [CrossRef]
28. Wild, D.; Grove, A.; Martin, M.; Eremenco, S.; McElroy, S.; Verjee-Lorenz, A.; Erikson, P. Principles of good practice for the translation and cultural adaptation process for patient-reported outcomes (PRO) measures: Report of the ISPOR task force for translation and cultural adaptation. *Value Health* **2005**, *8*, 94–104. [CrossRef] [PubMed]
29. Beaton, D.E.; Bombardier, C.; Guillemin, F.; Ferraz, M.B. Guidelines for the process of cross-cultural adaptation of self-report measures. *Spine* **2000**, *25*, 3186–3191. [CrossRef]
30. Osler, M.; Heitmann, B.L. The Validity of a Short Food Frequency Questionnaire and its Ability to Measure Changes in Food Intake: A Longitudinal Study. *Int. J. Epidemiol.* **1996**, *25*, 1023–1029. [CrossRef] [PubMed]
31. Cooper, R.; Al-Alami, U. Food consumption patterns of female undergraduate students in the United Arab Emirates. *West Afr. J. Med.* **2011**, *30*, 42–46. [CrossRef] [PubMed]
32. Musaiger, A.O.; Abuirmeileh, N.M. Food consumption patterns of adults in the United Arab Emirates. *J. R. Soc. Promot. Health* **1998**, *118*, 146–150. [CrossRef]
33. Streiner, D.L. Starting at the Beginning: An Introduction to Coefficient Alpha and Internal Consistency. *J. Personal. Assess.* **2003**, *80*, 99–103. [CrossRef]
34. Panagiotakos, D.B.; Pitsavos, C.; Stefanadis, C. Dietary patterns: A Mediterranean diet score and its relation to clinical and biological markers of cardiovascular disease risk. *Nutr. Metab. Cardiovasc. Dis.* **2006**, *16*, 559–568. [CrossRef]
35. Bhutani, S.; Cooper, J.A. COVID-19 related home confinement in adults: Weight gain risks and opportunities. *Obesity* **2020**. [CrossRef]
36. Di Renzo, L.; Gualtieri, P.; Pivari, F.; Soldati, L.; Attinà, A.; Cinelli, G.; Leggeri, C.; Caparello, G.; Barrea, L.; Scerbo, F.; et al. Eating habits and lifestyle changes during COVID-19 lockdown: An Italian survey. *J. Transl. Med.* **2020**, *18*, 229. [CrossRef] [PubMed]
37. Husain, W.; Ashkanani, F. Does COVID-19 Change Dietary Habits and Lifestyle Behaviours in Kuwait? *Environ. Health Prev. Med.* **2020**. [CrossRef] [PubMed]

38. ALMughamis, N.S.; AlAsfour, S.; Mehmood, S. Poor Eating Habits and Predictors of Weight Gain During the COVID-19 Quarantine Measures in Kuwait: A Cross Sectional Study. *Res. Sq.* **2020**. [CrossRef]
39. Moynihan, A.B.; Van Tilburg, W.A.; Igou, E.R.; Wisman, A.; Donnelly, A.E.; Mulcaire, J.B. Eaten up by boredom: Consuming food to escape awareness of the bored self. *Front. Psychol.* **2015**, *6*, 369. [CrossRef] [PubMed]
40. Gardner, B.; Rebar, A.L. Habit Formation and Behavior Change. In *Oxford Research Encyclopedia of Psychology*; Oxford University Press: Oxford, UK, 2019.
41. Mattioli, A.V.; Puviani, M.B.; Nasi, M.; Farinetti, A. COVID-19 pandemic: The effects of quarantine on cardiovascular risk. *Eur. J. Clin. Nutr.* **2020**. [CrossRef]
42. Sulaiman, N.; Elbadawi, S.; Hussein, A.; Abusnana, S.; Madani, A.; Mairghani, M.; Alawadi, F.; Sulaiman, A.; Zimmet, P.; Huse, O. Prevalence of overweight and obesity in United Arab Emirates Expatriates: The UAE national diabetes and lifestyle study. *Diabetol. Metab. Syndr.* **2017**, *9*, 88. [CrossRef]
43. Razzak, H.A.; El-Metwally, A.; Harbi, A.; Al-Shujairi, A.; Qawas, A. The prevalence and risk factors of obesity in the United Arab Emirates. *Saudi J. Obes.* **2017**, *5*, 57. [CrossRef]
44. Belal, A.M. Nutrition-related chronic diseases Epidemic in UAE: Can we stand to STOP it? *Sudan. J. Public Health* **2009**, *4*, 383–392.
45. Makansi, N.; Allison, P.; Awad, M.; Bedos, C. Fruit and vegetable intake among Emirati adolescents: A mixed methods study. *East. Mediterr. Health J.* **2018**, *24*. [CrossRef]
46. Díez, J.; Bilal, U.; Franco, M. Unique features of the Mediterranean food environment: Implications for the prevention of chronic diseases Rh: Mediterranean food environments. *Eur. J. Clin. Nutr.* **2019**, *72*, 71–75. [CrossRef]
47. Martínez-González, M.A.; Gea, A.; Ruiz-Canela, M. The Mediterranean diet and cardiovascular health: A critical review. *Circ. Res.* **2019**, *124*, 779–798. [CrossRef]
48. Becerra-Tomás, N.; Blanco Mejía, S.; Viguiliouk, E.; Khan, T.; Kendall, C.W.; Kahleova, H.; Rahelić, D.; Sievenpiper, J.L.; Salas-Salvadó, J. Mediterranean diet, cardiovascular disease and mortality in diabetes: A systematic review and meta-analysis of prospective cohort studies and randomized clinical trials. *Crit. Rev. Food Sci. Nutr.* **2020**, *60*, 1207–1227. [CrossRef] [PubMed]
49. Godos, J.; Zappala, G.; Bernardini, S.; Giambini, I.; Bes-Rastrollo, M.; Martinez-Gonzalez, M. Adherence to the Mediterranean diet is inversely associated with metabolic syndrome occurrence: A meta-analysis of observational studies. *Int. J. Food Sci. Nutr.* **2017**, *68*, 138–148. [CrossRef] [PubMed]
50. Germani, A.; Vitiello, V.; Giusti, A.M.; Pinto, A.; Donini, L.M.; del Balzo, V. Environmental and economic sustainability of the Mediterranean Diet. *Int. J. Food Sci. Nutr.* **2014**, *65*, 1008–1012. [CrossRef] [PubMed]
51. Giugliano, D.; Esposito, K. Mediterranean diet and metabolic diseases. *Curr. Opin. Lipidol.* **2008**, *19*, 63–68. [CrossRef] [PubMed]
52. Hassapidou, M.; Tziomalos, K.; Lazaridou, S.; Pagkalos, I.; Papadimitriou, K.; Kokkinopoulou, A.; Tzotzas, T. The Nutrition Health Alliance (NutriHeAl) Study: A Randomized, Controlled, Nutritional Intervention Based on Mediterranean Diet in Greek Municipalities. *J. Am. Coll. Nutr.* **2020**, *39*, 338–344. [CrossRef] [PubMed]
53. Sánchez-Villegas, A.; Bes-Rastrollo, M.; Martínez-González, M.A.; Serra-Majem, L. Adherence to a Mediterranean dietary pattern and weight gain in a follow-up study: The SUN cohort. *Int. J. Obes.* **2006**, *30*, 350–358. [CrossRef]
54. Serra-Majem, L.; Roman-Vinas, B.; Sanchez-Villegas, A.; Guasch-Ferre, M.; Corella, D.; La Vecchia, C. Benefits of the Mediterranean diet: Epidemiological and molecular aspects. *Mol. Asp. Med.* **2019**, *67*, 1–55. [CrossRef]
55. Martínez-González, M.A.; Salas-Salvadó, J.; Estruch, R.; Corella, D.; Fitó, M.; Ros, E. Benefits of the Mediterranean Diet: Insights From the PREDIMED Study. *Prog. Cardiovasc. Dis.* **2015**, *58*, 50–60. [CrossRef]
56. Turk-Adawi, K.; Sarrafzadegan, N.; Fadhil, I.; Taubert, K.; Sadeghi, M.; Wenger, N.K.; Tan, N.S.; Grace, S.L. Cardiovascular disease in the Eastern Mediterranean region: Epidemiology and risk factor burden. *Nat. Rev. Cardiol.* **2018**, *15*, 106–119. [CrossRef]
57. Mahmoud, I.; Sulaiman, N. Dyslipidaemia prevalence and associated risk factors in the United Arab Emirates: A population-based study. *BMJ Open* **2019**, *9*, e031969. [CrossRef]
58. Taha, Z.; Eltom, S.E. The Role of Diet and Lifestyle in Women with Breast Cancer: An Update Review of Related Research in the Middle East. *Biores. Open Access* **2018**, *7*, 73–80. [CrossRef] [PubMed]

59. Musaiger, A.O.; Al-Hazzaa, H.M. Prevalence and risk factors associated with nutrition-related noncommunicable diseases in the Eastern Mediterranean region. *Int. J. Gen. Med.* **2012**, *5*, 199–217. [CrossRef]
60. Galal, O. Nutrition-related health patterns in the Middle East. *Asia Pac. J. Clin. Nutr.* **2003**, *12*, 337–343.
61. Gombart, A.F.; Pierre, A.; Maggini, S. A review of micronutrients and the immune System–Working in harmony to reduce the risk of infection. *Nutrients* **2020**, *12*, 236. [CrossRef] [PubMed]
62. Ipsos. 5 Ways COVID-19 Has Impacted MENA's Food Habits. Available online: https://www.ipsos.com/sites/default/files/ct/news/documents/2020-06/5_ways_covid-19_impacted_menas_food_habits_-_ipsos_mena_0.pdf (accessed on 16 August 2020).
63. Ammar, A.; Brach, M.; Trabelsi, K.; Chtourou, H.; Boukhris, O.; Masmoudi, L.; Bouaziz, B.; Bentlage, E.; How, D.; Ahmed, M. Effects of COVID-19 home confinement on physical activity and eating behaviour Preliminary results of the ECLB-COVID19 international online-survey. *medRxiv* **2020**. [CrossRef]
64. Abbas, A.M.; Fathy, S.K.; Fawzy, A.T.; Salem, A.S.; Shawky, M.S. The mutual effects of COVID-19 and obesity. *Obes. Med.* **2020**. [CrossRef] [PubMed]
65. Burtscher, J.; Burtscher, M.; Millet, G.P. (Indoor) isolation, stress and physical inactivity: Vicious circles accelerated by Covid-19? *Scand. J. Med. Sci. Sports* **2020**. [CrossRef]
66. Jiménez-Pavón, D.; Carbonell-Baeza, A.; Lavie, C.J. Physical exercise as therapy to fight against the mental and physical consequences of COVID-19 quarantine: Special focus in older people. *Prog. Cardiovasc. Dis.* **2020**. [CrossRef] [PubMed]
67. Czosnek, L.; Lederman, O.; Cormie, P.; Zopf, E.; Stubbs, B.; Rosenbaum, S. Health benefits, safety and cost of physical activity interventions for mental health conditions: A meta-review to inform translation efforts. *Ment. Health Phys. Act.* **2019**, *16*, 140–151. [CrossRef]
68. Shigemura, J.; Ursano, R.J.; Morganstein, J.C.; Kurosawa, M.; Benedek, D.M. Public responses to the novel 2019 coronavirus (2019-nCoV) in Japan: Mental health consequences and target populations. *Psychiatry Clin. Neurosci.* **2020**, *74*, 281–282. [CrossRef] [PubMed]
69. Wang, C.; Pan, R.; Wan, X.; Tan, Y.; Xu, L.; Ho, C.S.; Ho, R.C. Immediate psychological responses and associated factors during the initial stage of the 2019 coronavirus disease (COVID-19) epidemic among the general population in China. *Int. J. Environ. Res. Public Health* **2020**, *17*, 1729. [CrossRef]
70. Zandifar, A.; Badrfam, R. Iranian mental health during the COVID-19 epidemic. *Asian J. Psychiatry* **2020**, *51*. [CrossRef] [PubMed]
71. World Health Organization. *Mental Health and Psychosocial Considerations during the COVID-19 Outbreak, 18 March 2020*; World Health Organization: Geneva, Switzerland, 2020.
72. Cinelli, M.; Quattrociocchi, W.; Galeazzi, A.; Valensise, C.M.; Brugnoli, E.; Schmidt, A.L.; Zola, P.; Zollo, F.; Scala, A. The covid-19 social media infodemic. *arXiv* **2020**, arXiv:2003.05004. [CrossRef] [PubMed]
73. Gao, J.; Zheng, P.; Jia, Y.; Chen, H.; Mao, Y.; Chen, S.; Wang, Y.; Fu, H.; Dai, J. Mental health problems and social media exposure during COVID-19 outbreak. *PLoS ONE* **2020**, *15*, e0231924. [CrossRef]
74. Xiao, H.; Zhang, Y.; Kong, D.; Li, S.; Yang, N. The effects of social support on sleep quality of medical staff treating patients with coronavirus disease 2019 (COVID-19) in January and February 2020 in China. *Med. Sci. Monit. Int. Med. J. Exp. Clin. Res.* **2020**, *26*, e923549. [CrossRef]
75. Zhou, X.; Snoswell, C.L.; Harding, L.E.; Bambling, M.; Edirippulige, S.; Bai, X.; Smith, A.C. The role of telehealth in reducing the mental health burden from COVID-19. *Telemed. e-Health* **2020**, *26*, 377–379. [CrossRef]
76. Rosato, V.; Temple, N.J.; La Vecchia, C.; Castellan, G.; Tavani, A.; Guercio, V. Mediterranean diet and cardiovascular disease: A systematic review and meta-analysis of observational studies. *Eur. J. Nutr.* **2019**, *58*, 173–191. [CrossRef]
77. Salvatore, F.P.; Relja, A.; Filipčić, I.Š.; Polašek, O.; Kolčić, I. Mediterranean diet and mental distress:"10,001 Dalmatians" study. *Br. Food J.* **2019**, *121*, 1314–1326. [CrossRef]
78. Godos, J.; Ferri, R.; Caraci, F.; Cosentino, F.I.I.; Castellano, S.; Galvano, F.; Grosso, G. Adherence to the mediterranean diet is associated with better sleep quality in Italian adults. *Nutrients* **2019**, *11*, 976. [CrossRef]

79. Muñoz, M.A.; Fíto, M.; Marrugat, J.; Covas, M.I.; Schröder, H. Adherence to the Mediterranean diet is associated with better mental and physical health. *Br. J. Nutr.* **2008**, *101*, 1821–1827. [CrossRef]
80. Smith, G. *Does Gender Influence Online Survey Participation: A Record-Linkage Analysis of University Faculty Online Survey Response Behavior*; ERIC Document Reproduction Service No. ED 501717; San Jose State University, ScholarWorks: San Jose, CA, USA, 2008.

nutrients

MDPI

Article

Adherence to Mediterranean Diet and Selected Lifestyle Elements among Young Women with Type 1 Diabetes Mellitus from Northeast Poland: A Case-Control COVID-19 Survey

Monika Grabia †, Anna Puścion-Jakubik †, Renata Markiewicz-Żukowska *, Joanna Bielecka, Anita Mielech, Patryk Nowakowski and Katarzyna Socha

Department of Bromatology, Faculty of Pharmacy with the Division of Laboratory Medicine, Medical University of Białystok, Mickiewicza 2D Street, 15-222 Białystok, Poland; monika.grabia@umb.edu.pl (M.G.); anna.puscion-jakubik@umb.edu.pl (A.P.-J.); joanna.bielecka@umb.edu.pl (J.B.); anita.mielech@umb.edu.pl (A.M.); patryk.nowakowski@umb.edu.pl (P.N.); katarzyna.socha@umb.edu.pl (K.S.)
* Correspondence: renmar@poczta.onet.pl; Tel.: +48-85-748-5469
† These authors contributed equally to this work.

Abstract: An appropriate balanced diet and dietary patterns are important at every stage of life, but in the case of young patients with type 1 diabetes mellitus (T1DM), it is especially crucial during the COVID-19 pandemic. The aim of the study was to assess health and nutritional behaviors, mainly adherence to the Mediterranean diet (MD), during the second wave of the COVID-19 pandemic in Poland among women with T1DM, and to compare them with a healthy population. This survey (based on a questionnaire) was conducted in December 2020 and included 219 young women, healthy (n = 106) and with T1DM (n = 113), from northeast Poland. Over 30% of the study group admitted that they did not engage in any physical activity. A large proportion declared that their screen time was 5–7 h a day (48% in control and 40% in T1DM group). High intakes of sweet-beverages, sweets and red meat, but also low intakes of olive oil, fish and nuts were observed. The vast majority of participants (60% vs. 71%) were moderately adherent to the Mediterranean Diet Adherence Screener (MEDAS). The study demonstrated that despite the similarity between the behaviors of healthy people and those with T1DM, negative health and nutritional practices, such as low physical activity, long screen time, medium and high levels of stress and inappropriate eating habits were observed.

Keywords: diabetes mellitus; Mediterranean diet; COVID-19; dietary pattern; metabolic disease; women; nutritional habits; health behaviors; lifestyle; obesity

Citation: Grabia, M.; Puścion-Jakubik, A.; Markiewicz-Żukowska, R.; Bielecka, J.; Mielech, A.; Nowakowski, P.; Socha, K. Adherence to Mediterranean Diet and Selected Lifestyle Elements among Young Women with Type 1 Diabetes Mellitus from Northeast Poland: A Case-Control COVID-19 Survey. *Nutrients* **2021**, *13*, 1173. https://doi.org/10.3390/nu13041173

Academic Editors: Michael Chourdakis and Emmanuella Magriplis

Received: 16 March 2021
Accepted: 31 March 2021
Published: 2 April 2021

1. Introduction

Type 1 diabetes mellitus (T1DM) is an insulin-dependent, multifactorial autoimmune disease, which results in degradation of the beta cells of the islets of Langerhans, which causes impaired insulin production and secretion. The treatment method consists of functional intensive insulin therapy delivered by multiple daily injections (MDIs) using an insulin pen, or a device called personal insulin pump, enabling continuous subcutaneous insulin infusion (CSII), which better mimics the physiological rhythm of insulin secretion [1].

COVID-19 (coronavirus disease 2019) is an acute infectious respiratory disease caused by the SARS-CoV-2 virus (severe acute respiratory syndrome coronavirus). It was first recognized and described in November 2019 in central China (Hubei province). It is considered that the origin of this virus was a seafood market where other animals such as snakes, frogs and bats were also sold. The genome of SARS-CoV-2 is known to be similar to the bat coronavirus and one unrecognized coronavirus, probably the pangolin coronavirus [2].

The Mediterranean diet (MD) is a dietary pattern, the benefits of which are supported by a large body of scientific evidence that highlights the potential health benefits of adherence. Nowadays, the MD pattern should be considered not only from a nutritional perspective but also in the light of environmental, economic as well as sociocultural factors. MD is related to a lower risk of developing several chronic diseases, such as type 2 diabetes mellitus (T2DM), heart disease and cancer [3,4]. MD has also been shown to improve cognitive functions [5]. The recently updated MD model highlights the need for a sustainable approach to this diet, with special emphasis on decreased consumption of meat, high fat dairy products and processed foods, and increased intake of locally grown fruits, vegetables, legumes, olive oil, whole grains and nuts. Fish, poultry and red wine should be consumed in moderate amounts. Moreover, the MD may provide considerable amounts of antioxidants, polyphenols, carotenoids (such as lycopene and β-carotene), as well as dietary fiber [3,4,6,7]. Also, because of the high consumption of olive oil, especially extra virgin and nuts, it is rich in monounsaturated and polyunsaturated fatty acids. Many studies have linked their high consumption with an improvement in insulin sensitivity, blood lipid profile, and a reduction in systolic and diastolic blood pressure levels, in line with the standards of medical care established by the American Diabetes Association [7–9].

The aim of the study was to assess health and nutritional behaviors, mainly adherence to MD, during the second wave of the COVID-19 pandemic in Poland among women with T1DM, and to compare them with a healthy population. It was undertaken due to the fact that a number of studies have shown a beneficial effect of the MD in people with diabetes mellitus (DM). This is of particular importance in times of the COVID-19 pandemic. Our research is designed to identify the problem, the solution to which may be inclusion of preventive and educational programs aimed at rectifying possible unhealthy habits. Studies assessing health habits (mainly concerned glycemic management) during the COVID-19 pandemic in healthy people; there are few studies among people with DM, and even fewer among those with T1DM.

2. Materials and Methods

2.1. Participants

This case-control survey was conducted among 219 young Polish women. The study group consisted of 113 persons with T1DM (52% used MDIs and 48% used CSII) and the control group contained 106 healthy individuals. The median ages in T1DM and healthy groups were 22 and 25 years, respectively. The online survey was carried out in December 2020, during the peak of the second wave of the COVID-19 pandemic, through private groups on social media platforms. The main criterion for inclusion in the study group was young age (between 16 and 35 years) and residence in Warmian-Masurian or Podlaskie Voivodeships. Responses from participants residing abroad, a different type of DM than the type 1 and people who had ever tested positive for the new coronavirus have been rejected. At the same time, a survey was conducted among healthy volunteers who expressed their willingness to participate in our study. Each person was informed that the completed questionnaire was anonymous and confidential. The questionnaire could be completed only once and it was possible to withdraw from the survey at any given moment, then the answers were not saved. By completing and sending the questionnaire, respondents confirmed consent to participate in the study. No personal data were required. The study had obtained the consent of the Bioethical Commission of the Medical University of Bialystok No. R-I-002/587/2019.

2.2. Questionnaire

The initial part of the questionnaire included questions that allowed for a reliable selection of study participants, dividing them into groups. The questions concerned the existing diseases, duration of the T1DM and type of treatment, sex, age, place of residence. The body weight and height (self-reported) results were used to calculate the body mass index (BMI), which reflected the general nutritional status of the patient. It was calculated as: weight in kg divided by height in meters squared. In children and adolescents under 18 years of age, it is interpreted according to national standards, and the limits of underweight, overweight and obesity are defined as the 10th, 85th and 97th centiles, respectively [10]. For adults, the values established by the World Health Organization were applied: a person whose BMI is below 18.5 kg/m^2 is considered underweight, the normal value is 18.5–24.9 kg/m^2, whereas in overweight and obese persons the values are 25.0–29.9 kg/m^2 and over 30.0 kg/m^2, respectively [11]. The results of glycated hemoglobin (HbA1c) from the last 3 months (self-reported) were obtained in a laboratory at the request of the attending physician.

The next part of the survey included questions about lifestyle (sleep time, screen time, stress levels), physical activity and eating habits, including the Mediterranean Diet Adherence Screener (MEDAS), which consists of 14 questions about eating behaviors typical of a MD (Table 1). Each question could earn a point; the maximum number of points to be earned was 14. The responses were to refer to the last month preceding the completion of the questionnaire. Based on the total scores, participants were divided into three levels: low (score 0–5), medium (6–9 points) and high (≥10 points) MD adherence.

Table 1. Interpretation of Mediterranean Diet Adherence Screener.

Question	Answer: Yes [Points]	Answer: No [Points]
1. Is olive oil the major dietary fat in your diet?	1	0
2. Do you consume at least 4 tablespoons of vegetable oil every day?	1	0
3. Do you eat at least 2 servings (about 400 g) of vegetables every day?	1	0
4. Do you eat at least 3 servings (about 240 g) of fruit every day?	1	0
5. Do you eat less than 1 serving of red meat/other meat products every day?	1	0
6. Do you eat less than 1 serving of butter, margarine or cream every day?	1	0
7. Do you consume less than 1 serving of sweet or sugar-sweetened fizzy drinks every day?	1	0
8. Do you consume more than 3 glasses (approx. 400 mL) of wine per week per week?	1	0
9. Do you eat at least 3 servings (approx. 450 g) of legume seeds (peas, beans, broad beans, lentils, chickpeas) per week?	1	0
10. Do you eat at least 3 servings (approx. 300 g) of fish or seafood weekly?	1	0
11. Do you consume less than 3 servings of sweets (bought, homemade) weekly?	1	0
12. Do you eat at least 30 g of nuts per week?		
13. Do you choose chicken, turkey or rabbit instead of veal, pork or sausage?	1	0
14. Do you eat pasta, vegetable or rice dishes with garlic, tomatoes, leeks or onions more than twice a week?	1	0
TOTAL	14	0

Category: low (score 0–5), medium (6–9 points) and high (≥10 points) Mediterranean Diet adherence.

The entire questionnaire consisted of questions that had appeared in our previously published study and other authors' work [12,13]. Questions in foreign languages were translated into Polish and assessed by a native speaker of the Polish language in order to exclude any bias in the translation. The translated questionnaire was tested on a small sample of respondents in order to avoid formal and substantive errors.

2.3. Statistical Analysis

Statistical analysis of the results was performed using Statistica software (TIBCO Software Inc., Palo Alto, CA, USA). The Shapiro–Wilk test was applied to check the normal distribution of the variables. According to the test outcomes, Student's *t*-test (parametric variables), the Mann–Whitney U and Kruskal–Wallis ANOVA tests (non-parametric variables) were used. The Chi-square independence test evaluated the relationships between qualitative features. Before the survey, a required minimum sample size was estimated. It was useful for calculating the total participants of our study with a specified confidence interval (95%) and a maximum bias (10%). Values at $p < 0.05$ were considered statistically significant. The supplementary material contains additional characteristics of the most significant results divided according to variables (place of residence, age group).

3. Results

The characteristics of the groups are summarized in Table 2. The distribution of study participants according to insulin therapy was almost equal (52% MDIs vs. 48% CSII users). The majority of patients with T1DM had well-controlled diabetes (glycated hemoglobin —7%). Most of the study respondents (60%) had a normal BMI, 25% and 9%, respectively, were overweight or obese, while 6% were underweight. There were statistically significant differences in body weight and BMI between the healthy and the T1DM groups. People with T1DM had excess body weight and higher BMI more often than healthy persons. The same trend was noticed when the groups were distinguished according to the insulin therapy used. Additionally, in those using pens both parameters were higher compared to users of insulin pumps and healthy persons.

Table 2. Baseline characteristic of study groups.

Studied Parameters	T1DM			Healthy (n = 106)
	Total (n = 113)	CSII (n = 54)	MDIs (n = 59)	
Age (years)	25 (20–29)	21 (18–25)	28 (23–32)	22 (21–23)
Body weight (kg) A**, B*, C**	71 (61–79)	68 (61–78)	72 (62–80)	60 (56–68)
Height (cm)	170 (165–174)	170 (165–175)	169 (163–174)	168.5 (163–173)
Body mass index (kg/m^2) A**, C**	24.4 (21.6–27.7)	23.6 (21.7–27.0)	25.4 (22.4–28.4)	21.9 (19.6–24.1)
HbA1c (%) F	7.1 (6.5–8.0)	7.0 (6.6–7.8)	7.3 (6.4–8.2)	-
		Place of residence		
Village	15%	15%	15%	24%
City (≤150 k inhabitants)	29%	24%	32%	27%
City (150–250 k inhabitants)	27%	30%	25%	8%
City (≥250 k inhabitants)	29%	31%	27%	42%
		Duration of disease E**		
Up to 5 years	18%	28%	8%	-
5–10 years	26%	35%	17%	-
More than 10 years	56%	37%	75%	-
		Body Mass Index D**		
Underweight	5%	7%	3%	8%
Normal	50%	56%	45%	72%
Overweight	32%	32%	32%	17%
Obesity	13%	5%	20%	3%

Values are expressed as median, lower, and upper quartile (Me (Q1–Q3)) or percentage of respondents (%). Abbreviations: continuous subcutaneous insulin infusion (CSII), multiple daily injections (MDIs), number of respondents (n), type 1 diabetes mellitus (T1DM). A Statistically significant difference between the medians, T1DM vs. Healthy (the Mann–Whitney U test). Statistically significant difference between the medians: B CSII vs. MDIs, C MDIs vs. Healthy (the ANOVA Kruskal–Wallis test). Statistically significant dependence between variables: D T1DM vs. Healthy, E CSII vs. MDIs (the Chi-square test). F Results of the glycated hemoglobin (HbA1c) test were collected from 79% of respondents. * $p < 0.01$ and ** $p < 0.001$.

There was a significant dependence ($p < 0.01$) of the frequency of physical activity between the main groups (T1DM vs. healthy). The frequency of physical activity did not affect the type of insulin therapy used—31% of the study group admitted that they did not engage in any physical activity, 38% (39% of CSII and 37% of MDIs users) exercised once or twice a week, 25% (22% and 27%, respectively) exercised three to four times a week, while 6% (7% and 5%, respectively) more than five times a week. Comparing these results to the control group, it was respectively: 15%, 37%, 35% and 13%.

Figure 1 shows the type of physical activity chosen by all the study participants. At that time, the most popular pursuits, in both the healthy and TD1DM groups, were walking (over 80% and 40%, respectively) and home gymnastics (62% in control vs. 35% in T1DM group, $p < 0.001$).

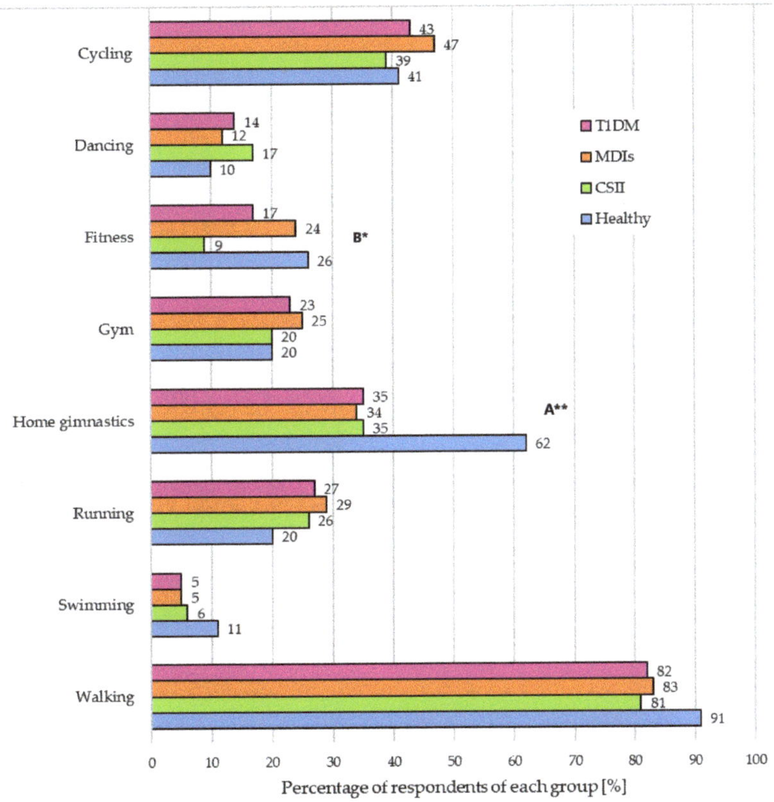

Figure 1. Type of physical activity chosen by study participants during the second wave of the COVID-19 pandemic. Abbreviations: continuous subcutaneous insulin infusion (CSII), multiple daily injections (MDIs), type 1 diabetes mellitus (T1DM). Statistically significant dependence between variables: ^{A} T1DM vs. Healthy, ^{B} CSI vs. MDIs (the Chi-square test), * $p < 0.05$ and ** $p < 0.001$.

Most respondents devoted 5–8 h per day to sleep: 73% of healthy and 46% T1DM persons (a similar percentage was found in both groups on insulin therapy). Over 8 h of sleep was declared by 23% and 46%, respectively (Table 3).

Almost one-third of the respondents in both groups replied that they spent 2–4 h a day in front of a computer or TV. However, in most cases the declared screen time was 5–7 h a day (48% in control and 40% in T1DM group) (Table 3).

Also, there was a characteristic variation in the number of meals for the T1DM group (Table 3). Statistically significantly ($p < 0.001$), people from this group ate more frequently (41% and 54% ate more than five meals or three to four meals a day, while in the group of healthy people it was 20% and 66%, respectively).

Table 3. Frequency of selected healthy behaviors.

Studied Parameters	T1DM			Healthy (n = 106)
	Total (n = 113)	CSII (n = 54)	MDIs (n = 59)	
		Sleep length [A**]		
<5 h	8%	8%	8%	4%
5–8 h	46%	46%	46%	73%
>8 h	46%	46%	46%	23%
		Screen time [B*]		
<2 h	10%	3%	17%	5%
2–4 h	26%	26%	27%	28%
5–7 h	40%	54%	27%	48%
≥8 h	24%	17%	29%	18%
		Number of meals [A**]		
1–2 times/day	5%	8%	3%	14%
3–4 times/day	54%	46%	61%	66%
≥5 times/day	41%	46%	36%	20%

Values are expressed as percentage of respondents (%). Abbreviations: continuous subcutaneous insulin infusion (CSII), multiple daily injections (MDIs), number of respondents (n), type 1 diabetes mellitus (T1DM). Statistically significant dependence between variables: [A] T1DM vs. Healthy, [B] CSII vs. MDIs (the Chi-square test), * $p < 0.01$ and ** $p < 0.001$.

Figure 2 shows stress level percentage distribution in the study cohort during the second wave of COVID-19. The vast majority (44%) declared that they experienced medium stress. Slightly fewer (32% of healthy people and 23% of diabetics) said they still felt highly stressed.

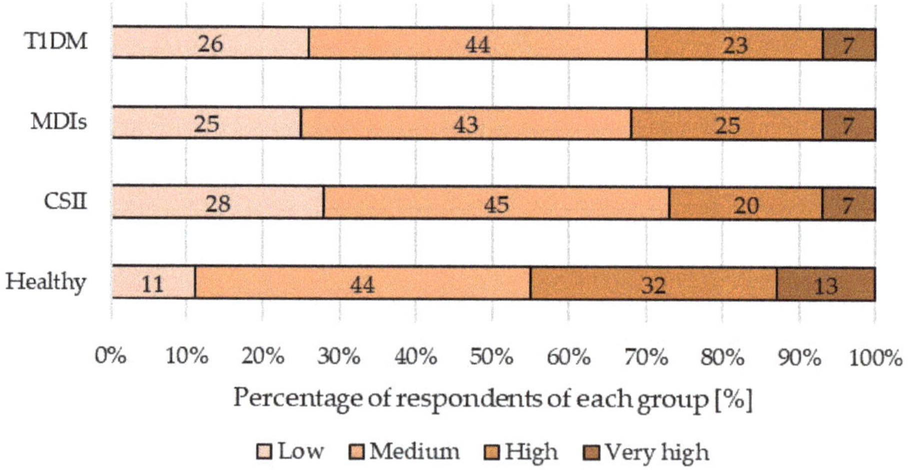

Figure 2. Stress level distribution of study cohort during the second wave of the COVID-19 pandemic. Abbreviations: continuous subcutaneous insulin infusion (CSII), multiple daily injections (MDIs), type 1 diabetes mellitus (T1DM). Statistically significant ($p < 0.001$) dependence between T1DM and healthy (the Chi-square test).

The respondents were asked whether they consumed a specific number of servings of a given product or group of products characteristic of the MD according to the MEDAS. Figure 3 presents the percentage of people who declared that they consumed this number of portions of a given food. Statistically significant differences between the responses in the main groups (healthy vs. T1DM) were observed for the servings of vegetables, olive oil, fruits, meat, butter/margarine/cream and fish/seafood consumed. There was also a significant relationship between subgroups using different types of insulin therapy (CSII vs. MDIs) as regards the amount of wine consumed (Figure 3). The vast majority were moderately adherent to MEDAS—60% of healthy and 71% of diabetics (Figure 4).

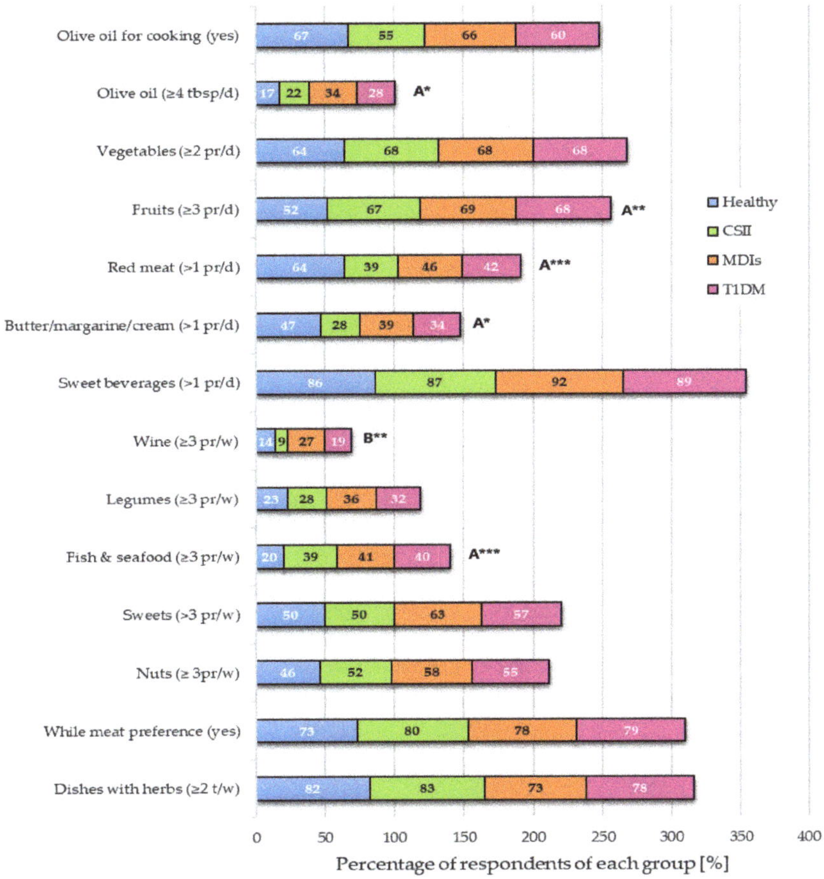

Figure 3. Percentage of respondents consuming certain portion sizes of product groups characteristic of the Mediterranean diet. Values are expressed as percentage of respondents (%). Abbreviations: continuous subcutaneous insulin infusion (CSII), multiple daily injections (MDIs), Mediterranean Diet Adherence Screener (MEDAS), Mediterranean Diet (MD), number of respondents (n), daily (d), weekly (w), portion (pr), tablespoon (tbsp), times (t), type 1 diabetes mellitus (T1DM). Statistically significant dependence between variables: [A] T1DM vs. Healthy, [B] CSII vs. MDIs (the Chi-square test), * $p < 0.05$, ** $p < 0.01$, *** $p < 0.001$. The size of portion: vegetables 200 g, sweet or beverages 200 mL, meat and fish 100–150 g, legumes 150 g, wine 125 mL, fruits 100 g, nuts 10 g, butter/margarine/cream 12 g.

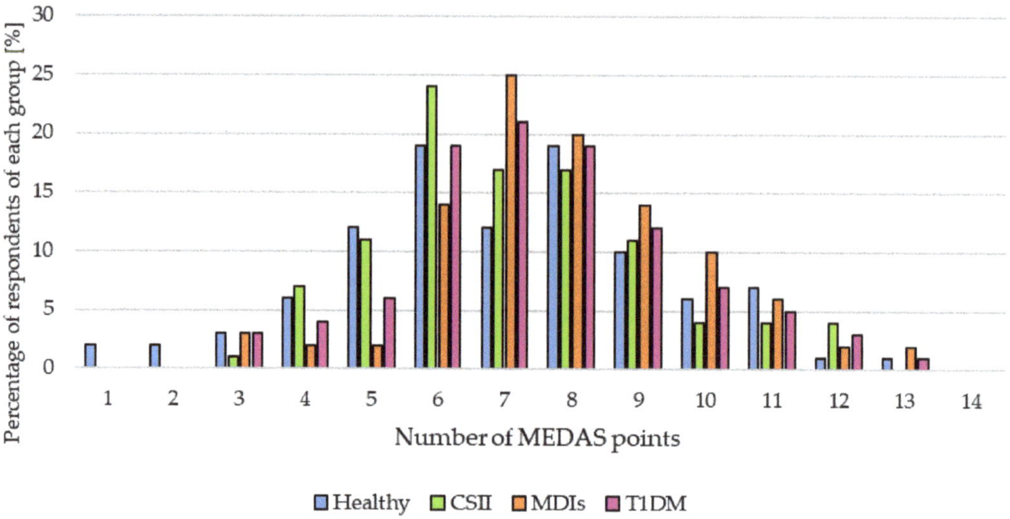

Figure 4. Adherence to the Mediterranean diet in the study cohort. Abbreviations: continuous subcutaneous insulin infusion (CSII), multiple daily injections (MDIs), Mediterranean Diet Adherence Screener (MEDAS), type 1 diabetes mellitus (T1DM).

It was observed that diabetic women in the group with high adherence to MEDAS, compared to women with low adherence to MEDAS, more often slept for more than 8 h (50% vs. 40%), spent less time in front of a TV or computer ($\geq$5 h of screen time: 49% vs. 87%) and consumed $\geq$5 meals a day (44% vs. 27%) (Table 4).

The above results (frequency of physical activity, number of meals, screen and sleep time and stress level) were divided into variables (place of residence, age group) and included in Supplementary Tables S1 and S2.

Table 4. Health behaviors depending on the Mediterranean Diet Adherence Screener (MEDAS) score category.

Studied Parameters	Low Medas (n = 41)				Medium Medas (n = 144)				High Medas (n = 34)			
	T1DM			Healthy (n = 26)	T1DM			Healthy (n = 64)	T1DM			Healthy (n = 16)
	Total (n = 15)	CSII (n = 11)	MDIs (n = 4)		Total (n = 80)	CSII (n = 37)	MDIs (n = 43)		Total (n = 18)	CSII (n = 6)	MDIs (n = 12)	
Weekly activity												
No activity	40%	46%	25%	35%	25%	24%	26%	9%	50%	50%	50%	6%
1–2 times/week	33%	27%	50%	31%	40%	46%	35%	41%	42%	17%	42%	31%
3–4 times/week	27%	27%	25%	27%	26%	20%	32%	36%	8%	33%	8%	44%
≥5 times/week	-	-	46%	7%	9%	10%	7%	14%	-	-	-	19%
Sleep length												
<5 h	60%	64%	50%	12%	8%	8%	7%	2%	17%	17%	17%	81%
5–8 h	-	-	-	81%	45%	41%	49%	67%	33%	50%	33%	-
>8 h	40%	36%	50%	7%	47%	51%	44%	31%	50%	33%	50%	19%
Screen time												
<2 h	-	-	-	12%	10%	2%	17%	2%	22%	17%	25%	12.5%
2–4 h	13%	9%	25%	15%	26%	22%	30%	34%	39%	83%	17%	25%
5–7 h	47%	55%	25%	58%	45%	62%	30%	44%	11%	-	17%	50%
≥8 h	40%	36%	50%	15%	19%	14%	23%	20%	28%	-	41%	12.5%
Stress level												
Low	47%	37%	75%	12%	25%	30%	21%	10%	39%	37%	75%	13%
Medium	20%	27%	-	42%	44%	49%	4%	45%	17%	27%	-	42%
High	13%	18%	-	19%	25%	16%	32%	34%	27%	18%	-	18%
Very high	20%	18%	25%	27%	6%	5%	7%	11%	17%	18%	25%	27%
Number of meals												
1–2 times/day	20%	18%	25%	19%	39%	5%	67%	14%	28%	67%	8%	6%
3–4 times/day	53%	55%	50%	54%	19%	41%	-	69%	28%	-	42%	75%
≥5 times/day	27%	27%	25%	27%	42%	54%	33%	17%	44%	33%	50%	19%

Values are expressed as percentage of respondents (%). Abbreviations: continuous subcutaneous insulin infusion (CSII), multiple daily injections (MDIs), Mediterranean Diet Adherence Screener (MEDAS), number of respondents (n), type 1 diabetes mellitus (T1DM). Category: low (score 0–5), medium (6–9 points), and high (≥10 points) Mediterranean Diet adherence.

4. Discussion

A properly balanced diet and appropriate dietary patterns are important at every stage of life, but in the case of young patients with T1DM, it is especially crucial since it can prevent or delay the symptoms of many diabetes-related conditions.

The survey was conducted in December 2020, and respondents were asked provide information regarding the previous month. The number of COVID-19 cases recorded in Poland on 1 November was 17,717, and on 23 December—12,358, which was the second peak of the pandemic [14].

Our study showed a high percentage of patients with T1DM who were overweight (32%) or obese (13%). Factors such as increased body weight, low physical activity, long screen time and exposure to stressful situations may lead to diabetic complications. Adherence to the MD has a crucial role in reducing the risk of health consequences.

The restrictions introduced due to the COVID-19 crisis affect various aspects of life. For instance, our research on a group of diabetics, assessing the health consequences of the first wave of the pandemic, showed that the body weight of 31% of respondents had increased by less than 5 kg, while in 11% of the cases—by more than 5 kg [12]. Another study conducted in Poland showed that during the first lockdown, 48.8% of overweight and 55.3% of obese people declared that they ate more, 55.3% and 61.7%, respectively, indicated that they ate more snacks, while 63.3% and 62.6%, respectively, said they cooked more [15]. The research conducted in this study, concerning the period of the second wave, showed BMI above the norm in as many as 45% of respondents with T1DM, which indicates a disturbing trend caused by restrictions on, for example, access to gyms. Research conducted among healthy population, during the first rise in COVID-19 incidence, also showed significant differences in the number of meals consumed. It was shown that during isolation there was an 11.2% increase in the percentage of people who ate five or more meals (from 19.9 to 31.1%) [16]. Being overweight or obese is an increasingly frequent risk factor among people with T1DM, not only in Poland, but also all over the world. It has been demonstrated that in Australia as many as 33% of adolescents under the age of 16 are overweight or obese, and among persons over 18 years of age: 38.3% and 17.2%, respectively [17,18]. Data from Sweden also indicate a large percentage of people over 18 years of age with excess body weight (35.1% of overweight people and 8.9% of obese people) [19]. Our study also showed significant differences in the number of meals consumed by healthy women and those with T1DM. Consumption of five or more meals was declared by 20% and 41%, respectively ($p < 0.001$). At its onset, the pandemic enforced certain social behaviors, such as excessive buying of food and hygiene products for the purpose of creating stocks. The resultant large amounts of products stored at home could be associated with excessive calorie consumption—it has been proven that the number of meals eaten at home increased by 38%. Stressful factors can trigger negative eating behavior, such as snacking between meals, leading to increased caloric value of the diet, and thus obesity [20].

Physical activity is another important element in the prevention of obesity and diabetes complications. Our previous study revealed that during the first wave of the COVID-19 pandemic, the percentage of respondents exercising one to two times a week had increased from 36% (before the pandemic) to 41%. On the other hand, the percentage of people exercising more often had decreased: three to four times a week—from 31% to 19%, more than five times a week—from 12% to 6%. The most common activities were walking and cycling [12]. Our current study found that walking was the physical activity that both people with T1DM (82%) and healthy ones (91%) chose most frequently. Patients with DM also chose cycling (43%) and exercising at home (35%). Regular physical activity improves, among others, sleep quality. There have been reports that during the lockdown period, physical activity, because of its numerous benefits, should be promoted in the same way as other public health related behaviors (including disinfection and distancing). Exercise can be a way to improve both physical and mental health [20,21].

Sleep duration was another factor that was analyzed. We showed that 46% of our respondents slept for more than 8 h—the differences between T1DM and healthy people were statistically significant ($p < 0.001$). Reduction of sleep time has been revealed to play a significant role in the pathogenesis of many chronic diseases. People have more flexibility as regards their sleep hours when they spend more time at home. Usually they fall asleep later and the quality of their sleep is worse: an increase in nocturnal awakenings is observed even when the length of nighttime rest is adequate. Sleep disorders may adversely affect homeostasis, consequently leading to disorders of mood, impaired well-being, worse eating habits, loss of motivation to take up physical activity, eventually resulting in hormonal disorders in obesity and DM [20,22–24].

As regards screen time, we have shown significant differences ($p < 0.01$) between patients with CSII and MDIs. It is a concern that as many as 40% of the diabetics involved in our study spent 5 to 7 h in front of a computer or TV, and 24%—8 h or more.

Stress is another factor that may exacerbate the course of many diseases, including T1DM, and trigger the development of long-term complications. The timing of the pandemic resulted in different patterns of coping with stress. Our previous research aiming to assess changes in social behavior among the DM population found that prior to the pandemic, none of the respondents had described their stress levels as 'very high'. At the beginning of the pandemic, the percentage of people who claimed to be highly stressed was around 32%, while during the study, 4% of respondents rated their stress levels as 'very high' and 17% as 'high' [12]. Our current results have revealed a tendency towards better control of negative emotions and greater capacity to learn to function in a changed reality. The highest percentage of people assessing their stress level as 'very high' was found among healthy people (13%), while among all diabetics, both in the CSII and MDIs groups, the figure was 7%. This may be due to the fact that having been exposed to stress for an extended period of time, they now perceive the new threats differently and are better equipped to face them.

None of the subjects included in our study received the maximum number of points on the MEDAS scale. The most frequent scores were the medium values: from six to nine. The highest percentage of people with MDIs obtained seven points (25%), while the highest percentage of patients with CSII: six points (24%). In the healthy group, 19% of respondents obtained six and eight points each, which proves the need for educational activities that must be carried out in the field of pro-health prophylaxis of patients with T1DM, but also among healthy people.

Metabolic syndrome (MetS) can be another consequence of an improper lifestyle, including inappropriate diet. The impact of cardiovascular disease (CVD) risk factors in adolescents with T1DM is not completely explained. Mayer-Davis et al. conducted a study on a group of 1198 diabetic patients at an average age of 14.83 $\pm$ 3.13 years. They showed that CVD risk factors were increased: blood pressure (incidence: 27%), obesity (21%) and high lipid level (18%). The authors concluded that there was little evidence that only a single factor underlay the pattern of CVD risk factors in adolescents with DM [25].

Vidal-Peracho et al. conducted a study to assess compliance with the MD among the inhabitants of Spain—also women with T1DM in the older age group (44.13 $\pm$ 12.0 years). The authors, similarly to our study, showed that the average index of the MD among those patients was medium (69%). Interestingly, among the subjects who strictly complied with the recommendations, women constituted a significantly lower percentage than men (22.4% vs. 30.2%). The smallest percentage of women (around 10%) did not follow the recommendation to drink more than seven servings of wine, while the largest proportion complied with the recommendation to use olive oil (around 90%) [26].

The specific components that should be present in the menu of patients following the MD are characterized by multidirectional prophylactic properties and have a positive effect on the parameters of the MetS.

In our study, 46% of healthy people, 52% of CSII and 58% of MDIs patients consumed more than three servings of nuts per week. Although for the majority of diabetic patients oil was the main fat (55% of CSII and 66% of MDIs users), only 22% and 34% of the respondents declared daily consumption of more than four tablespoons. It is worth emphasizing the statistically significant difference (17% vs. 28%, $p < 0.01$) in the frequency of consumption of olive oil between healthy people and those with T1DM. Studies by Grando-Casas et al. showed a positive tendency: patients with T1DM consumed significantly more fatty fish (36.2 vs. 29.2, $p = 0.009$) and nuts (14.7 vs. 9.0, $p = 0.011$) than healthy people [27]. The literature emphasizes the synergistic anti-inflammatory effect of nuts and olive oil, which helps to reduce the health consequences of diabetes. The consumption of fatty acids, including eicosapentaenoic acid (EPA) and docosahexaenoic acid (DHA), contributes to the reduction of inflammation and has cardioprotective action [28].

The main sources of dietary fiber in the MD are: whole grains, vegetables, fruits and nuts. In our study, consumption of three or more servings of legumes per week was reported by 28% of patients with CSII and 36% of patients with MDIs. Vegetables were consumed twice a day or more often by 68% of patients with CSII and MDIs, while fruit was eaten three or more times a day by a similar number of people: 67% of CSII and 69% of MDIs. In patients with T1DM, adherence to the guidelines of the MD has a beneficial effect on the intestinal microflora. This is an important mechanism because T1DM is an autoimmune disease. Proper microflora decreases the permeability of the intestines and modulates the immune system, whereas low consumption of fiber is related to the development of inflammatory diseases [29].

Products recommended by the MD, such as fruits (e.g., berries) and vegetables, are rich in polyphenolic compounds. Their supporting role is especially emphasized in the context of chronic diseases. Cocoa flavan-3-oils are associated with a reduction in the risk of insulin resistance, systemic inflammation, and DM, as well as improved lipid levels, endothelial blood flow, and blood pressure control. Resveratrol and quercetin also play an important part in cardiometabolic protection. Polyphenols can influence the composition of the intestinal microflora and can also be metabolized to bioactive compounds by intestinal bacteria [30]. The mechanism of action of polyphenols is based on inhibition of intestinal glucose absorption by sodium-dependent glucose transporter 1 (SGLT1), increasing insulin secretion and insulin-dependent glucose uptake, and decreasing hepatic glucose production [31]. There are also reports in the literature that it might be possible to treat DM with polyphenols influencing the AMP-activated protein kinase pathway [32].

We have observed high figures as regards to consumption of sweet beverages of more than one serving per day in 87% of diabetics with CSII and in 92% of diabetics with MDIs. Consuming less than three servings of sweets in a week was reported by 50% of the members of the CSII group and 47% of patients with MDIs. Granado-Casas et al. assessed the compliance with the MD recommendations among patients with T1DM and healthy subjects and showed that diabetic patients consumed significantly fewer sweets (17.4 g vs. 38.5 g, $p < 0.001$) [27]. Patients with insulin resistance and DM are aware of the health consequences of consuming sweet snacks, i.e., excessive body weight and increased insulin resistance, leading to glucotoxicity and accelerated apoptosis of B lymphocytes. Subsequently, immunogenicity is increased, and then symptomatic diabetes develops. In insulin resistance, there is an overload of β cells, which accelerates apoptosis and immune damage [33–36]. It has been shown that obesity and deteriorated self-management that occur in patients with T1DM are significantly associated with the risk of hospitalization for heart failure, as well as retinopathies and macrovascular diseases [17,19,37]. Obese people have three times higher incidence of low-cholesterol high-density lipoprotein (HDL-C) hypolipidemia and four times higher incidence of hypertension compared to normal body weight [38].

The recommendations of the MD include drinking good-quality red wine in moderate amounts. Valerio et al. assessed the relationship between alcohol consumption as well as cigarette smoking and CVD risk factors in adolescents with T1DM. It was shown that 10% of respondents consumed alcohol and smoked cigarettes. Adolescents who drank alcohol and smoked had higher triglyceride levels compared to those who did not (86.9 vs. 63.9 mg/dL, $p = 0.01$) and lower compliance to MD (6 vs. 7) [39].

Other authors who studied adherence to the MD recommendations among people with T1DM also assessed anthropometric and biochemical parameters. Fortin et al. conducted a 6-month nutritional intervention based on the use of an MD and a low-fat diet in patients with T1DM. Changes in anthropometric parameters were observed in the MD group: waist circumference decreased by 1.5 cm and BMI by 0.7 kg/m^2. There was also a reduction in systolic blood pressure (from 137 $\pm$ 20 to 134 $\pm$ 17 mmHg), diastolic blood pressure (from 79 $\pm$ 9 to 77 $\pm$ 10 mmHg), LDL-cholesterol (from 1.92 $\pm$ 0.67 to 1.81 $\pm$ 0.61 mmol/L) and triglycerides (from 1.14 $\pm$ 0.069 to 0.93 $\pm$ 0.44 mmol/L), but these differences were not statistically significant. The need for long-term use of the above-mentioned diet is emphasized in order to obtain greater improvement in parameters [40].

The study by Zhong et al. was designed to determine the relationship between adherence to the MD and glycemic control in adolescents (<20 years of age) with T1DM. It should be stressed that at the beginning of the study only 3% of the 793 participants obtained a high result (score $\geq$ 8) regarding the compliance with the MD, 46%—a medium (score from 4 to 7) result, and 51.5%—a low result. People with a high index of the quality of the MD had significantly lower total cholesterol compared to those with a low and medium index (143.6 vs. 161.6 and 157.7 mg/dL) and LDL cholesterol (77.1 vs. 95.5 and 91.8 mg/dL) [41].

One of the consequences of DM is cognitive impairment, especially in terms of verbal memory. Kössler et al. assessed the impact of adherence to the MD in patients with T1DM and T2DM. A beneficial effect on cognitive functions was found in patients with T2DM only, which requires further research [42].

Our study has several limitations. Being retrospective, like many studies from the COVID-19 pandemic period, we left it to the patients to estimate the portions consumed, and they may have been biased. Our survey was conducted only among the inhabitants of northeast Poland; therefore, subsequent studies should be based on a broader population sample from other regions of the country with a large number of cases. The study was conducted among women because they are willing to take part in various types of research far more often than men. Moreover, in Poland the percentage of young women with T1DM is much higher than that of men [43]. However, this can be considered an advantage of this study because we had a group that was homogeneous in terms of age and gender (only women) and resided in neighboring provinces, which provided an overview of a larger region—northeast Poland.

5. Conclusions

Despite the similarities between the behaviors of healthy people and those with T1DM, undesirable nutritional and health habits were observed during the second wave of the COVID-19 pandemic in both groups. The nutritional patterns of those groups were moderately consistent with the MD. Therefore, it is advisable to promote nutritional and health education in order to increase the awareness of the issue among healthy individuals and those with chronic diseases such as DM. The impact of the aforementioned interventions, with particular emphasis on the above results, would have a positive impact on behavior change, but also on improving treatment results. In the times of the COVID-19 pandemic, new guidelines should be developed based on, for example, the MD pyramid combined with local products.

Supplementary Materials: The following are available online at https://www.mdpi.com/article/10.3390/nu13041173/s1, Table S1. Health behaviors depending on the age group; Table S2. Health behaviors depending on the place of residence.

Author Contributions: Conceptualization, M.G., A.P.-J. and R.M.-Ż.; formal analysis, M.G.; investigation, M.G. and A.P.-J.; methodology, M.G., A.P.-J. and R.M.-Ż.; project administration, A.M. and P.N.; supervision, R.M.-Ż. and K.S.; validation, J.B.; visualization, M.G.; writing—original draft, M.G., A.P.-J. and R.M.-Ż.; writing—review and editing, M.G. and A.P.-J. All authors have read and agreed to the published version of the manuscript.

Funding: This research received no external funding.

Institutional Review Board Statement: The study was conducted according to the guidelines of the Declaration of Helsinki and approved by the Ethics Committee of the Medical University of Bialystok (R-I-002/587/2019).

Informed Consent Statement: Informed consent was obtained from all subjects involved in the study.

Data Availability Statement: The datasets generated and analyzed during the current study are available from the corresponding author on reasonable request.

Acknowledgments: The authors thank the participants of the study.

Conflicts of Interest: The authors declare no conflict of interest.

References

1. Alberti, K.G.; Zimmet, P.Z. Definition, diagnosis and classification of diabetes mellitus and its complications. Part 1: Diagnosis and classification of diabetes mellitus provisional report of a WHO consultation. *Diabet. Med.* **1998**, *15*, 539–553. [CrossRef]
2. Khan, M.; Adil, S.F.; Alkhathlan, H.Z.; Tahir, M.N.; Saif, S.; Khan, M.; Khan, S.T. COVID-19: A Global Challenge with Old History, Epidemiology and Progress So Far. *Molecules* **2021**, *26*, 39. [CrossRef] [PubMed]
3. Fernandez, M.L.; Raheem, D.; Ramos, F.; Carrascosa, C.; Saraiva, A.; Raposo, A. Highlights of Current Dietary Guidelines in Five Continents. *Int. J. Environ. Res. Public Health* **2021**, *18*, 2814. [CrossRef]
4. Serra-Majem, L.; Tomaino, L.; Dernini, S.; Berry, E.M.; Lairon, D.; de la Cruz, J.N.; Bach-Faig, A.; Donini, L.M.; Medina, F.-X.; Belahsen, R.; et al. Updating the Mediterranean Diet Pyramid towards Sustainability: Focus on Environmental Concerns. *Int. J. Environ. Res. Public Health* **2020**, *17*, 8758. [CrossRef]
5. Valls-Pedret, C.; Sala-Vila, A.; Serra-Mir, M.; Corella, D.; de la Torre, R.; Martínez-González, M.; Martínez-Lapiscina, E.H.; Fitó, M.; Pérez-Heras, A.; Salas-Salvadó, J.; et al. Mediterranean Diet and Age-Related Cognitive Decline: A Randomized Clinical Trial. *JAMA Intern. Med.* **2015**, *175*, 1094–1103. [CrossRef]
6. Franquesa, M.; Pujol-Busquets, G.; García-Fernández, E.; Rico, L.; Shamirian-Pulido, L.; Aguilar-Martínez, A.; Medina, F.X.; Serra-Majem, L.; Bach-Faig, A. Mediterranean Diet and Cardiodiabesity: A Systematic Review through Evidence-Based Answers to Key Clinical Questions. *Nutrients* **2019**, *11*, 655. [CrossRef]
7. Pérez-Martínez, P.; Mikhailidis, D.P.; Athyros, V.G.; Bullo, M.; Couture, P.; Covas, M.I.; de Koning, L.; Delgado-Lista, J.; Díaz-López, A.; Drevon, C.A.; et al. Lifestyle recommendations for the prevention and management of metabolic syndrome: An international panel recommendation. *Nutr. Rev.* **2017**, *75*, 307–326. [CrossRef]
8. Gaforio, J.J.; Visioli, F.; Alarcón-de-la-Lastra, C.; Castañer, O.; Delgado-Rodríguez, M.; Fitó, M.; Hernández, A.F.; Huertas, J.R.; Martínez-González, M.A.; Menendez, J.A.; et al. Virgin Olive Oil and Health: Summary of the III International Conference on Virgin Olive Oil and Health Consensus Report, JAEN (Spain) 2018. *Nutrients* **2019**, *11*, 2039. [CrossRef]
9. Comprehensive Medical Evaluation and Assessment of Comorbidities: Standards of Medical Care in Diabetes—2021. *Diabetes Care* **2021**, *44*, S40–S52. [CrossRef]
10. Kulaga, Z.; Litwin, M.; Tkaczyk, M.; Różdżyńska, A.; Barwicka, K.; Grajda, A.; Świąder, A.; Gurzkowska, B.; Napieralska, E.; Pan, H. The height-, weight-, and BMI-for-age of Polish school-aged children and adolescents relative to international and local growth references. *BMC Public Health* **2010**, *10*, 109. [CrossRef]
11. World Health Organisation. The problem of overweight and obesity. In *Obesity: Preventing and Managing the Global Epidemic*; World Health Organisation: Geneva, Switzerland, 2000; Volume 894, pp. 5–13.
12. Grabia, M.; Markiewicz-Żukowska, R.; Puścion-Jakubik, A.; Bielecka, J.; Nowakowski, P.; Gromkowska-Kępka, K.; Mielcarek, K.; Socha, K. The Nutritional and Health Effects of the COVID-19 Pandemic on Patients with Diabetes Mellitus. *Nutrients* **2020**, *12*, 3013. [CrossRef] [PubMed]
13. Di Renzo, L.; Gualtieri, P.; Pivari, F.; Soldati, L.; Attinà, A.; Cinelli, G.; Leggeri, C.; Caparello, G.; Barrea, L.; Scerbo, F.; et al. Eating habits and lifestyle changes during COVID-19 lockdown: An Italian survey. *J. Transl. Med.* **2020**, *18*, 229. [CrossRef] [PubMed]
14. Polish Ministry of Health. Available online: https://www.gov.pl/web/koronawirus/wykaz-zarazen-koronawirusem-sars-cov-2 (accessed on 14 March 2021).
15. Sidor, A.; Rzymski, P. Dietary Choices and Habits during COVID-19 Lockdown: Experience from Poland. *Nutrients* **2020**, *12*, 1657. [CrossRef] [PubMed]
16. Błaszczyk-Bębenek, E.; Jagielski, P.; Bolesławska, I.; Jagielska, A.; Nitsch-Osuch, A.; Kawalec, P. Nutrition Behaviors in Polish Adults before and during COVID-19 Lockdown. *Nutrients* **2020**, *12*, 3084. [CrossRef] [PubMed]
17. Price, S.A.; Gorelik, A.; Fourlanos, S.; Colman, P.G.; Wentworth, J.M. Obesity is associated with retinopathy and macrovascular disease in type 1 diabetes. *Obes. Res. Clin. Pract.* **2014**, *8*, e178–e182. [CrossRef]
18. Islam, S.T.; Abraham, A.; Donaghue, K.C.; Chan, A.K.; Lloyd, M.; Srinivasan, S.; Craig, M.E. Plateau of adiposity in Australian children diagnosed with Type 1 diabetes: A 20-year study. *Diabet. Med.* **2014**, *31*, 686–690. [CrossRef]

19. Vestberg, D.; Rosengren, A.; Olsson, M.; Gudbjörnsdottir, S.; Svensson, A.M.; Lind, M. Relationship between overweight and obesity with hospitalization for heart failure in 20,985 patients with type 1 diabetes: A population-based study from the Swedish National Diabetes Registry. *Diabetes Care* **2013**, *36*, 2857–2861. [CrossRef]
20. Arora, T.; Grey, I. Health behaviour changes during COVID-19 and the potential consequences: A mini-review. *J. Health Psychol.* **2020**, *25*, 1155–1163. [CrossRef]
21. Matias, T.; Dominski, F.H.; Marks, D.F. Human needs in COVID-19 isolation. *J. Health Psychol.* **2020**, *25*, 871–882. [CrossRef]
22. Von Ruesten, A.; Weikert, C.; Fietze, I.; Boeing, H. Association of sleep duration with chronic diseases in the European Prospective Investigation into Cancer and Nutrition (EPIC)-Potsdam study. *PLoS ONE* **2012**, *7*, e30972. [CrossRef]
23. Spiegel, K.; Knutson, K.; Leproult, R.; Tasali, E.; Van Cauter, E. Sleep loss: A novel risk factor for insulin resistance and Type 2 diabetes. *J. Appl. Physiol.* **2005**, *99*, 2008–2019. [CrossRef] [PubMed]
24. Spiegel, K.; Tasali, E.; Penev, P.; Van Cauter, E. Brief communication: Sleep curtailment in healthy young men is associated with decreased leptin levels, elevated ghrelin levels, and increased hunger and appetite. *Ann. Intern. Med.* **2004**, *141*, 846–850. [CrossRef] [PubMed]
25. Mayer-Davis, E.J.; Ma, B.; Lawson, A.; D'Agostino, R.B.; Liese, A.D.; Bell, R.A.; Dabelea, D.; Dolan, L.; Pettitt, D.J.; Rodriguez, B.L.; et al. Cardiovascular disease risk factors in youth with type 1 and type 2 diabetes: Implications of a factor analysis of clustering. *Metab. Syndr. Relat. Disord.* **2009**, *7*, 89–95. [CrossRef] [PubMed]
26. Vidal-Peracho, C.; Tricás-Moreno, J.M.; Lucha-López, A.C.; Lucha-López, M.O.; Camuñas-Pescador, A.C.; Caverni-Muñoz, A.; Fanlo-Mazas, P. Adherence to Mediterranean Diet Pattern among Spanish Adults Attending a Medical Centre: Nondiabetic Subjects and Type 1 and 2 Diabetic Patients. *J. Diabetes Res.* **2017**, *2017*, 5957821. [CrossRef]
27. Granado-Casas, M.; Alcubierre, N.; Martín, M.; Real, J.; Ramírez-Morros, A.M.; Cuadrado, M.; Alonso, N.; Falguera, M.; Hernández, M.; Aguilera, E.; et al. Improved adherence to Mediterranean Diet in adults with type 1 diabetes mellitus. *Eur. J. Nutr.* **2019**, *58*, 2271–2279. [CrossRef]
28. Yang, B.; Shi, L.; Wang, A.M.; Shi, M.Q.; Li, Z.H.; Zhao, F.; Guo, X.J.; Li, D. Lowering Effects of n-3 Fatty Acid Supplements on Blood Pressure by Reducing Plasma Angiotensin II in Inner Mongolia Hypertensive Patients: A Double-Blind Randomized Controlled Trial. *J. Agric. Food Chem.* **2019**, *67*, 184–192. [CrossRef]
29. Calabrese, C.M.; Valentini, A.; Calabrese, G. Gut Microbiota and Type 1 Diabetes Mellitus: The Effect of Mediterranean Diet. *Front. Nutr.* **2021**, *7*. [CrossRef]
30. Fraga, C.G.; Croft, K.D.; Kennedy, D.O.; Tomás-Barberán, F.A. The effects of polyphenols and other bioactives on human health. *Food Funct.* **2019**, *10*, 514–528. [CrossRef]
31. Kim, Y.; Keogh, J.B.; Clifton, P.M. Polyphenols and Glycemic Control. *Nutrients* **2016**, *8*, 17. [CrossRef]
32. Momtaz, S.; Salek-Maghsoudi, A.; Abdolghaffari, A.H.; Jasemi, E.; Rezazadeh, S.; Hassani, S.; Ziaee, M.; Abdollahi, M.; Behzad, S.; Nabavi, S.M. Polyphenols targeting diabetes via the AMP-activated protein kinase pathway; future approach to drug discovery. *Crit. Rev. Clin. Lab. Sci.* **2019**, *56*, 472–492. [CrossRef] [PubMed]
33. Polsky, S.; Ellis, S.L. Obesity, insulin resistance, and type 1 diabetes mellitus. *Curr. Opin. Endocrinol. Diabetes Obes.* **2015**, *22*, 277–282. [CrossRef]
34. Wilkin, T.J. The accelerator hypothesis: Weight gain as the missing link between Type I and Type II diabetes. *Diabetologia* **2001**, *44*, 914–922. [CrossRef]
35. Islam, S.T.; Srinivasan, S.; Craig, M.E. Environmental determinants of type 1 diabetes: A role for overweight and insulin resistance. *J. Paediatr. Child Health* **2014**, *50*, 874–879. [CrossRef] [PubMed]
36. Dahlquist, G. Can we slow the rising incidence of childhood-onset autoimmune diabetes? The overload hypothesis. *Diabetologia* **2006**, *49*, 20–24. [CrossRef]
37. Kaštelan, S.; Salopek Rabatić, J.; Tomić, M.; Gverović Antunica, A.; Ljubić, S.; Kaštelan, H.; Novak, B.; Orešković, D. Body Mass Index and Retinopathy in Type 1 Diabetic Patients. *Int. J. Endocrinol.* **2014**, *2014*, 387919. [CrossRef] [PubMed]
38. Pinhas-Hamiel, O.; Levek-Motola, N.; Kaidar, K.; Boyko, V.; Tisch, E.; Mazor-Aronovitch, K.; Graf-Barel, C.; Landau, Z.; Lerner-Geva, L.; Frumkin Ben-David, R. Prevalence of overweight, obesity and metabolic syndrome components in children, adolescents and young adults with type 1 diabetes mellitus. *Diabetes Metab. Res. Rev.* **2015**, *31*, 76–84. [CrossRef] [PubMed]
39. Valerio, G.; Mozzillo, E.; Zito, E.; Nitto, E.D.; Maltoni, G.; Marigliano, M.; Zucchini, S.; Maffeis, C.; Franzese, A. Alcohol consumption or cigarette smoking and cardiovascular disease risk in youth with type 1 diabetes. *Acta Diabetol.* **2019**, *56*, 1315–1321. [CrossRef]
40. Fortin, A.; Rabasa-Lhoret, R.; Lemieux, S.; Labonté, M.E.; Gingras, V. Comparison of a Mediterranean to a low-fat diet intervention in adults with type 1 diabetes and metabolic syndrome: A 6-month randomized trial. *Nutr. Metab. Cardiovasc. Dis.* **2018**, *28*, 1275–1284. [CrossRef] [PubMed]
41. Zhong, V.W.; Lamichhane, A.P.; Crandell, J.L.; Couch, S.C.; Liese, A.D.; The, N.S.; Tzeel, B.A.; Dabelea, D.; Lawrence, J.M.; Marcovina, S.M.; et al. Association of adherence to a Mediterranean diet with glycemic control and cardiovascular risk factors in youth with type I diabetes: The SEARCH Nutrition Ancillary Study. *Eur. J. Clin. Nutr.* **2016**, *70*, 802–807. [CrossRef]
42. Kössler, T.; Weber, K.S.; Wölwer, W.; Hoyer, A.; Strassburger, K.; Burkart, V.; Szendroedi, J.; Roden, M.; Müssig, K.; Roden, M.; et al. Associations between cognitive performance and Mediterranean dietary pattern in patients with type 1 or type 2 diabetes mellitus. *Nutr. Diabetes* **2020**, *10*, 10. [CrossRef]
43. Narodowy Fundusz Zdrowia. NFZ o Zdrowiu: Cukrzyca. Centrala Narodowego Funduszu Zdrowia. Available online: https://www.nfz.gov.pl/ (accessed on 5 October 2020).

nutrients

MDPI

Systematic Review

Impact of the Level of Adherence to Mediterranean Diet on the Parameters of Metabolic Syndrome: A Systematic Review and Meta-Analysis of Observational Studies

Dimitra Rafailia Bakaloudi †, Lydia Chrysoula †, Evangelia Kotzakioulafi, Xenophon Theodoridis and Michail Chourdakis *

Laboratory of Hygiene, Social & Preventive Medicine and Medical Statistics, School of Medicine, Faculty of Health Sciences, Aristotle University of Thessaloniki, 54124 Thessaloniki, Greece; dmpakalo@auth.gr (D.R.B.); chrysoulal@auth.gr (L.C.); evelinakotzak@hotmail.com (E.K.); xenophontheodoridis@gmail.com (X.T.)

* Correspondence: mhourd@gapps.auth.gr

† These authors contributed equally to this work.

Abstract: High adherence to the Mediterranean diet (MD) has been associated with a lower prevalence of Metabolic Syndrome (MetS). The present study aimed to investigate the impact of MD adherence on parameters of MetS. A systematic literature search was performed in PubMed, Cochrane Central Registry of Clinical Trials (CENTRAL), Scopus, EMBASE, Web of Science and Google Scholar databases. Observational studies that recorded adherence to MD and components/measures of the MetS, such as waist circumference (WC), blood pressure (BP), fasting blood glucose (FBG), high-density lipoprotein (HDL) cholesterol and triglycerides (TG), were included in this study. A total of 58 studies were included in our study. WC and TG were significantly lower in the high adherence MD group (SMD: −0.20, (95%CI: −0.40, −0.01), SMD: −0.27 (95%CI: −0.27, −0.11), respectively), while HDL cholesterol was significantly higher in the same group (SMD: −0.28 (95%CI: 0.07, 0.50). There was no difference in FBG and SBP among the two groups (SMD: −0.21 (95%CI: −0.54, 0.12) & SMD: −0.15 (95%CI: −0.38, 0.07), respectively). MD may have a positive impact on all parameters of MetS. However, further research is needed in this field.

Keywords: metabolic syndrome; Mediterranean diet adherence; Mediterranean dietary pattern

Citation: Bakaloudi, D.R.; Chrysoula, L.; Kotzakioulafi, E.; Theodoridis, X.; Chourdakis, M. Impact of the Level of Adherence to Mediterranean Diet on the Parameters of Metabolic Syndrome: A Systematic Review and Meta-Analysis of Observational Studies. *Nutrients* **2021**, *13*, 1514. https://doi.org/10.3390/nu13051514

Academic Editor: Dolores Corella

Received: 30 March 2021
Accepted: 28 April 2021
Published: 30 April 2021

1. Introduction

Metabolic Syndrome (MetS), also known as the syndrome X, belongs to the group of non-communicable diseases (NCDs) [1]. The prevalence of MetS has been closely related to socioeconomic factors, as well as lifestyle changes deriving from the impact of westernization on diet and health behavior [1]. Thereby, this transition has led to an increase in morbidity and mortality rates, forcing health systems to introduce more effective strategies so as to prevent the expansion of this epidemic [2]. According to the National Health and Nutrition Examination Survey (NHNES), the prevalence of MetS in US adults reached 34.2% during 2007–2012, with the highest rates observed in non-Hispanic white males and elderly >70 years of age [3]. A large analysis of cohort studies in European countries from 2000 to 2013 revealed that the prevalence of MetS ranged from 42.7%–78.2% for males and 24%–68.4% for females [4].

Metabolic syndrome has been characterized by health professionals and scientists as a cluster of predefined metabolic conditions, namely, hyperglycemia, dyslipidemia, hypertension and central obesity [5]. Chronic low-grade inflammation is considered another important risk factor present in the pathogenesis of MetS [6]. Increased adipose tissue and circulation of inflammatory mediators triggered by excess intake of specific micronutrients comprise the two primary components, which induce proinflammatory responses [6]. Consequently, MetS has been linked to not only the development but also to the progression of other NCDs, such as cardiovascular disease (CVD), type 2 diabetes mellitus (T2DM), chronic respiratory diseases, etc. [7,8]. More specifically, it has been demonstrated that metabolic syndrome can increase the risk of CVD and mortality by 78% [9].

Currently, the most popular criteria used for the diagnosis of the MetS come from three different organizations, the World Health Organization (WHO) [10], the National Cholesterol Education Program in Adult Treatment Panel III (NCEP-ATP III), established slightly different criteria for the identification of MetS, excluding insulin resistance and using waist circumference, which are the most commonly applied criteria in clinical practice [11], and the International Diabetes Federation (IDF) that has also published similar definitions with regards to the MetS, however, diagnosis relies mainly on central obesity [12]. A summary of the diagnostic criteria of MetS can be found in Table 1.

Table 1. Published definitions and criteria for the diagnoses of MetS by the WHO, NCEP-ATP III and IDF.

Organization	Criteria
WHO (1998) [10]	Impaired glucose intolerance or diabetes and insulin resistance *Two or more of the following risk markers:* • BP $\geq$ 160/90 mmHg • Serum TG concentration >150 mg/dL • HDL cholesterol concentration <35 mg/dL (males) and <39 mg/dL (females) • Abdominal obesity: waist to hip ratio >0.90 (males) and >0.85 • (females) and/or BMI > 30 kg/m^2 • Microalbuminuria $\geq$ 20 μg/min
NCEP-ATP III (2002) [11]	*Three or more of the following risk markers:* • Abdominal obesity: WC > 102 cm (males) and >88 cm (females) • Serum TG $\geq$ 150 mg/dL • HDL cholesterol <40 mg/dL (males) and <50 mg/dL (females) • BP $\geq$ 130/85 mmHg • FBG $\geq$ 110 mg/dL
IDF (2006) [12]	Central adiposity [a] *Plus two or more of the following markers* • FBG > 100 mg/dL or diagnosed diabetes • HDL cholesterol <40 mg/dL (males) and <50 mg/dL (females) or treatment for low HDL concentration • Serum TG > 150 mg/dL or treatment for hypertriglyceridemia • BP > 130/85 mmHg or treatment for hypertension

WHO: World Health Organization, NCEP-ATP III: National Cholesterol Education Program in Adult Treatment Panel III, IDF: International Diabetes Federation, HDL: High-Density Lipoprotein, TG: Triglycerides and FBG: Fasting Blood Glucose. [a] Ethnic-specific WC values: Europe $\geq$94 cm for males and $\geq$80 cm for females; South Asia and China $\geq$90 cm for males and $\geq$80 cm for females; Japan $\geq$85 cm for males and $\geq$90 cm for females.

Lifestyle modifications, focusing on dietary patterns and physical activity, may improve markers of MetS and further reduce the risk of development of NCDs [13]. Among various types of dietary treatments, there has been a great deal of evidence with regards to the potential benefits of the Mediterranean diet (MD) in the field of nutritional epidemiology [14]. The traditional MD can be characterized as a plant-based diet containing high amounts of monosaturated fats, omega-3 fatty acids, polyphenols, vitamins and antioxidants, and low amounts of saturated fats and ethanol. With respect to nutrient content, the MD provides approximately 35%–45% fats (of which about 20% derives from monounsaturated fatty acids (MUFAs), 5% from polyunsaturated fatty acids (PUFAs) and 9% from saturated fatty acids (SFAs)), 15% protein and 45% carbohydrates [15]. However, what makes the MD distinct from other dietary patterns is the presence of various food components, including unrefined cereals, legumes, fish, vegetables, fruit, nuts, moderate amounts of wine and, most importantly, olive oil, which is considered the traditional symbol of MD [16].

Over the years, different dietary index scores have been developed for assessing the degree of adherence to the MD [17]. These composite scores aim to measure overall dietary quality with the use of validated food frequency questionnaires (FFQs) [17,18]. Data obtained from FFQs are combined within specific groups, food combinations or nutrients found typically in the MD, in which a specific value is assigned based on a predefined calculation [19]. Ratings resulting from MD scores (MDSs) from all groups are often categorized as low, moderate or high, reflecting the adherence level to MD for each subject [17,18]. As there is no specific rule or consensus as to how the adherence level of different MDSs should be interpreted, low scores indicate poor adherence, whereas higher scores indicate good adherence to MD or otherwise described by the authors. In general, high adherence is the result of frequent consumption in adequate quantities of beneficial components, such as fruits, vegetables, legumes, fish, nuts, whole grain products and olive oil, whereas there is a low intake of alcohol, meat and SFA [20,21].

Several studies have revealed an inverse association between adherence to MD and risk of obesity, CVDs, T2DM as well as all-cause mortality [22–27]. The potential advantages relate to the synergic effect and mechanisms of specific nutrients that have a direct impact on all risk markers of MetS, namely, WC, HDL, TG, FBG, BP, as well as systemic inflammation [28]. Even though the positive impact of MD on risk and occurrence of MetS has been previously confirmed [29,30], there have not been any analyses evaluating how different levels of adherence to MD could favorably impact each parameter of MetS.

Therefore, the purpose of this study was to examine the impact of low and high adherence to MD on the parameters of MetS.

2. Materials and Methods

This study is a systematic review and a meta-analysis which was conducted according to the Meta-analyses Of Observational Studies in Epidemiology (MOOSE) statement (Supplementary File S1). The protocol of this systematic review and meta-analysis was submitted in the OSF platform (https://osf.io/n4ja8/ accessed on 5 March 2021).

2.1. Literature Search

A systematic literature search was conducted in the following electronic databases PubMed, EMBASE, Google Scholar, Scopus, Web of Science and Cochrane Central Registry of Clinical Trials (until 11 January 2021) in all fields option using the following search string: ("Mediterranean diet") AND (Adherence) for the PubMed database, which was modified accordingly for the other search engines (search terms and keywords of our search strategy can be found in Supplementary File S2). Additional relevant studies were searched by references screening of the articles retrieved.

2.2. Study Selection-Eligibility Criteria

Eligible studies for inclusion to systematic review were original observational studies that investigated the impact of MD adherence on three or more parameters of MetS (WC, HDL, TG, SBP and FBG), according to the revised criteria NCEP ATP III [11], in the adult population, using a validated tool or scoring algorithm. MDSs developed by Panagiotakos et al. [31], Sofi et al. [32] and Trichopoulou et al. [21], as well as the PREDIMED MD Adherence Screener (MEDAS) score [33], the short MDS produced by Martinez Gonzalez et al. [34] the serving MDS [35], the Mediterranean-Style Dietary Pattern Score (MSDPS) by Rumawas et al. [36], the MD quality index [37], the relative MD system [38], and modified versions of MDSs [39–49], were used in our included studies. A summary of the diagnostic criteria of MetS can be found in Table 1. Studies that were not published as original papers (e.g., abstracts, conference papers, editorials and commentaries, etc.) were excluded. Additionally, manuscripts that did not provide adequate data regarding low and high adherence to MD were also excluded from this analysis. Only studies in English and Spanish language were part of our review.

2.3. Data Extraction

Records of our search results were imported into a reference management software (Endnote X9 for windows-by Clarivate Analytics USA) and two reviewers (LC, DB), after the removal of duplicates, assessed the studies for eligibility. Any disagreements were solved by a third reviewer (EK). Data extraction was performed independently by the above-mentioned two reviewers using a pre-specified standardized Microsoft® excel form and was checked for accuracy by a third reviewer (EK). In cases of missing data, corresponding authors were contacted by email in order to retrieve any additional data.

The primary outcome of our study was to investigate the impact of high adherence to MD compared to low adherence to MD on the five parameters of MetS according to the NCEP ATP III [11] revised criteria for diagnosis.

2.4. Quality Assessment of Included Studies

The quality of the eligible studies was assessed using the Newcastle Ottawa Scale (NOS) adjusted version for cross-sectional studies by two independent authors (LC and DB) [50]. Any disagreements that arose were solved by consensus and by the involvement of a third author (EK). Sensitivity analysis was further performed after the exclusion of low-quality studies (NOS < 7).

2.5. Statistical Analysis

Means and standard deviations (SD) from eligible studies reported high and low MD adherence for each parameter of MetS were used. Wherever it was necessary, and data were presented as median, minimum or maximum values or 95% confidence intervals (CI), conversion to mean and SD was performed [51–54]. When values of FBG, TG and HDL cholesterol were presented as mmol/L, conversion to mg/dL was employed using the Omni calculator [55]. The inverse variance method was used in order to estimate the weight of each study. The random effects model was used due to higher methodological heterogeneity among the included studies [56,57]. Moreover, Hedge's g was used as effect size and standardized mean difference (SMD) as a summary statistic model due to the heterogenous scores using in included studies for the definition of low and high adherence to MD [56]. Estimation of heterogeneity was performed with Cochrane Q test ($p < 0.1$: existence of heterogeneity) and I^2 statistic [56,57]. I^2 values >50% indicated substantial heterogeneity across studies. Publication bias was assessed with funnel plots and Egger's test [53]. All statistical analyses were performed using the R software developed at Bell Laboratories (formerly AT&T, now Lucent Technologies version 4.0.2).

3. Results

3.1. Search Results

A total of 9933 studies were identified through the literature search. After removing 3654 duplicates, 6279 studies were detailed screened for eligibility. The process of eligibility of our included studies can be found in the flow diagram in Figure 1. Not relevant to the topic examined studies, studies including population <18 years old, studies in which validated tool for assessment of MD were not used and in which the level of adherence was not clearly described were excluded. Overall, 58 studies were characterized as acceptable for the systematic review [39,40,43–47,49,58–107] and 41 for the meta-analysis [45–47,49,58–88,90–94]. Authors of studies in which data were not adequate for our systematic review or/and meta-analysis were contacted by email requesting supplemental data without any response received.

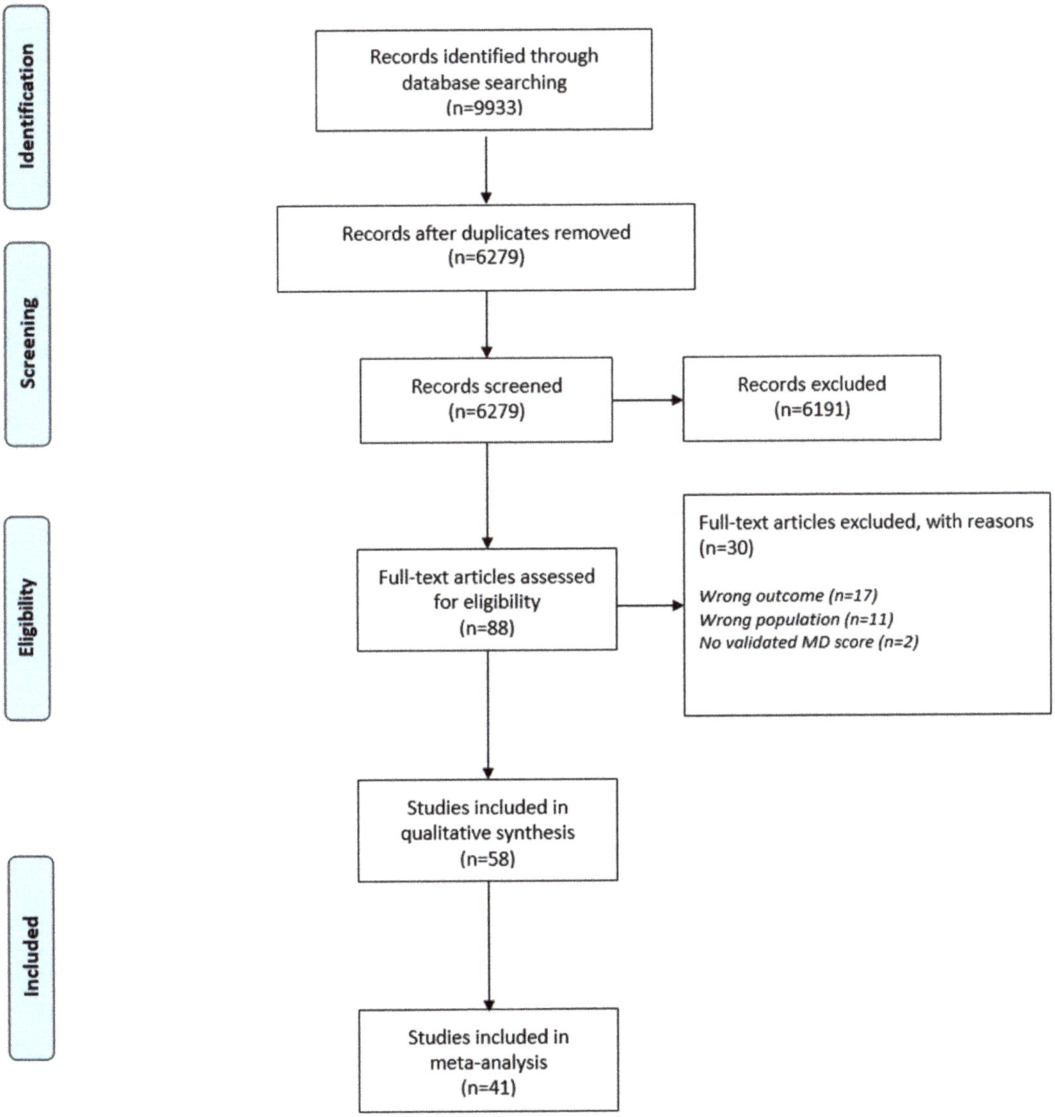

Figure 1. Flow diagram of the eligibility process of included studies.

3.2. Quality Assessment

The quality of the 58 included studies was examined according to the NOS [50]. Five studies were characterized as unsatisfactory due to their ratings (2–4 stars) [43,67,75,80,107], whereas for 17 studies the quality was only satisfactory (5–6 stars) [39,49,61,63,71,86,92–94,96, 97,100,104,105]. The majority of the included studies (n = 28) [40,44,45,47,58–60,62,65,68–70,72,74,76,77,79,81–85,87,88,95,101,103,106] were good quality studies (7–8 stars), and eight studies were at the top of quality studies scoring 9 stars [46,64,66,73,91,98,99,102]. More information regarding the assessment of quality according to the NOS can be found in Supplementary File S3.

3.3. Publication Bias

Funnel plots of studies included in our meta-analysis regarding each parameter of MetS can be found in Supplementary Figure S1a–e. Both the symmetry of funnel plots and Egger's test results confirm the absence of publication bias in all parameters of MetS except TG. Eggers's test results were $p = 0.8325$ referred to WC, $p = 0.2177$ referred to HDL, $p = 0.04598$ referred to TG, $p = 0.8533$ referred to SBP, and $p = 0.4677$ referred to FGL.

3.4. Study Characteristics

Characteristics of the included studies can be found in Table 2 for studies included in the systematic review and Table 3 for studies included in the meta-analysis, in which the country origin, the number, the mean age as well as the specific group of participants, and the MD assessment tool are included. In total, 74,058 adult subjects from all over the world (Australia, Chile, Finland, France, Greece, Iran, Italy, Korea, Morocco, The Netherlands, Poland, Spain, Sweden, Taiwan, Turkey, UK and USA) who followed an MD were examined.

3.5. Result on Components of MetS

3.5.1. Waist Circumference (WC)

In three studies in which OR of the prevalence of WC >102 cm for males and >88 cm for females was used as a measure of the effect, low odds for this outcome were observed in the groups of high adherence to MD [39,99,104]. Moreover, in the study by Mirmiran et al. [103], in which the incidence of abnormalities during 3 years follow-up was examined and expressed as OR, a lower incidence was found in the high adherence group, but this was not significant ($p > 0.05$). In Aridi et al. [95] and Mattei et al. [101], a significantly lower mean WC was found in the high adherence groups, as well as in 3 more studies [98,102,107] in which follow-up results were obtained. In Rumavas et al. [106], a significantly lower geometric mean of WC in the high adherence group was reported ($p < 0.001$), and in Steffen et al., the prevalence of subjects reporting an unhealthy WC was significantly lower in the high adherence group [44]. Only in one study, WC did not differ between the low and the high adherence group [40].

The meta-analysis results showed a lower WC in the low adherence group [SMD: −0.20, (95%CI: −0.40, −0.01)] with a high heterogeneity among studies ($I^2 = 95\%$) as presented in Figure 2. In order to explore the heterogeneity, a subgroup analysis of higher quality (NOS > 7) and lower quality (NOS < 7) studies was performed, which led to not significant results (SMD: −0.19 (95%CI: −0.48, 0.10)) and $I^2 = 96\%$ as can be seen in Supplementary Figure S2.

Table 2. Characteristics of studies included only in the systematic review.

Study ID (Country)	No of Participants (F/M)	Mean Age (Years)	Population	MD Assessment Tool	WC (cm)	HDL Cholesterol (mg/dL)	TG (mg/dL)	FBG (mg/dL)	SBP (mmHg)	Measure of Effect
Alvarez-Leon 2006 (Canary Islands) [39]	578 (329/249)	≥18 [1]	General population	Semi-quant FFQ 81 to calculate Specific food item score (10-item) [39]	L = 1 H = 0.77 [0.38–1.56]	L = 1 H = 0.90 [0.56–1.42]	L = 1 H = 1.05 [0.63–1.75]	L = 1 H = 2.46 [1.13–5.37] *	L = 1 H = 0.58 [0.34–0.99] *	OR [95%CI]
Aridi 2020 (Australia) [95]	3245 (1753/1492)	48.6 (17.6)	General population	Trichopoulou MDS [21]	L = 94.5 (14.7) H = 90.7 (13.3) *	L = 88.7% H= 89.9%	L = 83.1% H = 85.8%	L = 6.1% H = 5.7%	L = 123.6 (18.8) H = 122.1 (18.4)	Mean (SD)/ %Prevalence
Barnaba 2020 (Italy) [96]	349 (228/121)	18–86 [1]	General population	MD serving score [35]	No info	L + M = 52.2 (11.1) H = 52.2 (13.4)	L + M = 107.5 (54.4) H = 110 (43.42)	L + M = 98.1 (12.2) H = 103.5 (11.76)	No info	Mean (SD)
Huang 2013 (Sweden) [40]	187 (0/187)	70	Elderly population with CKD	Modified Trichopoulou MDS 14-item [21]	L = 97 (10) H = 97 (11)	L = 47 (14) H = 48 (14)	L = 127.8 (59.9) H = 122.2 (70.8)	L = 103 (20) H = 106 (28)	L = 149 (19) H = 148 (19)	Mean (SD)
Karayiannis 2017 (Greece) [97]	142 (0/142)	37.8 (5.4)	Subjects without systemic diseases, cryptorchidism or varicocele, microorchidism, vasectomy or hormonal treatment in the last six months	MDS by Panagiotakos 0–55 points [31]	No info	L = 49.4 (11.3) H = 50.4 (10.6)	L = 107.9 (39.3) H = 84.3 (27.1)	L = 89.6 (9.1) H = 86.4 (8.3)	No info	Mean (SD)
Kesse-Geyot 2013 (France) [98]	1881 (668/1213)	49.7 (6.2)	General population	Trichopoulou MDS—9 points [21]	L = 84.21 (0.9) H = 82.8 (0.96)	L = 58 (1.19) H = 58.8 (1.2)	L = 88.5 (35.4) H = 84.07 (2.65)	L = 90.7 (0.4) H = 90.4 (0.7)	L = 128.7 (1.4) H = 127.67 (1.42)	Mean (SD)
Kim 2018 (Korea) [99]	2349 (1159/1190)	19–65 [1]	General population	Modified MDS -9 points [41]	L = 1 H = 0.45 [0.31–0.66] *	L = 1 H = 0.89 [0.70–1.13] *	L = 1 H = 0.72 [0.55–0.94] *	L = 1 H = 0.83 [0.63–1.10] *	L = 1 H = 0.99 [0.74–1.34] *	OR
Mahdavi-Roshnan 2017 (Iran) [100]	344 (154/190)	L = 59.0 (8.30) H = 58.0 (9.36)	Subjects with CVD risk factors	PREDIMED MEDAS score -14 points [33]	No info	L = 42.81 (8.34) H = 43.3 (8.23)	L = 209.61 (399.33) H = 155.83 (87.63)	L = 116.4 (66.9) H = 105.9 (66.1)	No info	OR/ Mean (SD)
Mattei 2017 (US) [101]	1194 (No info)	L = 56.6 (7.9) H = 57.2 (7.7)	Subjects with no severe health conditions or cognitive impairments	Trichopoulou MDS—9 points [21]	L = 103 (14) H = 102 (13) *	L = 46.3 (12.5) H = 45.96 (12.3)	L = 163 (93) H = 165 (127)	L = 115 (53) H = 112 (36) *	L = 135 (19) H = 137 (20)	Mean (SD)
Mayr 2019 (Australia) [102]	37 (No info)	No info	Patients with coronary heart disease	PREDIMED MEDAS score 14—item [33]	L = 103.5 (3.4) H = 100.7 (3.3) *	L = 48.7 (6.5) H = 46.02 (6.1)	L = 102.75 (33.9) H = 115.15 (36.8)	L = 91.6 (13.40) H = 99 (13.30)	L = 136.5 (10.4) H = 133.4 (10.2)	Mean (SD)
Mirmiran 2015 (Iran) [103]	1683 (927/756)	L = 36.3 (13.3) H = 41.3 (13.8)	General population	Trichopoulou MDS—8 points [21]	L = 1 H = 0.74 [0.48–1.13]	L = 1 H = 0.82 [0.48–1.40] *	L = 1 H = 0.81 [0.56–1.17] *	L = 1 H = 1.01 [0.73–1.39]	L = 1 H = 0.86 [0.64–1.22]	OR
Mziwira 2015 (Morocco) [104]	90 (90/0)	39.9 (0.66)	General non-pregnant population	Specific MDS-0%–100% [42]	L = 1 H = 0.54 [0.13–2.27]	L = 1 H = 0.29 [0.02–3.02]	L = 1 H = 0.47 [0.04–4.94]	L = 1 H = 0.27 [0.05–1.49]	L = 1 H = 0.77 [0.19–3.15]	OR

Table 2. *Cont.*

Study ID (Country)	No of Participants (F/M)	Mean Age (Years)	Population	MD Assessment Tool	WC (cm)	HDL Cholesterol (mg/dL)	TG (mg/dL)	FBG (mg/dL)	SBP (mmHg)	Measure of Effect
Roldan 2019 (Spain) [105]	107 (58/49)	61.16 (23)	Overweight/Obese T2DM patients with poor glycemic control	PREDIMED MEDAS score—14 points [33]	No info	L = 48.29 H = 52.45 *	L = 223.56 H = 171.23 **	L = 201.14 H = 132.88 *	No info	Mean
Rumawas 2009 (US) [106]	1069 (608/461)	L = 52.4 (9.9) H = 54.8 (9.6)	Non-diabetic general population	The MSDPS—100 points [36]	L = 98.5 H = 97.1 **	L = 53.3 H = 54 *	L = 114 H = 103 **	L= 98.5 H = 97.1 *	L = 122 H = 121	Geometric mean
Steffen 2014 (US) [44]	865 (511/354)	L = 24.3 H = 25.7	General population	Modified Trichopoulou MDS—22 points [21]	L = 59.4% H = 41.9% **	L = 68.4% H = 59.3% *	L = 37.3% H = 21.6% **	L= 21.3% H = 19.1% *	L= 49.2% H = 40.4% *	%Prevalence
Tortosa 2007 (Spain) [107]	1040 (No info)	No info	Graduate students	Trichopoulou MDS—9 points [21]	L = 82.5 (12) H = 82 (12) *	L = 63.8 (15) H = 64.1 (19) *	L = 80.0 (38) H = 78 (40)	L = 86.1 (11) H = 87.3 (17)	L = 112.5 (14) H = 113.3 (13)	Mean (SD)
Yang 2014 (US) [43]	395 (0/395)	L = 38.2 (8.6) H = 37.1 (8.4)	General population	Study Specific MDS—42 points [43]	No info	L = 41.7 (1.3) H = 46.6 (1.3)	L = 140.4 (1.8) H = 115.8 (1.8)	L = 93.2 (1.2) H = 91.1 (1.2)	L = 122.4 (12.6) H = 122.8 (13.3)	Geometric mean (SD)

* $p < 0.05$, ** $p < 0.001$. [1]: Age range. Variables are displayed as mean (SD), OR [95% Confidence Interval]. CKD: Chronic Kidney Disease, F: Female, FBG: Fasting Blood Glucose, FFQ: Food Frequency Questionnaire, H: High Adherence, HDL: High-Density Lipoprotein, L: Low Adherence, M: Male, M: Moderate Adherence, MD: Mediterranean Diet, MEDAS: Mediterranean Diet Adherence Screener, MDS: Mediterranean Diet Score, MSDPS: Mediterranean-Style Dietary Pattern Score, OR: Odds Ratio, SBP: Systolic Blood Pressure, SD: Standard Deviation, T2DM: Type 2 Diabetes Mellitus, TG: Triglycerides and WC: Waist circumference.

Table 3. Characteristics of studies included in the meta-analysis.

Study ID (Country)	No Participants (F/M)	Age (Years)	Population	MD Assessment Tool
Abiemo 2013 (US) [45]	2440 (1305/1135)	L = 60.0 (10.3) H = 63.0 (10.3)	General population	Study Specific Alternate MDS—10 points [45]
Ahmad 2018 (US) [58]	16,623 (16,623/0)	L = 52.6 (6.7) H = 54.9 (8.1)	General population	Trichopoulou MDS—9 points [21]
Ahmed 2020 (US) [59]	224 (133/91)	L = 56.2 (12.6) H = 66.7 (11.6)	Community-dweling adults	Sofi MDS—12 points [32]
Asghari 2016 (Iran) [60]	622 (308/314)	L = 43.0 (9.1) H = 43.7 (9.7)	Subjects without CKD	Trichopoulou MDS—8 points [108]
Baratta 2017 (Italy) [61]	148 (47/101)	L = 51.7 (11.3) H = 57.7 (11.9)	Outpatients presenting with T2DM, HBP, Overweight/Obese, Dyslipedemia or MetS	Short MDS—9 points [34]
Bondia-Pons 2009 (Spain) [62]	70 (41/29)	47 (15.3)	General population	MD Quality Index—14 point % adherence [37]
Campanella 2020 (Italy) [63]	2387 (1183/1204)	L = 45.5(15.5) H = 54.6 (15.5)	General population	Relative MD system—18 points [38]
Dai 2008 (US) [64]	194 (0/194)	L = 53.8 (0.3) H = 54.8 (0.3)	Middle aged twins who have served in the Vietman War	Trichopoulou MDS—9 points [21]
Esposito 2009 (Italy) [65]	475 (232/243)	L = 58.0 (7.0) H = 58.3 (7.0)	T2DM patients	Trichopoulou MDS—9 points [21]
Gardener 2015 (US) [66]	543 (308/235)	L = 69.0 (8.0) H = 65.0 (9.0)	Population never diagnosed with stroke	Trichopoulou MDS—9 points [21]
Giraldi 2020 (Italy) [67]	209 (61/148)	L = 41.7 (13.3) H = 49.9 (16.4)	Patients with NAFLD	Sofi MDS—12 points [32]
Giugliano 2010a (Italy) [69]	315 (315/0)	L = 57.7 (6.7) H = 58.0 (6.8)	T2DM patients	Trichopoulou MDS—9 points [21]
Giugliano 2010b (Italy) [68]	288 (0/288)	L = 54.7 (6.9) H = 58.7 (7.0)	T2DM patients	Trichopoulou MDS- 9 points [21]
Granado-Casas 2020 (Spain) [70]	92 (52/40)	L = 41.9 (10.6) H = 45.1 (10.9)	T1DM patients	Trichopoulou MDS—9 points [21]

Table 3. *Cont.*

Study ID (Country)	No Participants (F/M)	Age (Years)	Population	MD Assessment Tool
Grosso 2015 (Poland) [46]	4678 (2408/2270)	45–69 *	General population	Modified Panagiotakos MDS—60 points [31]
Hu 2013 (Spain) [71]	7305 (4188/3117)	L = 67.2 (6.2) H = 67.0 (6.2)	Adults with high risk of CVD, with T2DM or at least 3/6 CVD risk factors	PREDIMED MEDAS Score—14 points [33]
Izadi 2016 (Iran) [72]	325 (325/0)	L = 28.0 (6.2) H = 27.2 (5.2)	Pregnant carrying singleton fetuses with/without GDM	Trichopoulou MDS—9 points [21]
Jalilpiran 2020 (Iran) [73]	357 (0/357)	L = 66.5 (6.7) H = 63.3 (5.8)	General population	Trichopoulou MDS—9 points [21]
Jayedi 2019 (Iran) [74]	131 (131/0)	L = 54.7 (6.8) H = 54.9 (7.5)	Females with prevalent T2DM or with history of 3–10 yrs T2DM and with/without DN	Trichopoulou MDS—9 points [21]
Köroğlu 2020 (Turkey) [75]	25 (0/25)	18–65 *	Patients with lower limb amputation	PREDIMED MEDAS Score—14 points [33]
Kwon 2020 (Korea) [76]	148 (84/64)	L = 43.6 (9.1) H = 53.3 (8.3)	General Population	PREDIMED MEDAS Score—14 points [33]
Lavados 2020 (Leu) [77]	368 (158/210)	L = 67.2 (18.7) H = 69.9 (16.9)	Patients with acute ischemic stroke	PREDIMED MEDAS Score—14 points [33]
Leu 2019 (Taiwan) [78]	1400 (807/593)	L = 48.4 (12.7) H = 50.6 (11.4)	General Population	Trichopoulou MDS—9 points [21]
Mateo-Gallego 2017 (Spain) [79]	1016 (54/962)	L = 50.9 (4.0) H = 51.7 (3.7)	Employees of car assembly plant	Trichopoulou MDS—9 points [21]
Molina-Leyva 2018 (Spain) [80]	25 (No info)	L = 43.7 (10.9) H = 50.8 (13.5)	Patients with psoriasis	PREDIMED MEDAS Score—14 points [33]
Moradi 2020 (Iran) [81]	153 (95/58)	L = 64.7 (9.3) H = 67.2 (9.8)	Diabetic patients with nephropathy	Trichopoulou MDS—9 points [21]
Mosconi 2014 (US) [82]	52 (37/15)	L = 53.0 (13) H = 55.0 (12)	Cognitive-normal individuals	Study Specific MDS—9 points [82]

Table 3. *Cont.*

Study ID (Country)	No Participants (F/M)	Age (Years)	Population	MD Assessment Tool
Park 2016 (US) [83]	1034 (572/462)	L = 40.8 (0.9) H = 40.8 (1.3)	Metabolicaly healthy and unhealthy obese population	Panagiotakos MDS—55 points [31]
Peñalvo 2015 (Spain) [84]	516 (18/498)	L = 50.8 (3.8) H = 51.5 (3.4)	General population	MEDAS Score [33] Alternative MD index [41]
Pocovi-Gerardino 2020 (Spain) [85]	159 (143/16)	L = 38.6 (9.7) H = 28.3 (12.8)	Patients with SLE	PREDIMED MEDAS Score—14 points [33]
Ruiz-Cabello 2016 (Spain) [86]	118 (118/0)	L = 52.0 (4.8) H = 52.9 (4.1)	Peri- and menopausal females	Panagiotakos MDS—55 points [31]
Salas-Huetos 2019 (Spain) [87]	57 (0/57)	L = 24.1 (4.5) H = 26.3 (4.8)	Healthy subjects	Trichopoulou MDS—9 points [21]
Sotos-Prieto 2014 (UK) [88]	10,359 (5593/4766)	L = 59.0 (9.4) H = 59.3 (9.3)	General population	Trichopoulou MDS—9 points [21]
Tuttolomondo 2015 (Italy) [89]	288 (162/126)	L = 72.9 (14.8) H = 72.4 (13.2)	Patients with ischemic heart disease	Trichopoulou MDS—9 points [21]
Tuttolomondo 2020 (Italy) [90]	409 (250/159)	L = 70.2 (12.6) H = 72.0 (10.4)	Patients with congestive heart failure	Trichopoulou MDS—9 points [21]
Tzima 2007 (Greece) [91]	1040 (333/707)	L = 55.0 (13) H = 35.0 (10)	Obese and Overweight population	Panagiotakos MDS—55 points [31]
Veglia 2019 (Finland, Sweden, Netherlands, France, Italy) [47]	1835 (980/855)	L = 64.8 (5.4) H = 63.9 (5.7)	Patients with >3 vascular risk factors	Study Specific MDS—7 points [47]
Veissi 2016 (Iran) [92]	157 (104/53)	L = 54.3 (9.9) H = 54.6 (8.9)	T2DM patients	Study Specific MDS—4 points [92]
Viscogliosi 2013 (Italy) [93]	55 (33/22)	L = 59.6 (10.2) H = 60.0 (9.4)	High CVD risk population	PREDIMED MEDAS Score—14 points [33]
Vitale 2018 (Italy) [49]	1539 (606/933)	No info	T2DM patients with HbA1c 7%–9%	Modified Trichopoulou MDS—18 points [21]
Zupo 2020 (Italy) [94]	324 (228/96)	L = 38.0 (13.1) H = 42.5 (13.1)	General population	PREDIMED MEDAS Score—14 points [33]

* Age range. Variables are displayed as mean (SD). CKD: Chronic Kidney Disease, CVD: Cardiovascular Diseases, DN: Diabetic Nephropathy, F: Female, GDM: Gestational Diabetes Mellitus, H: High Adherence, HBP: High Blood Pressure, L: Low Adherence: M: Male, MDS: Mediterranean Diet Score, MEDAS: Mediterranean Diet Adherence Screener, MetS: Metabolic Syndrome, NAFLD: Non-Alcoholic Fatty Liver Disease, SLE: Systemic Lupus Erythematosus, T1DM: Type 1 Diabetes Mellitus and T2DM: Type 2 Diabetes Mellitus.

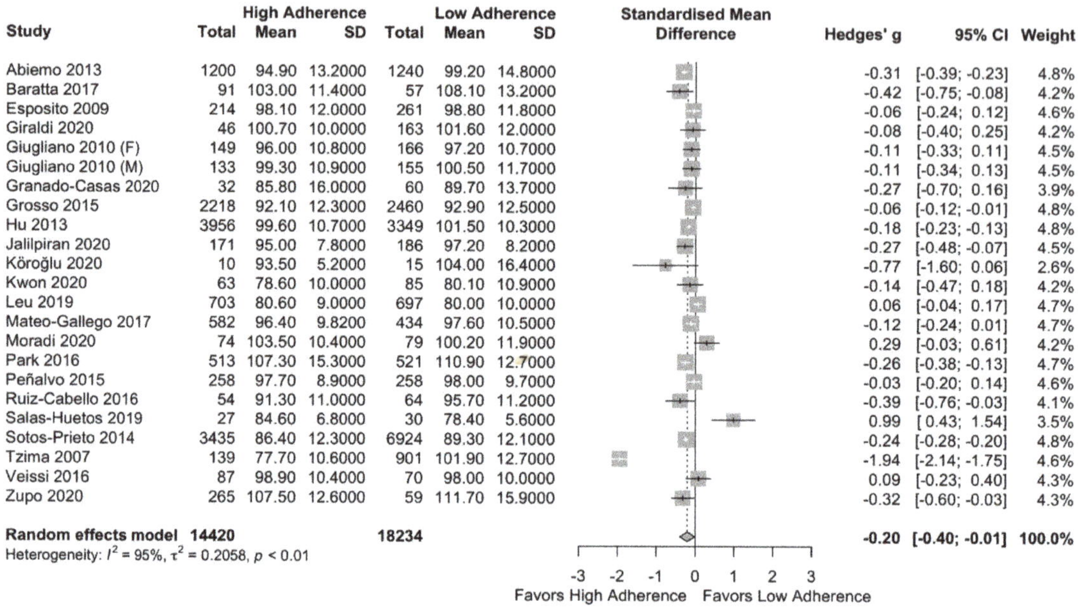

Figure 2. Forest plot of the impact of level of adherence to MD on WC (cm).

3.5.2. HDL Cholesterol

In subjects reporting high adherence to MD, the ORs of HDL cholesterol <40 mg/dL for males and <50 mg/dL for females were lower, compared to low adherers but not significantly [39,99,104], even after three years of follow-up [103]. Mean and geometric mean HDL cholesterol concentrations were increased in the high adherence groups [40,97,98,100,105–107]. A significantly increased ($p = 0.0258$) HDL cholesterol concentration in the high adherence group was reported by Yang et al. [43]. In Aridi et al. [95] and Steffen et al. [44], the percentage of subjects with increased HDL cholesterol was higher in the high MD adherence group compared to the low adherence group. On the contrary, in two studies, the mean HDL cholesterol concentration was higher in low adherence compared to high adherence groups [101,102]. Only in Barnaba et al., no difference regarding the mean HDL concentration was found between the moderate-high adherence group and the low adherence to MD group [96].

Results of our meta-analysis can be found in the forest plot of Figure 3. Significant higher HDL cholesterol concentration in the high adherence to MD group was observed (SMD: 0.28 (95%CI: 0.07, 0.50)) with high heterogeneity among the included studies $I^2 = 96\%$.

Study	High Adherence Total	High Adherence Mean	High Adherence SD	Low Adherence Total	Low Adherence Mean	Low Adherence SD	Hedges' g	95% CI	Weight
Abiemo 2013	1200	53.00	15.3000	1240	50.90	14.8000	0.14	[0.06; 0.22]	2.7%
Ahmad 2018	6483	54.20	14.6000	10140	51.80	13.9000	0.17	[0.14; 0.20]	2.7%
Ahmed 2020	77	58.60	15.6000	147	51.70	15.3000	0.45	[0.17; 0.73]	2.6%
Asghari 2016	204	42.10	10.0000	418	41.60	10.2000	0.05	[-0.12; 0.22]	2.7%
Baratta 2017	91	49.10	12.3000	57	46.60	10.7000	0.21	[-0.12; 0.54]	2.6%
Bondia-Pons 2009	59	54.10	5.4000	11	45.20	7.7000	1.52	[0.82; 2.21]	2.1%
Campanella 2020	1001	52.60	13.9000	1386	50.70	13.1000	0.14	[0.06; 0.22]	2.7%
Dai 2008	90	37.70	9.5000	104	38.90	9.1000	-0.13	[-0.41; 0.15]	2.6%
Esposito 2009	214	42.50	8.9000	261	42.50	8.9000	0.00	[-0.18; 0.18]	2.7%
Gardener 2015	372	46.00	14.0000	171	45.00	14.0000	0.07	[-0.11; 0.25]	2.7%
Giraldi 2020	46	48.60	14.5000	163	46.50	16.4000	0.13	[-0.20; 0.46]	2.6%
Giugliano 2010 (F)	149	47.00	9.0000	166	44.00	9.0000	0.33	[0.11; 0.56]	2.6%
Giugliano 2010 (M)	133	47.00	9.0000	155	44.00	9.0000	0.33	[0.10; 0.57]	2.6%
Granado-Casas 2020	32	67.50	10.7000	60	59.50	18.0000	0.50	[0.06; 0.94]	2.4%
Grosso 2015	2218	55.70	14.3000	2460	55.30	14.7000	0.03	[-0.03; 0.08]	2.7%
Hu 2013	2471	53.40	12.8000	1853	52.50	12.8000	0.07	[0.01; 0.13]	2.7%
Izadi 2016	165	47.70	8.9000	160	45.70	9.3000	0.22	[0.00; 0.44]	2.6%
Jalilpiran 2020	171	51.90	7.8000	186	47.10	8.2000	0.60	[0.39; 0.81]	2.6%
Jayedi 2019	78	44.70	8.8000	53	45.50	8.9000	-0.09	[-0.44; 0.26]	2.5%
Köroğlu 2020	10	38.00	6.1000	15	40.60	8.0000	-0.34	[-1.15; 0.46]	2.0%
Kwon 2020	63	59.20	14.0000	85	60.00	14.9000	-0.05	[-0.38; 0.27]	2.6%
Lavados 2020	151	48.60	14.8000	217	47.20	15.2000	0.09	[-0.11; 0.30]	2.6%
Leu 2019	703	41.90	12.3000	697	43.20	13.2000	-0.10	[-0.21; 0.00]	2.7%
Mateo-Gallego 2017	582	55.40	11.9000	434	51.90	11.7000	0.30	[0.17; 0.42]	2.7%
Molina-Leyva 2018	14	58.90	9.7000	11	51.40	19.9000	0.48	[-0.32; 1.29]	2.0%
Park 2016	513	47.10	23.1000	521	43.10	13.3000	0.21	[0.09; 0.33]	2.7%
Peñalvo 2015	258	54.80	11.5000	258	51.50	11.5000	0.29	[0.11; 0.46]	2.7%
Pocovi-Gerardino 2020	143	59.10	17.1000	16	54.60	17.7000	0.26	[-0.26; 0.78]	2.3%
Ruiz-Cabello 2016	54	64.50	17.6000	64	57.90	19.2000	0.35	[-0.01; 0.72]	2.5%
Salas-Huetos 2019	27	54.20	8.6000	30	59.70	9.0000	-0.62	[-1.15; -0.08]	2.3%
Sotos-Prieto 2014	3435	53.40	11.6000	6924	51.80	16.2000	0.11	[0.07; 0.15]	2.7%
Tuttolomondo 2015	180	47.50	18.3000	108	48.50	15.9000	-0.06	[-0.30; 0.18]	2.6%
Tuttolomondo 2020	179	45.50	17.7000	230	47.10	16.2000	-0.09	[-0.29; 0.10]	2.7%
Tzima 2007	139	47.60	0.4000	901	45.30	0.6000	3.98	[3.73; 4.23]	2.6%
Veglia 2019	737	51.00	0.4000	1098	47.60	13.9000	0.32	[0.22; 0.41]	2.7%
Veissi 2016	87	44.80	10.0000	70	43.30	9.4000	0.15	[-0.16; 0.47]	2.6%
Viscogliosi 2013	18	60.00	14.6000	37	48.00	13.3000	0.86	[0.27; 1.45]	2.3%
Vitale 2018	705	46.80	12.4000	834	45.30	11.6000	0.13	[0.02; 0.23]	2.7%
Zupo 2020	265	52.10	13.4000	59	48.50	14.3000	0.26	[-0.02; 0.55]	2.6%
Random effects model	**23517**			**31800**			**0.28**	**[0.07; 0.50]**	**100.0%**

Heterogeneity: $I^2 = 96\%$, $\tau^2 = 0.4499$, $p < 0.01$

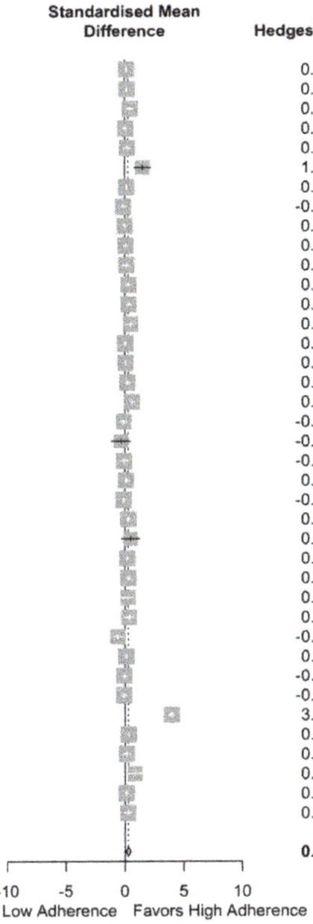

Figure 3. Forest plot of the impact of level of adherence to the MD on HDL cholesterol (mg/dL).

In the subgroup analysis (based on the quality of studies per NOS), the significantly increased HDL cholesterol concentration was remained after excluding the low-quality studies (SMD: 0.36 (95% CI: 0.03, 0.68)) with $I^2 = 98\%$ as can be seen in Supplementary Figure S3.

3.5.3. Serum Triglycerides

Regarding the studies which used OR as a measure of effect, in three studies [99,103,104], the ORs of having TG concentration above 150 mg/dL were lower for the high adherence group, and in only one study, the OR was higher [39]. Means and geometric means TG concentration were observed to be lower in high adherence groups [40,43,98,100,102,105–107] compared to the low adherence groups. Similarly, in Steffen et al. [44], a significantly lower percentage was reported for increased TG concentration in the high adherence to MD group compared to the low adherence group. In contrast, in two studies led by Barnaba and by Matei, a higher concentration of TG was reported in the high-moderate adherence group and in the high adherence group, respectively, compared to the low adherence group [96,101]. Additionally, in the study led by Aridi, a higher, but not significant, percentage reported increased TG concentration in the high adherence to MD group compared to the low adherence group [95].

After performing the meta-analysis, TG concentration was found to be lower in the high adherence to MD group compared to the low adherence group (SMD: −0.27 (95%CI: −0.44, −0.11)) with a high heterogeneity among the studies $I^2 = 95\%$ as is presented in Figure 4. In the subgroup analysis of low- and high-quality studies, the same results also remained after excluding the low-quality studies (SMD: −0.29 (95% CI: −0.52, −0.05)) with I^2 = 97% (Supplementary Figure S4).

Study	High Adherence Total	High Adherence Mean	High Adherence SD	Low Adherence Total	Low Adherence Mean	Low Adherence SD	Hedges' g	95% CI	Weight
Abiemo 2013	1200	118.00	66.0000	1240	131.00	75.0000	-0.18	[-0.26; -0.10]	2.7%
Ahmad 2018	6483	123.30	63.8000	10140	125.40	65.9000	-0.03	[-0.06; 0.00]	2.7%
Ahmed 2020	77	117.80	60.2000	147	135.50	70.5000	-0.26	[-0.54; 0.01]	2.6%
Asghari 2016	204	158.00	91.7000	418	153.80	97.5000	0.04	[-0.12; 0.21]	2.7%
Baratta 2017	91	127.70	42.2000	57	167.20	92.8000	-0.59	[-0.93; -0.25]	2.5%
Bondia-Pons 2009	59	91.20	17.7000	11	106.30	17.7000	-0.84	[-1.50; -0.18]	1.9%
Campanella 2020	1001	120.50	80.6000	1386	121.40	91.2000	-0.01	[-0.09; 0.07]	2.7%
Dai 2008	90	182.50	99.6000	104	176.60	102.0000	0.06	[-0.22; 0.34]	2.5%
Esposito 2009	214	159.40	61.1000	261	168.30	58.5000	-0.15	[-0.33; 0.03]	2.7%
Gardener 2015	372	135.00	79.0000	171	146.00	79.0000	-0.14	[-0.32; 0.04]	2.7%
Giraldi 2020	46	142.00	79.0000	163	158.10	83.8000	-0.19	[-0.52; 0.13]	2.5%
Giugliano 2010 (F)	149	156.00	60.0000	166	172.00	65.0000	-0.25	[-0.48; -0.03]	2.6%
Giugliano 2010 (M)	133	153.00	59.0000	155	168.00	58.0000	-0.26	[-0.49; -0.02]	2.6%
Grosso 2015	2218	137.30	64.7000	2460	141.70	69.0000	-0.07	[-0.12; -0.01]	2.7%
Granado-Casas 2020	32	57.90	16.6000	60	67.50	23.3000	-0.45	[-0.88; -0.01]	2.3%
Izadi 2016	165	131.70	55.9000	160	161.50	67.4000	-0.48	[-0.70; -0.26]	2.6%
Jalilpiran 2020	171	123.70	39.2000	186	136.70	39.6000	-0.33	[-0.54; -0.12]	2.6%
Jayedi 2019	78	163.10	70.7000	53	169.90	58.0000	-0.10	[-0.45; 0.25]	2.5%
Köroğlu 2020	10	134.30	46.6000	15	265.80	184.5000	-0.87	[-1.71; -0.02]	1.6%
Kwon 2020	63	101.90	60.4000	85	110.10	58.9000	-0.14	[-0.46; 0.19]	2.5%
Lavados 2020	151	130.70	111.9000	217	138.40	82.6000	-0.08	[-0.29; 0.13]	2.6%
Leu 2019	703	103.70	65.7000	697	105.60	75.4000	-0.03	[-0.13; 0.08]	2.7%
Mateo-Gallego 2017	582	146.00	104.0000	434	154.00	92.3000	-0.08	[-0.20; 0.04]	2.7%
Molina-Leyva 2018	14	116.30	55.7000	11	124.00	48.1000	-0.14	[-0.93; 0.65]	1.7%
Moradi 2020	74	254.30	59.2000	79	258.70	57.5000	-0.08	[-0.39; 0.24]	2.5%
Mosconi 2014	20	96.00	49.0000	32	86.00	34.0000	0.24	[-0.32; 0.80]	2.1%
Park 2016	513	164.80	176.6000	521	174.30	109.0000	-0.06	[-0.19; 0.06]	2.7%
Peñalvo 2015	258	145.00	98.3000	258	156.00	98.3000	-0.11	[-0.28; 0.06]	2.7%
Pocovi-Gerardino 2020	143	91.60	43.9000	16	128.30	49.8000	-0.82	[-1.35; -0.30]	2.2%
Ruiz-Cabello 2016	54	88.70	66.9000	64	112.80	68.0000	-0.35	[-0.72; 0.01]	2.4%
Salas-Huetos 2019	27	71.40	22.7000	30	70.80	19.5000	0.03	[-0.49; 0.55]	2.2%
Sotos-Prieto 2014	3435	134.60	53.1000	6924	139.00	37.2000	-0.10	[-0.14; -0.06]	2.7%
Tuttolomondo 2015	180	122.60	101.5000	108	134.60	79.9000	-0.13	[-0.37; 0.11]	2.6%
Tuttolomondo 2020	179	116.00	56.6000	230	128.50	53.1000	-0.23	[-0.42; -0.03]	2.7%
Tzima 2007	139	129.00	11.0000	901	146.00	4.0000	-3.10	[-3.33; -2.88]	2.6%
Veglia 2019	737	117.60	58.7000	1098	123.00	63.8000	-0.09	[-0.18; 0.01]	2.7%
Veissi 2016	87	160.10	99.3000	70	150.90	68.7000	0.11	[-0.21; 0.42]	2.5%
Viscogliosi 2013	18	95.50	50.7000	37	168.20	89.3000	-0.91	[-1.50; -0.32]	2.0%
Vitale 2018	705	146.70	71.0000	834	156.20	78.6000	-0.13	[-0.23; -0.03]	2.7%
Zupo 2020	265	105.80	62.5000	59	109.80	60.5000	-0.06	[-0.35; 0.22]	2.5%
Random effects model	**21140**			**30058**			**-0.27**	**[-0.44; -0.11]**	**100.0%**

Heterogeneity: I^2 = 95%, τ^2 = 0.2614, $p < 0.01$

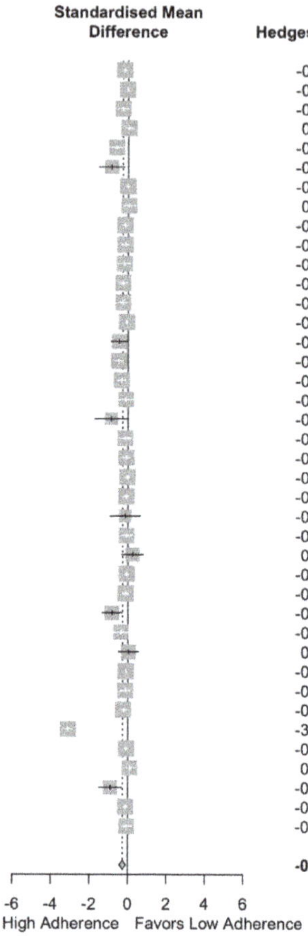

Figure 4. Forest plot of the impact of level of adherence to the MD on serum TG (mg/dL).

3.5.4. Fasting Blood Glucose

In 2 studies by Alvarez-Leon et al. [39] and Mirmiran et al. [103], ORs of having FBG >180 mg/dL were higher in the high adherence group to MD in comparison to the low adherence group, whereas in 2 other studies were opposite (ORs were lower regarding in the high adherence group) [99,104]. Means and geometric means concentration of FBG were lower in high adherers compared to low MD adherers [43,97,98,100,105,106]. According to Aridi et al. and Steffen et al. studies, a lower percentage of subjects presented FBG concentration >110 mg/dL in the high adherence group compared to the low adherence to MD group [44,95]. However, the mean concentration of FBG was increased in high adherers compared to low adherers [40,102,107] and low-moderate adherers [96].

The meta-analysis results can be found in Figure 5. There was no difference in FBG between the two groups (SMD: −0.21 (95%CI: −0.54, 0.12)). The above did not change after performing a subgroup analysis per the NOS classification (SMD: −0.24 (95%CI: −0.70, 0.22) for the high-quality studies) as can be seen in Supplementary Figure S5.

Study	High Adherence Total	High Adherence Mean	High Adherence SD	Low Adherence Total	Low Adherence Mean	Low Adherence SD	Hedges' g	95% CI	Weight
Abiemo 2013	1200	89.40	8.8300	1240	89.90	8.9000	-0.06	[-0.14; 0.02]	3.2%
Ahmed 2020	77	93.50	15.8000	147	99.50	26.1000	-0.26	[-0.54; 0.02]	3.2%
Asghari 2016	204	95.50	27.4000	418	90.50	19.2000	0.22	[0.06; 0.39]	3.2%
Baratta 2017	91	100.20	16.6000	57	108.20	42.0000	-0.27	[-0.61; 0.06]	3.1%
Bondia-Pons 2009	59	93.60	14.4000	11	102.60	27.0000	-0.53	[-1.18; 0.12]	2.9%
Campanella 2020	1001	106.00	27.4000	1386	104.80	24.1000	0.05	[-0.03; 0.13]	3.2%
Dai 2008	90	103.30	18.0000	104	98.20	18.4000	0.28	[0.00; 0.56]	3.2%
Esposito 2009	214	154.80	46.8000	261	153.00	39.6000	0.04	[-0.14; 0.22]	3.2%
Gardener 2015	372	108.00	52.0000	171	101.00	41.0000	0.14	[-0.04; 0.32]	3.2%
Giraldi 2020	46	99.90	43.4000	163	98.70	37.3000	0.03	[-0.30; 0.36]	3.1%
Giugliano 2010 (F)	149	157.00	34.0000	166	155.00	34.0000	0.06	[-0.16; 0.28]	3.2%
Giugliano 2010 (M)	133	154.00	34.0000	155	149.00	34.0000	0.15	[-0.09; 0.38]	3.2%
Grosso 2015	2218	96.10	25.6000	2460	96.70	25.4000	-0.02	[-0.08; 0.03]	3.2%
Izadi 2016	165	95.20	40.8000	160	118.80	54.4000	-0.49	[-0.71; -0.27]	3.2%
Jalilpiran 2020	171	104.70	18.3000	186	101.70	19.1000	0.16	[-0.05; 0.37]	3.2%
Jayedi 2019	78	160.40	54.4000	53	165.00	45.3000	-0.09	[-0.44; 0.26]	3.1%
Köroğlu 2020	10	80.50	5.8000	15	96.40	19.8000	-0.97	[-1.82; -0.12]	2.7%
Kwon 2020	63	97.40	19.0000	85	97.40	19.0000	0.00	[-0.33; 0.33]	3.1%
Leu 2019	703	98.90	22.9000	697	100.60	29.3000	-0.06	[-0.17; 0.04]	3.2%
Mateo-Gallego 2017	582	98.90	16.4000	434	97.70	14.9000	0.08	[-0.05; 0.20]	3.2%
Molina-Leyva 2018	14	93.40	22.4000	11	87.80	7.6000	0.31	[-0.49; 1.10]	2.7%
Moradi 2020	74	130.80	27.1000	79	129.10	26.1000	0.06	[-0.25; 0.38]	3.1%
Mosconi 2014	20	81.00	15.0000	32	76.00	9.0000	0.42	[-0.14; 0.99]	3.0%
Park 2016	513	101.30	18.8000	521	101.80	38.4000	-0.02	[-0.14; 0.11]	3.2%
Peñalvo 2015	258	99.90	18.2000	258	98.70	15.8000	0.07	[-0.10; 0.24]	3.2%
Ruiz-Cabello 2016	54	88.40	16.2000	64	85.60	16.8000	0.17	[-0.19; 0.53]	3.1%
Salas-Huetos 2019	27	88.50	9.1000	30	88.00	9.3000	0.05	[-0.47; 0.57]	3.0%
Tzima 2007	139	92.00	2.0000	901	98.00	1.0000	-5.07	[-5.35; -4.79]	3.2%
Veglia 2019	737	97.70	20.7000	1098	112.70	32.8000	-0.52	[-0.62; -0.43]	3.2%
Veissi 2016	87	162.40	82.7000	70	151.50	55.9000	0.15	[-0.16; 0.47]	3.1%
Viscogliosi 2013	18	93.00	9.3000	37	111.00	20.2000	-1.02	[-1.61; -0.42]	2.9%
Zupo 2020	265	89.80	12.8000	59	88.70	10.1000	0.09	[-0.19; 0.37]	3.2%
Random effects model	**9832**			**11529**			**-0.21**	**[-0.54; 0.12]**	**100.0%**

Heterogeneity: $I^2 = 98\%$, $\tau^2 = 0.8724$, $p < 0.01$

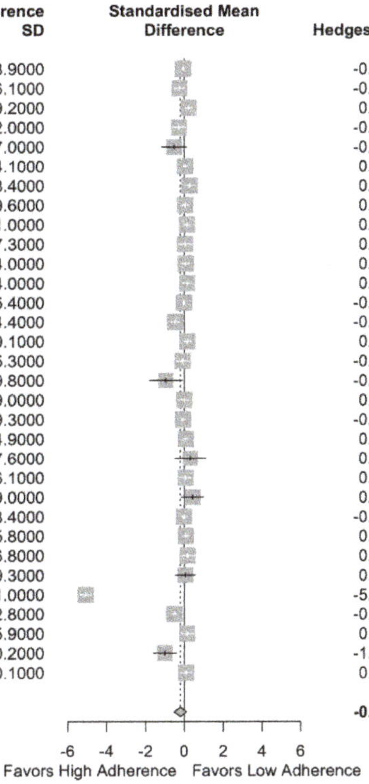

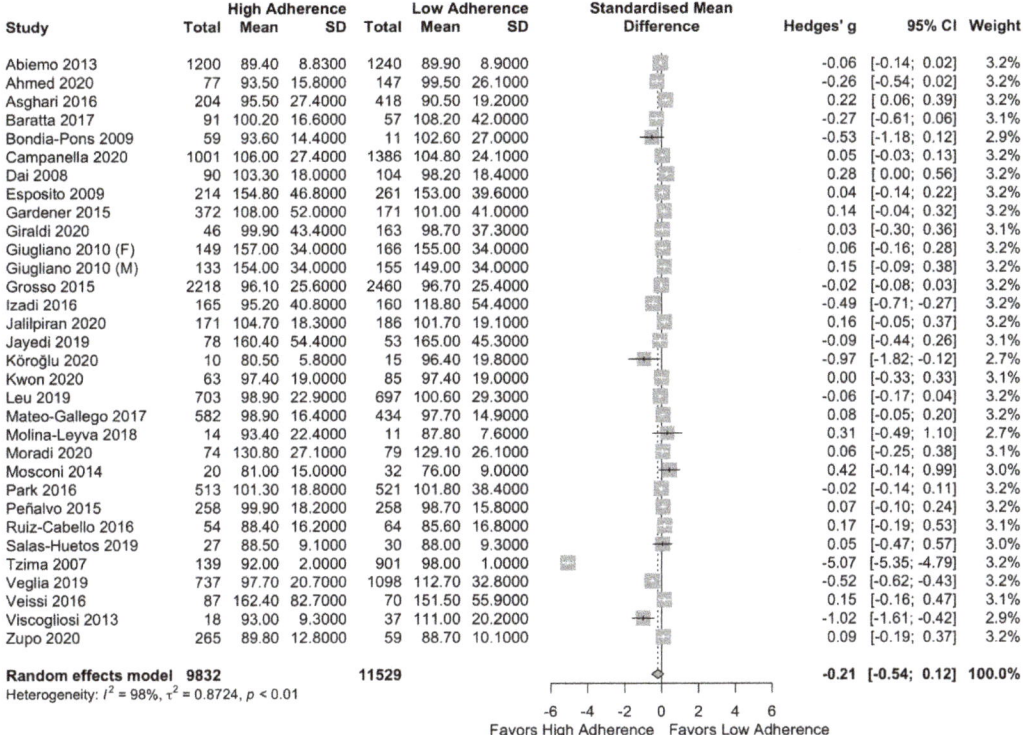

Figure 5. Forest plot of the impact of level of adherence to MD on FBG (mg/dL).

3.5.5. Systolic Blood Pressure (SBP)

Regarding the SBP, in four studies, the ORs of a measuring SBP >130 mmHg were lower in subjects reporting high adherence to MD compared to low adherers [39,99,103,104]. Moreover, means and geometric means of SBP were lower in the high adherence group compared to the low adherence group [40,98,102,106]. According to Aridi et al. [95] and Steffen et al. [44], lower percentages of subjects presented SBP >130 mmHg from the high adherence to MD group compared to the low adherence group. Three studies reported the opposite (higher SBP was observed in higher adherence to MD) [43,101,107].

Meta-analysis results can be found in Figure 6. Lower SBP was observed in the high adherence group but not significant (SMD:−0.15 (95% CI: −0.38, 0.07)) with high heterogeneity across the included studies ($I^2 = 97\%$). This result did not change after the performance of a subgroup analysis based on the quality of studies (SMD: −0.25 (95%CI: −0.60, 0.10), $I^2 = 98\%$) as can be seen in Supplementary Figure S6.

Study	High Adherence Total	High Adherence Mean	High Adherence SD	Low Adherence Total	Low Adherence Mean	Low Adherence SD	Hedges' g	95% CI	Weight
Abiemo 2013	1200	126.00	21.0000	1240	124.00	22.0000	0.09	[0.01; 0.17]	3.3%
Ahmad 2018	6483	121.50	7.4000	10140	125.00	14.8000	-0.28	[-0.31; -0.25]	3.3%
Ahmed 2020	77	130.40	25.7000	147	132.90	21.1000	-0.11	[-0.39; 0.17]	3.2%
Asghari 2016	204	114.20	16.9000	418	110.60	16.0000	0.22	[0.05; 0.39]	3.3%
Baratta 2017	91	130.00	15.1000	57	130.00	15.2000	0.00	[-0.33; 0.33]	3.1%
Bondia-Pons 2009	59	116.30	10.9000	11	139.80	13.4000	-2.06	[-2.79; -1.32]	2.5%
Campanella 2020	1001	127.90	17.1000	1386	120.90	16.5000	0.42	[0.34; 0.50]	3.3%
Dai 2008	90	129.30	15.2000	104	130.30	16.3000	-0.06	[-0.35; 0.22]	3.2%
Gardener 2015	372	142.00	19.0000	171	145.00	22.0000	-0.15	[-0.33; 0.03]	3.3%
Grosso 2015	2218	136.90	20.8000	2460	138.70	20.9000	-0.09	[-0.14; -0.03]	3.3%
Hu 2013	3956	148.40	19.1000	3349	148.90	19.0000	-0.03	[-0.07; 0.02]	3.3%
Izadi 2016	165	12.50	1.7000	160	12.50	1.8000	0.00	[-0.22; 0.22]	0.0%
Jalilpiran 2020	171	12.80	1.3000	186	13.00	1.4000	-0.15	[-0.36; 0.06]	0.0%
Jayedi 2019	78	132.00	114.5000	53	126.30	14.6000	0.06	[-0.29; 0.41]	3.1%
Köroğlu 2020	10	115.80	6.5000	15	120.00	17.2000	-0.29	[-1.09; 0.52]	2.3%
Kwon 2020	63	119.20	12.1000	85	116.90	12.7000	0.18	[-0.14; 0.51]	3.1%
Lavados 2020	151	148.00	25.0000	217	151.00	26.2000	-0.12	[-0.32; 0.09]	3.3%
Leu 2019	703	119.70	18.1000	697	117.50	17.3000	0.12	[0.02; 0.23]	3.3%
Mateo-Gallego 2017	582	125.00	14.2000	434	125.00	14.5000	0.00	[-0.12; 0.12]	3.3%
Molina-Leyva 2018	14	135.40	18.3000	11	127.50	8.3000	0.52	[-0.29; 1.32]	2.3%
Moradi 2020	74	104.20	21.2000	79	105.70	20.4000	-0.07	[-0.39; 0.25]	3.1%
Mosconi 2014	20	122.00	12.0000	32	117.00	15.0000	0.35	[-0.21; 0.92]	2.8%
Park 2016	513	129.90	21.5000	521	125.90	14.2000	0.22	[0.10; 0.34]	3.3%
Peñalvo 2015	258	126.00	14.6000	258	125.00	14.0000	0.07	[-0.10; 0.24]	3.3%
Pocovi-Gerardino 2020	143	118.70	19.4000	16	115.40	14.9000	0.17	[-0.34; 0.69]	2.8%
Ruiz-Cabello 2016	54	121.10	16.2000	64	123.40	16.0000	-0.14	[-0.50; 0.22]	3.1%
Salas-Huetos 2019	27	127.00	11.0000	30	126.30	11.4000	0.06	[-0.46; 0.58]	2.8%
Tuttolomondo 2015	180	138.60	24.7000	108	143.10	27.6000	-0.17	[-0.41; 0.07]	3.2%
Tuttolomondo 2020	179	132.60	20.5000	230	133.90	18.3000	-0.07	[-0.26; 0.13]	3.3%
Tzima 2007	139	125.00	1.0000	901	128.00	1.0000	-3.00	[-3.22; -2.78]	3.2%
Veglia 2019	737	135.00	18.0000	1098	147.00	18.0000	-0.67	[-0.76; -0.57]	3.3%
Veissi 2016	87	129.20	18.3000	70	131.70	19.8000	-0.13	[-0.45; 0.18]	3.1%
Vitale 2018	705	133.30	23.7000	834	135.30	14.9000	-0.10	[-0.20; 0.00]	3.3%
Zupo 2020	265	128.60	16.1000	59	129.20	18.1000	-0.04	[-0.32; 0.25]	3.2%
Random effects model	**21069**			**25641**			**-0.15**	**[-0.38; 0.07]**	**100.0%**

Heterogeneity: $I^2 = 97\%$, $\tau^2 = 0.3933$, $p < 0.01$

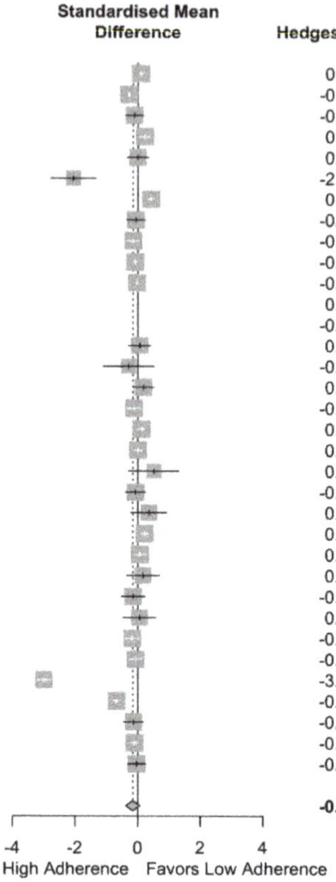

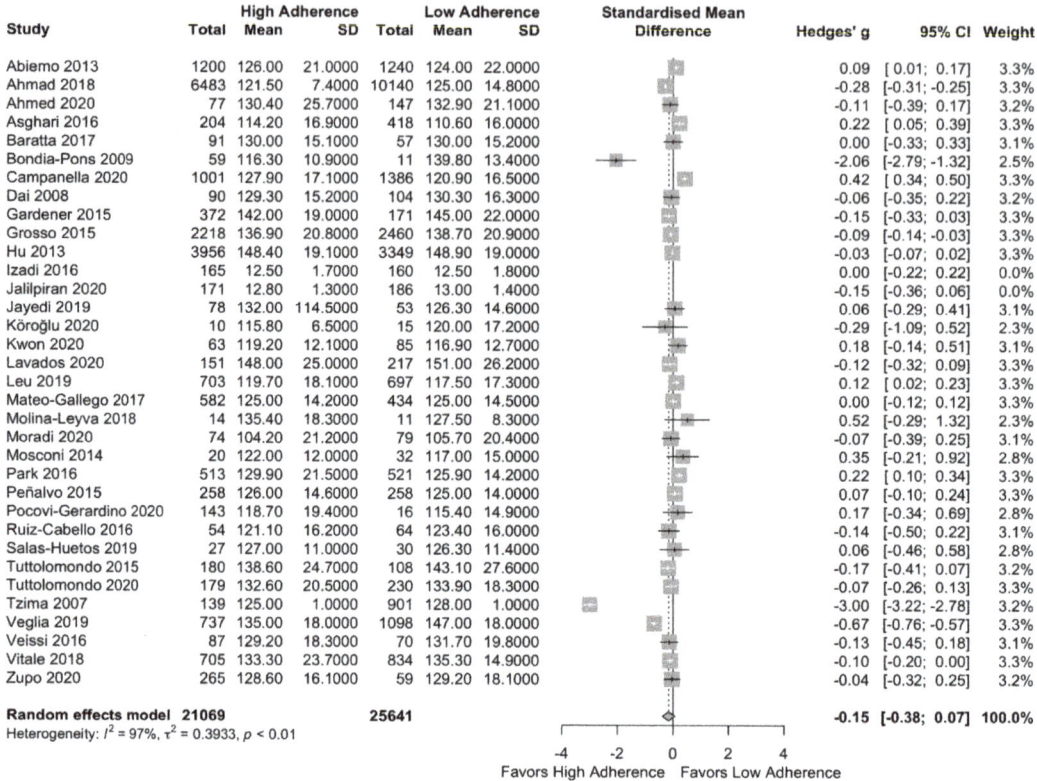

Figure 6. Forest plot of the impact of level of adherence to the MD on SBP (mg/dL)—n = 25,641.

4. Discussion

Our systematic review and meta-analysis aimed to investigate the association between a low and high level of adherence to MD and risk parameters of MetS, according to the NCEP-ATP III criteria. The present study, examining 41 observational studies, revealed a positive impact of MD on the five components of MetS, including WC, HDL, TG, FG and BP. Although a previous meta-analysis conducted by Kastorini et al. [30] explored the effect of MD on MetS prevalence, including its components, this is the first meta-analysis estimating the impact of the level of adherence to MD on each parameter of MetS according to evidence obtained by MD adherence scores.

With regards to abdominal obesity, our results showed a significant inverse association between WC and adherence to MD. Only one study [40] did not find any statistical difference in WC between the different levels of adherence to MD groups, which could be attributed to the underlying health condition of participants (CKD patients). Increased WC, which was detected in the low adherence to MD subjects, along with the accumulation of visceral fat, have been linked to the presence of low-grade systemic inflammation, increased oxidative stress and overexpression of pro-inflammatory cytokines, including CRP, IL-6 and TNF-a [109,110]. These metabolic abnormalities have a direct impact on other biochemical risk markers of MetS, and more specifically HDL, TG and FG, which consequently stimulate atherogenesis and mediate insulin resistance [111]. The high content of antioxidants, polyphenols and fiber found in MD have been previously associated with decreased systemic inflammation and central obesity, which could explain its beneficial effect [112,113]. Moreover, an enhanced with nuts MD was found to be helpful regarding the maintenance of body weight status [114,115].

A significantly positive correlation was also found between high adherence to MD and HDL cholesterol concentration. Our findings are consistent with previously reported data from randomized controlled trials (RCTs), in which a Mediterranean dietary pattern improved HDL cholesterol concentration and the overall lipid profile [116–118]. Increased intake of olive oil, polyphenols, antioxidants as well as an optimal ratio of MUFA:SFA, through the adherence to MD, seemed to have a synergistic effect on various mechanisms of lipid metabolism by promoting changes on the overall composition of HDL cholesterol particles, increased antioxidant and cholesterol efflux capacity [117,119]. Furthermore, a higher HDL concentration observed in high MD adherers could potentially be a secondary effect closely related to lower mean values of central obesity, as aforementioned, and improved cardiometabolic risk markers.

According to our results, an inverse significant association was observed between TGs concentration and adherence to MD. In a large network meta-analysis performed by Tsartsou et al. [108], the protective effect of MD on the overall lipid profile, including TGs, was also demonstrated. These findings were mainly attributed to the high content of olive oil polyphenols and oleic acid as part of the MD [108]. Another meta-analysis of RCTs, investigating the effect of plant oils on blood lipids, had also reported a decrease in TG concentration from the use of diets rich in olive oil [120]. Notwithstanding, it was demonstrated that oils rich in omega-3-fatty acids (n-3 FAs) caused a greater decrease in TGs than olive oil [120]. The metabolic mechanisms responsible for these changes are related to the types of fatty acids, i.e., MUFAS and n-3 FAs, which have the ability to suppress postprandial TGs, enhance TG clearance, decrease the activity of TG lipase and the overall TG synthesis [121–123].

Taking the above into consideration, where the mean values of WC, HDL cholesterol and serum TG concentration were significantly closer to normal in the high adherence to MD groups compared to the low adherence group, we conclude that the level of adherence to MD could play an important role to ameliorate the obesity level and the impaired lipid profile, in combination or not with appropriate pharmacological treatment.

With respect to FBG, an inverse correlation was demonstrated between MD levels of adherence and FBG, which, however, was not statistically significant. A possible explanation for that could be the high number of individuals diagnosed with diabetes or at diabetic risk who participated in the studies [49,61,65,68–71,74,81,92], along with other confounding factors (e.g., age, BMI, medication, etc.). However, the fact that mean values of FBG in both high and low adherers were within the normal range led us to the conclusion that MD adherence can have a positive impact on glycemic control regardless of the level of adherence. Sufficient evidence exists supporting the positive effect of adherence to MD so as to improve glycemic control and decrease the overall risk of T2DM [124]. A systematic review of 17 studies assessing the effect of MD on the incidence of T2DM revealed that high adherence to MD was significantly correlated with improved FBG concentration and HbA1c in diabetic patients [125]. Additionally, both RCTs and prospective cohort studies have also confirmed the benefits of MD on glycemic control over other diets among different subgroups of the population, including healthy individuals, individuals with high CVD/T2DM risk or diabetic patients [65,126,127]. These outcomes have been closely related to the composition of MD, which is rich in anti-inflammatory compounds, as well as to its enhanced activity of glucagon-like peptide (GLP-1) hormone and to changes in gut microbiome caused by MD [48]. Notwithstanding, a meta-analysis by Ajala et al. on 20 RCTs demonstrated that not only MD but also low-carbohydrate, low-glycemic-index and high protein diets could enhance the cardiometabolic profile [128].

Regarding SBP and adherence to MD level, we have also found an inverse but non-statistically significant association. Hypertension is considered a major risk factor for endothelial dysfunction and the development of CVDs [129]. It has been previously demonstrated that prolonged adherence to MD can decrease both SBP and DBP [130].

According to our included studies, in a vast majority, the mean SBP was <130 mmHg in both low and high adherence to MD groups. Consequently, we can conclude that even a poor adherence to MD can positively influence SBP. This conclusion is in accordance with existing data from previously published studies that have reported a significant inverse correlation between adherence of MD and BP [131,132]. Moreover, two recent meta-analyses showed that MD could significantly reduce BP when compared to control diets [133,134]. In addition, a greater decrease in BP was recorded for subjects presented with higher BP at baseline and in studies with a longer duration of the intervention [133]. Various nutrients included in MD exerted beneficial effects through improved vasodilation and endothelial function such as nitric oxides, flavonoids and minerals [135].

The benefits of MD adherence are not limited to the five parameters of MetS [136]. MiRNAs were found to be better regulated in obese patients following an MD [137]. Recent studies have shown that an MD reduces serum inflammatory markers as well as the incidence of stroke, CVD and breast cancer [138,139]. Moreover, MD was recommended as a diet that can help women with menopause-related symptoms and needs [140].

Our study can be characterized by several strengths. According to our knowledge, this is the first systematic review and meta-analysis that aimed to examine the impact of the level of adherence to an MD on the parameters of MetS. Moreover, the great number of the studies included and the subjects examined (n = 74,058), whose origin covered a significant part of the world, made our results quite representative. Furthermore, publication biases were not detected in our study, except from the studies included for the TG parameter in which the p-value of Egger's test was not rounded up 0.04598. In addition, the fact that we have included studies that used validated MD adherence scores in order to assess the level of adherence to MD increased the accuracy of our conclusions. The limitations of our study mainly concerned the heterogeneity in the included studies. High heterogeneity was detected for all parameters of MetS, which was potentially due to the different types of population (i.e., ethnicity) and health status (i.e., healthy, obese/overweight and diagnosed conditions) across all included studies, as well as to the difference between sample sizes and the use of a variety of MDS. The presence of high heterogeneity in population samples and the fact that subjects under pharmacological treatment were not excluded do not allow for inference of our results regarding the role of MD. Over and above, the variety of MDSs used to assess adherence among studies introduces biases due to the different ways of classification and quantification of food components. Furthermore, levels of adherence to MD may be perceived differently, depending on the geographical location and, thus, produce additional bias. For example, high adherers living in Mediterranean regions might have a greater intake of specific foods when compared to high adherers residing in non-Mediterranean regions. Moreover, the conversion of data whenever necessary for unification of the quantitative analysis adds to our study's limitations. Moreover, we have included studies published in English and Spanish; therefore, studies published in a different language were not a part of this study.

5. Conclusions

High adherence to MD can have a positive impact on all parameters of MetS. In addition, there is sufficient evidence suggesting that long-term consumption of MD can protect from obesity and improve cardiometabolic risk markers, including the markers used for the diagnosis of MetS. Although high heterogeneity was identified across the included studies, our results support previous findings and point to the potential biases that may derive from the use of MDSs. Furthermore, it remains still unclear whether MD exerts the same beneficial effect on both unhealthy and healthy populations; therefore, further research is needed in this field.

Supplementary Materials: The following are available online at https://www.mdpi.com/article/10.3390/nu13051514/s1, Supplementary File S1: MOOSE checklist, Supplementary File S2: Search Strategy, Supplementary File S3: Quality of Studies according to the New Castle Ottawa Scale, Supplementary Figure S1a–e: Funnel plots of studies included in our meta-analysis regarding each parameter of MetS, Supplementary Figure S2: Subgroup analysis based on the quality of studies regarding WC, Supplementary Figure S3: Subgroup analysis based on the quality of studies regarding HDL cholesterol, Supplementary Figure S4: Subgroup analysis based on the quality of studies regarding serum TG, Supplementary Figure S5: Subgroup analysis based on the quality of studies regarding FBG Supplementary Figure S6: Subgroup analysis based on the quality of studies regarding SBP.

Author Contributions: Conceptualization: L.C., D.R.B., E.K. and M.C.; methodology: X.T.; software: X.T.; validation: L.C., D.R.B. and E.K.; formal analysis: X.T.; investigation: L.C., D.R.B. and E.K.; data curation: L.C., D.R.B. and E.K.; writing—original draft preparation: L.C., D.R.B. and E.K.; writing—review and editing: L.C., D.R.B., E.K., X.T. and M.C.; visualization: X.T.; supervision, M.C.; project administration, M.C.; All authors have read and agreed to the published version of the manuscript.

Funding: This research received no external funding.

Institutional Review Board Statement: Not Applicable.

Informed Consent Statement: Not Applicable.

Data Availability Statement: Not Applicable.

Conflicts of Interest: The authors declare no conflict of interest.

Abbreviations

BP	Blood Pressure
CI	Confidence Interval
CVD	Cardiovascular Disease
DBP	Diastolic Blood Pressure
FFQs	Food Frequency Questionnaires
FG	Fasting Glucose
GLP-1	Glucagon-Like Peptide-1
HbA1c	Glycohemoglobin
HDL	High-Density Lipoprotein
IDF	International Diabetes Federation
MD	Mediterranean Diet
MDS	Mediterranean Diet Score
MEDAS	Mediterranean Diet Adherence Screener
MetS	Metabolic Syndrome
MSDPS	Mediterranean-Style Dietary Pattern Score
MOOSE	Meta-analyses Of Observational Studies in Epidemiology
N-3 FAs	Omga-3-Fatty Acids
NAFLD	Non-Alcoholic Fatty Liver Disease
NCDs	Non-Communicable Diseases
NCEP ATP III	National Cholesterol Program in Adult Treatment Panel III
NHNES	National Health and Nutrition Examination Survey
NOS	New Castle Ottawa Scale
OR	Odds Ration
RCT	Randomized Controlled Trial
SD	Standard Deviation
SBP	Systolic Blood Pressure
SMD	Standardized Mean Difference
T2DM	Type 2 Diabetes Mellitus
TG	Triglycerides
UK	United Kingdom
US	United States
WC	Waist Circumference
WHO	World Health Organization

References

1. Cordain, L.; Eaton, S.B.; Sebastian, A.; Mann, N.; Lindeberg, S.; Watkins, B.A.; O'Keefe, J.H.; Brand-Miller, J. Origins and evolution of the Western diet: Health implications for the 21st century. *Am. J. Clin. Nutr.* **2005**, *81*, 341–354. [CrossRef]
2. Misra, A.; Khurana, L. Obesity and the Metabolic Syndrome in Developing Countries. *J. Clin. Endocrinol. Metab.* **2008**, *93* (Suppl. 1), s9–s30. [CrossRef] [PubMed]
3. Moore, J.X.; Chaudhary, N.; Akinyemiju, T. Metabolic Syndrome Prevalence by Race/Ethnicity and Sex in the United States, National Health and Nutrition Examination Survey, 1988–2012. *Prev. Chronic Dis.* **2017**, *14*, E24. [CrossRef] [PubMed]
4. van Vliet-Ostaptchouk, J.V.; Nuotio, M.L.; Slagter, S.N.; Doiron, D.; Fischer, K.; Foco, L.; Gaye, A.; Gögele, M.; Heier, M.; Hiekkalinna, T.; et al. The prevalence of metabolic syndrome and metabolically healthy obesity in Europe: A collaborative analysis of ten large cohort studies. *BMC Endocr. Disord.* **2014**, *14*, 9. [CrossRef]
5. Kassi, E.; Pervanidou, P.; Kaltsas, G.; Chrousos, G. Metabolic syndrome: Definitions and controversies. *BMC Med.* **2011**, *9*, 48. [CrossRef]
6. Pérez-Martínez, P.; Mikhailidis, D.P.; Athyros, V.G.; Bullo, M.; Couture, P.; Covas, M.I.; De Koning, L.; Delgado-Lista, J.; Díaz-López, A.; Drevon, C.A.; et al. Lifestyle recommendations for the prevention and management of metabolic syndrome: An international panel recommendation. *Nutr. Rev.* **2017**, *75*, 307–326. [CrossRef] [PubMed]
7. Eckel, R.H.; Grundy, S.M.; Zimmet, P.Z. The metabolic syndrome. *Lancet* **2005**, *365*, 1415–1428. [CrossRef]
8. Steckhan, N.; Hohmann, C.-D.; Kessler, C.; Dobos, G.; Michalsen, A.; Cramer, H. Effects of different dietary approaches on inflammatory markers in patients with metabolic syndrome: A systematic review and meta-analysis. *Nutrients* **2016**, *32*, 338–348. [CrossRef] [PubMed]
9. Gami, A.S.; Witt, B.J.; Howard, D.E.; Erwin, P.J.; Gami, L.A.; Somers, V.K.; Montori, V.M. Metabolic syndrome and risk of incident cardiovascular events and death: A systematic review and meta-analysis of longitudinal studies. *J. Am. Coll. Cardiol.* **2007**, *49*, 403–414. [CrossRef] [PubMed]
10. Alberti, K.G.; Zimmet, P.Z. Definition, diagnosis and classification of diabetes mellitus and its complications. Part 1: Diagnosis and classification of diabetes mellitus provisional report of a WHO consultation. *Diabet Med.* **1998**, *15*, 539–553. [CrossRef]
11. National Cholesterol Education Program (U.S.). Expert Panel on Detection, Evaluation, and Treatment of High Blood Cholesterol in Adults. In *Third Report of the National Cholesterol Education Program (NCEP) Expert Panel on Detection, Evaluation, and Treatment of High Blood Cholesterol in Adults (Adult Treatment Panel III)*; The Program: Berkeley, CA, USA, 2002.
12. Alberti, K.G.M.M.; Zimmet, P.; Shaw, J. Metabolic syndrome-a new world-wide definition. A Consensus Statement from the International Diabetes Federation. *Diabet. Med.* **2006**, *23*, 469–480. [CrossRef] [PubMed]
13. Hoyas, I.; Leon-Sanz, M. Nutritional Challenges in Metabolic Syndrome. *J. Clin. Med.* **2019**, *8*, 1301. [CrossRef] [PubMed]
14. Lăcătușu, C.-M.; Grigorescu, E.-D.; Floria, M.; Onofriescu, A.; Mihai, B.-M. The Mediterranean Diet: From an Environment-Driven Food Culture to an Emerging Medical Prescription. *Int. J. Environ. Res. Public Health* **2019**, *16*, 942. [CrossRef] [PubMed]
15. Davis, C.R.; Bryan, J.; Hodgson, J.M.; Murphy, K.J. Definition of the Mediterranean Diet—A Literature Review. *Nutrients* **2015**, *7*, 9139–9153. [CrossRef]
16. Trichopoulou, A.; Lagiou, P. Healthy Traditional Mediterranean Diet: An Expression of Culture, History, and Lifestyle. *Nutr. Rev.* **1997**, *55*, 383–389. [CrossRef] [PubMed]
17. Zaragoza-Martí, A.; Cabañero-Martínez, M.J.; Hurtado-Sánchez, J.A.; Laguna-Pérez, A.; Ferrer-Cascales, R. Evaluation of Mediterranean diet adherence scores: A systematic review. *BMJ Open* **2018**, *8*, e019033. [CrossRef] [PubMed]
18. Bamia, C.; Martimianaki, G.; Kritikou, M.; Trichopoulou, A. Indexes for Assessing Adherence to a Mediterranean Diet from Data Measured through Brief Questionnaires: Issues Raised from the Analysis of a Greek Population Study. *Curr. Dev. Nutr.* **2017**, *1*, e000075. [CrossRef]
19. A Benítez-Arciniega, A.; Mendez, M.A.; Baena-Díez, J.M.; Martori, M.-A.R.; Soler, C.; Marrugat, J.; Covas, M.-I.; Sanz, H.; Llopis, A.; Schröder, H. Concurrent and construct validity of Mediterranean diet scores as assessed by an FFQ. *Public Health Nutr.* **2011**, *14*, 2015–2021. [CrossRef] [PubMed]
20. Willett, W.C.; Sacks, F.; Trichopoulou, A.; Drescher, G.; Ferro-Luzzi, A.; Helsing, E.; Trichopoulos, D. Mediterranean diet pyramid: A cultural model for healthy eating. *Am. J. Clin. Nutr.* **1995**, *61*, 1402S–1406S. [CrossRef]
21. Trichopoulou, A.; Costacou, T.; Bamia, C.; Trichopoulos, D. Adherence to a Mediterranean Diet and Survival in a Greek Population. *N. Engl. J. Med.* **2003**, *348*, 2599–2608. [CrossRef]
22. Martínez-González, M.; García-López, M.; Bes-Rastrollo, M.; Toledo, E.; Martínez-Lapiscina, E.; Delgado-Rodriguez, M.; Vazquez, Z.; Benito, S.; Beunza, J. Mediterranean diet and the incidence of cardiovascular disease: A Spanish cohort. *Nutr. Metab. Cardiovasc. Dis.* **2010**, *21*, 237–244. [CrossRef] [PubMed]
23. Tognon, G.; Lissner, L.; Sæbye, D.; Walker, K.Z.; Heitmann, B.L. The Mediterranean diet in relation to mortality and CVD: A Danish cohort study. *Br. J. Nutr.* **2013**, *111*, 151–159. [CrossRef] [PubMed]
24. Panagiotakos, D.; Georgousopoulou, E.; Pitsavos, C.; Chrysohoou, C.; Skoumas, I.; Pitaraki, E.; Georgiopoulos, G.; Ntertimani, M.; Christou, A.; Stefanadis, C. Exploring the path of Mediterranean diet on 10-year incidence of cardiovascular disease: The ATTICA study (2002–2012). *Nutr. Metab. Cardiovasc. Dis.* **2015**, *25*, 327–335. [CrossRef]
25. Martínez-González, M.Á.; De La Fuente-Arrillaga, C.; Nunez-Cordoba, J.M.; Basterra-Gortari, F.J.; Beunza, J.J.; Vazquez, Z.; Benito, S.; Tortosa, A.; Bes-Rastrollo, M. Adherence to Mediterranean diet and risk of developing diabetes: Prospective cohort study. *BMJ* **2008**, *336*, 1348–1351. [CrossRef]

26. Schwingshackl, L.; Missbach, B.; König, J.; Hoffmann, G. Adherence to a Mediterranean diet and risk of diabetes: A systematic review and meta-analysis. *Public Health Nutr.* **2015**, *18*, 1292–1299. [CrossRef]
27. Franquesa, M.; Pujol-Busquets, G.; García-Fernández, E.; Rico, L.; Shamirian-Pulido, L.; Aguilar-Martínez, A.; Medina, F.-X.; Serra-Majem, L.; Bach-Faig, A. Mediterranean Diet and Cardiodiabesity: A Systematic Review through Evidence-Based Answers to Key Clinical Questions. *Nutrients* **2019**, *11*, 655. [CrossRef]
28. Widmer, R.J.; Flammer, A.J.; Lerman, L.O.; Lerman, A. The Mediterranean Diet, its Components, and Cardiovascular Disease. *Am. J. Med.* **2015**, *128*, 229–238. [CrossRef] [PubMed]
29. Godos, J.; Zappalà, G.; Bernardini, S.; Giambini, I.; Bes-Rastrollo, M.; Martinez-Gonzalez, M. Adherence to the Mediterranean diet is inversely associated with metabolic syndrome occurrence: A meta-analysis of observational studies. *Int. J. Food Sci. Nutr.* **2017**, *68*, 138–148. [CrossRef]
30. Kastorini, C.M.; Milionis, H.J.; Esposito, K.; Giugliano, D.; Goudevenos, J.A.; Panagiotakos, D.B. The effect of Mediterranean diet on metabolic syndrome and its components: A meta-analysis of 50 studies and 534,906 individuals. *J. Am. Coll. Cardiol.* **2011**, *57*, 1299–1313. [CrossRef]
31. Panagiotakos, D.B.; Pitsavos, C.; Stefanadis, C. Dietary patterns: A Mediterranean diet score and its relation to clinical and biological markers of cardiovascular disease risk. *Nutr. Metab. Cardiovasc. Dis.* **2006**, *16*, 559–568. [CrossRef]
32. Sofi, F.; Macchi, C.; Abbate, R.; Gensini, G.F.; Casini, A. Mediterranean diet and health status: An updated meta-analysis and a proposal for a literature-based adherence score. *Public Health Nutr.* **2014**, *17*, 2769–2782. [CrossRef] [PubMed]
33. Schröder, H.; Fitó, M.; Estruch, R.; Martínez-González, M.A.; Corella, D.; Salas-Salvadó, J.; Lamuela-Raventós, R.; Ros, E.; Salaverría, I.; Fiol, M.; et al. A Short Screener Is Valid for Assessing Mediterranean Diet Adherence among Older Spanish Men and Women. *J. Nutr.* **2011**, *141*, 1140–1145. [CrossRef] [PubMed]
34. A Martínez-González, M.; Fernández-Jarne, E.; Serrano-Martínez, M.; Wright, M.; Gomez-Gracia, E. Development of a short dietary intake questionnaire for the quantitative estimation of adherence to a cardioprotective Mediterranean diet. *Eur. J. Clin. Nutr.* **2004**, *58*, 1550–1552. [CrossRef] [PubMed]
35. Monteagudo, C.; Mariscal-Arcas, M.; Rivas, A.; Lorenzo-Tovar, M.L.; Tur, J.A.; Olea-Serrano, F. Proposal of a Mediterranean Diet Serving Score. *PLoS ONE* **2015**, *10*, e0128594.
36. Rumawas, M.E.; Dwyer, J.T.; McKeown, N.M.; Meigs, J.B.; Rogers, G.; Jacques, P.F. The Development of the Mediterranean-Style Dietary Pattern Score and Its Application to the American Diet in the Framingham Offspring Cohort. *J. Nutr.* **2009**, *139*, 1150–1156. [CrossRef]
37. Patterson, R.E.; Haines, P.S.; Popkin, B.M. Diet quality index: Capturing a multidimensional behavior. *J. Am. Diet. Assoc.* **1994**, *94*, 57–64. [CrossRef]
38. Buckland, G.; González, C.A.; Agudo, A.; Vilardell, M.; Berenguer, A.; Amiano, P.; Ardanaz, E.; Arriola, L.; Barricarte, A.; Basterretxea, M.; et al. Adherence to the Mediterranean Diet and Risk of Coronary Heart Disease in the Spanish EPIC Cohort Study. *Am. J. Epidemiol.* **2009**, *170*, 1518–1529. [CrossRef] [PubMed]
39. León, E.Á.; Henríquez, P.; Serra-Majem, L. Mediterranean diet and metabolic syndrome: A cross-sectional study in the Canary Islands. *Public Health Nutr.* **2006**, *9*, 1089–1098. [CrossRef]
40. Huang, X.; Jiménez-Moleón, J.J.; Lindholm, B.; Cederholm, T.; Ärnlöv, J.; Risérus, U.; Sjögren, P.; Carrero, J.J. Mediterranean Diet, Kidney Function, and Mortality in Men with CKD. *Clin. J. Am. Soc. Nephrol.* **2013**, *8*, 1548–1555. [CrossRef]
41. Fung, T.T.; McCullough, M.L.; Newby, P.; Manson, J.E.; Meigs, J.B.; Rifai, N.; Willett, W.C.; Hu, F.B. Diet-quality scores and plasma concentrations of markers of inflammation and endothelial dysfunction. *Am. J. Clin. Nutr.* **2005**, *82*, 163–173. [CrossRef]
42. Sánchez-Villegas, A.; Martínez, J.A.; De Irala, J.; Martínez-González, M.A. Determinants of the adherence to an "a priori" defined Mediterranean dietary pattern. *Eur. J. Nutr.* **2002**, *41*, 249–257. [CrossRef]
43. Yang, J.; Farioli, A.; Korre, M.; Kales, S.N. Modified Mediterranean Diet Score and Cardiovascular Risk in a North American Working Population. *PLoS ONE* **2014**, *9*, e87539. [CrossRef] [PubMed]
44. Steffen, L.M.; Van Horn, L.; Daviglus, M.L.; Zhou, X.; Reis, J.P.; Loria, C.M.; Jacobs, D.R.; Duffey, K.J. A modified Mediterranean diet score is associated with a lower risk of incident metabolic syndrome over 25 years among young adults: The CARDIA (Coronary Artery Risk Development in Young Adults) study. *Br. J. Nutr.* **2014**, *112*, 1654–1661. [CrossRef] [PubMed]
45. Abiemo, E.E.; Alonso, A.; Nettleton, J.A.; Steffen, L.M.; Bertoni, A.G.; Jain, A.; Lutsey, P.L. Relationships of the Mediterranean dietary pattern with insulin resistance and diabetes incidence in the Multi-Ethnic Study of Atherosclerosis (MESA). *Br. J. Nutr.* **2012**, *109*, 1490–1497. [CrossRef]
46. Grosso, G.; Stepaniak, U.; Micek, A.; Topor-Mądry, R.; Stefler, D.; Szafraniec, K.; Bobak, M.; Pająk, A. A Mediterranean-type diet is associated with better metabolic profile in urban Polish adults: Results from the HAPIEE study. *Metabolism* **2015**, *64*, 738–746. [CrossRef]
47. Veglia, F.; Baldassarre, D.; De Faire, U.; Kurl, S.; Smit, A.J.; Rauramaa, R.; Giral, P.; Amato, M.; Di Minno, A.; Ravani, A.; et al. A priori-defined Mediterranean-like dietary pattern predicts cardiovascular events better in north Europe than in Mediterranean countries. *Int. J. Cardiol.* **2019**, *282*, 88–92. [CrossRef]
48. Martín-Peláez, S.; Fito, M.; Castaner, O. Mediterranean Diet Effects on Type 2 Diabetes Prevention, Disease Progression, and Related Mechanisms. A Review. *Nutrients* **2020**, *12*, 2236. [CrossRef]

49. Vitale, M.; Masulli, M.; Calabrese, I.; Rivellese, A.A.; Bonora, E.; Signorini, S.; Perriello, G.; Squatrito, S.; Buzzetti, R.; Sartore, G.; et al. Impact of a Mediterranean Dietary Pattern and Its Components on Cardiovascular Risk Factors, Glucose Control, and Body Weight in People with Type 2 Diabetes: A Real-Life Study. *Nutrients* **2018**, *10*, 1067. [CrossRef]
50. Wells, G.A.; Shea, B.; O'Connell, D.; Peterson, J.; Welch, V.; Losos, M.; Tugwell, P. *The Newcastle-Ottawa Scale (NOS) for Assessing the Quality of non Randomised Studies in Meta-Analyses*; University of Liverpool: Liverpool, UK, 2000.
51. Cox, D.R.; Snell, E.J. *Analysis of Binary Data*; CRC Press: Boca Raton, FL, USA, 1989.
52. da Costa, B.R.; Rutjes, A.W.; Johnston, B.C.; Reichenbach, S.; Nüesch, E.; Tonia, T.; Gemperli, A.; Guyatt, G.H.; Jüni, P. Methods to convert continuous outcomes into odds ratios of treatment response and numbers needed to treat: Meta-epidemiological study. *Int. J. Epidemiol.* **2012**, *41*, 1445–1459. [CrossRef] [PubMed]
53. Egger, M.; Smith, G.D.; Schneider, M.; Minder, C. Bias in meta-analysis detected by a simple, graphical test. *BMJ* **1997**, *315*, 629. [CrossRef] [PubMed]
54. Luo, D.; Wan, X.; Liu, J.; Tong, T. Optimally estimating the sample mean from the sample size, median, mid-range, and/or mid-quartile range. *Stat. Methods Med Res.* **2018**, *27*, 1785–1805. [CrossRef] [PubMed]
55. Omni Calculator. Available online: https://www.omnicalculator.com/ (accessed on 5 March 2021).
56. DerSimonian, R.; Laird, N. Meta-analysis in clinical trials. *Control Clin. Trials* **1986**, *7*, 177–188. [CrossRef]
57. Higgins, J.P.T.; Thompson, S.G.; Deeks, J.J.; Altman, D.G. Measuring inconsistency in meta-analyses. *BMJ* **2003**, *327*, 557–560. [CrossRef] [PubMed]
58. Ahmad, S.; Moorthy, M.V.; Demler, O.V.; Hu, F.B.; Ridker, P.M.; Chasman, D.I.; Mora, S. Assessment of Risk Factors and Biomarkers Associated With Risk of Cardiovascular Disease Among Women Consuming a Mediterranean Diet. *JAMA Netw. Open* **2018**, *1*, e185708. [CrossRef]
59. Ahmed, F.S.; Wade, A.T.; Guenther, B.A.; Murphy, K.J.; Elias, M.F. Adherence to a Mediterranean diet associated with lower blood pressure in a US sample: Findings from the Maine-Syracuse Longitudinal Study. *J. Clin. Hypertens.* **2020**, *22*, 2276–2284. [CrossRef] [PubMed]
60. Asghari, G.; Farhadnejad, H.; Mirmiran, P.; Dizavi, A.; Yuzbashian, E.; Azizi, F. Adherence to the Mediterranean diet is associated with reduced risk of incident chronic kidney diseases among Tehranian adults. *Hypertens. Res.* **2017**, *40*, 96–102. [CrossRef] [PubMed]
61. Baratta, F.; Pastori, D.; Polimeni, L.; Bucci, T.; Ceci, F.; Calabrese, C.; Ernesti, I.; Pannitteri, G.; Violi, F.; Angelico, F.; et al. Adherence to Mediterranean Diet and Non-Alcoholic Fatty Liver Disease: Effect on Insulin Resistance. *Am. J. Gastroenterol.* **2017**, *112*, 1832–1839. [CrossRef] [PubMed]
62. Bondia-Pons, I.; Mayneris-Perxachs, J.; Serra-Majem, L.; Castellote, A.I.; Mariné, A.; López-Sabater, M.C. Diet quality of a population sample from coastal north-east Spain evaluated by a Mediterranean adaptation of the Diet Quality Index (DQI). *Public Health Nutr.* **2009**, *13*, 12–24. [CrossRef] [PubMed]
63. Campanella, A.; Misciagna, G.; Mirizzi, A.; Caruso, M.G.; Bonfiglio, C.; Aballay, L.R.; Silveira, L.V.D.A.; Bianco, A.; Franco, I.; Sorino, P.; et al. The effect of the Mediterranean Diet on lifespan: A treatment-effect survival analysis of a population-based prospective cohort study in Southern Italy. *Int. J. Epidemiol.* **2021**, *50*, 245–255. [CrossRef]
64. Dai, J.; Miller, A.H.; Bremner, J.D.; Goldberg, J.; Jones, L.; Shallenberger, L.; Buckham, R.; Murrah, N.V.; Veledar, E.; Wilson, P.W.; et al. Adherence to the mediterranean diet is inversely associated with circulating interleukin-6 among middle-aged men: A twin study. *Circulation* **2008**, *117*, 169–175. [CrossRef]
65. Esposito, K.; Maiorino, M.I.; Di Palo, C.; Giugliano, D.; Campanian Postprandial Hyperglycemia Study Group. Adherence to a Mediterranean diet and glycaemic control in Type 2 diabetes mellitus. *Diabet. Med.* **2009**, *26*, 900–907. [CrossRef] [PubMed]
66. Gardener, H.; Wright, C.B.; Cabral, D.; Scarmeas, N.; Gu, Y.; Cheung, K.; Elkind, M.S.; Sacco, R.L.; Rundek, T. Mediterranean diet and carotid atherosclerosis in the Northern Manhattan Study. *Atheroscler.* **2014**, *234*, 303–310. [CrossRef] [PubMed]
67. Giraldi, L.; Miele, L.; Aleksovska, K.; Manca, F.; Leoncini, E.; Biolato, M.; Arzani, D.; Pirro, M.A.; Marrone, G.; Cefalo, C.; et al. Mediterranean diet and the prevention of non-alcoholic fatty liver disease: Results from a case-control study. *Eur. Rev. Med Pharmacol. Sci.* **2020**, *24*, 7391–7398. [PubMed]
68. Giugliano, F.; Maiorino, M.I.; Bellastella, G.; Autorino, R.; De Sio, M.; Giugliano, D.; Esposito, K. ERECTILE DYSFUNCTION: Adherence to Mediterranean Diet and Erectile Dysfunction in Men with Type 2 Diabetes. *J. Sex. Med.* **2010**, *7*, 1911–1917. [CrossRef]
69. Giugliano, F.; Maiorino, M.I.; Di Palo, C.; Autorino, R.; De Sio, M.; Giugliano, D.; Esposito, K. ORIGINAL RESEARCH—WOMEN'S SEXUAL HEALTH: Adherence to Mediterranean Diet and Sexual Function in Women with Type 2 Diabetes. *J. Sex. Med.* **2010**, *7*, 1883–1890. [CrossRef]
70. Granado-Casas, M.; Martin, M.; Martínez-Alonso, M.; Alcubierre, N.; Hernández, M.; Alonso, N.; Castelblanco, E.; Mauricio, D. The Mediterranean Diet is Associated with an Improved Quality of Life in Adults with Type 1 Diabetes. *Nutrients* **2020**, *12*, 131. [CrossRef]
71. Hu, E.; Toledo, E.; Diez-Espino, J.; Estruch, R.; Corella, D.; Salas-Salvado, J.; Vinyoles, E.; Gomez-Gracia, E.; Aros, F.; Fiol, M.; et al. Lifestyles and risk factors associated with baseline adherence to the mediterranean diet in the predimed trial. *Ann. Nutr. Metab.* **2013**, *63* (Suppl. 1), 912. [CrossRef]
72. Izadi, V.; Tehrani, H.; Haghighatdoost, F.; Dehghan, A.; Surkan, P.J.; Azadbakht, L. Adherence to the DASH and Mediterranean diets is associated with decreased risk for gestational diabetes mellitus. *Nutrients* **2016**, *32*, 1092–1096. [CrossRef]

73. Jalilpiran, Y.; Mofrad, M.D.; Mozaffari, H.; Bellissimo, N.; Azadbakht, L. Adherence to dietary approaches to stop hypertension (DASH) and Mediterranean dietary patterns in relation to cardiovascular risk factors in older adults. *Clin. Nutr. ESPEN* **2020**, *39*, 87–95. [CrossRef]
74. Jayedi, A.; Mirzaei, K.; Rashidy-Pour, A.; Yekaninejad, M.S.; Zargar, M.-S.; Eidgahi, M.R.A. Dietary approaches to stop hypertension, mediterranean dietary pattern, and diabetic nephropathy in women with type 2 diabetes: A case-control study. *Clin. Nutr. ESPEN* **2019**, *33*, 164–170. [CrossRef]
75. Köroğlu, Ö.; Adıgüzel, K.T. Cardiometabolic risk parameters of individuals with lower extremity amputation: What is the effect of adherence to DASH diet and Mediterranean diet? *Turk. J. Phys. Med. Rehabil.* **2020**, *66*, 291–298. [CrossRef]
76. Kwon, Y.-J.; Lee, H.; Yoon, Y.; Kim, H.M.; Chu, S.H.; Lee, J.-W. Development and Validation of a Questionnaire to Measure Adherence to the Mediterranean Diet in Korean Adults. *Nutrients* **2020**, *12*, 1102. [CrossRef]
77. Lavados, P.M.; Mazzon, E.; Rojo, A.; Brunser, A.M.; Olavarría, V.V. Pre-stroke adherence to a Mediterranean diet pattern is associated with lower acute ischemic stroke severity: A cross-sectional analysis of a prospective hospital-register study. *BMC Neurol.* **2020**, *20*, 1–8. [CrossRef] [PubMed]
78. Leu, H.-B.; Chung, C.-M.; Chen, J.-W.; Pan, W.-H. The Mediterranean diet reduces the genetic risk of chromosome 9p21 for myocardial infarction in an Asian population community cohort. *Sci. Rep.* **2019**, *9*, 1–8. [CrossRef]
79. Mateo-Gallego, R.; Uzhova, I.; Moreno-Franco, B.; León-Latre, M.; Casasnovas, J.A.; Laclaustra, M.; Peñalvo, J.L.; Civeira, F. Adherence to a Mediterranean diet is associated with the presence and extension of atherosclerotic plaques in middle-aged asymptomatic adults: The Aragon Workers' Health Study. *J. Clin. Lipidol.* **2017**, *11*, 1372–1382.e4. [CrossRef] [PubMed]
80. Molina-Leyva, A.; Cuenca-Barrales, C.; Vega-Castillo, J.; Ruiz-Carrascosa, J.; Ruiz-Villaverde, R. Adherence to Mediterranean diet in Spanish patients with psoriasis: Cardiovascular benefits? *Dermatol. Ther.* **2019**, *32*, e12810. [CrossRef] [PubMed]
81. Moradi, M.; Daneshzad, E.; Najafabadi, M.M.; Bellissimo, N.; Suitor, K.; Azadbakht, L. Association between adherence to the Mediterranean diet and renal function biomarkers and cardiovascular risk factors among diabetic patients with nephropathy. *Clin. Nutr. ESPEN* **2020**, *40*, 156–163. [CrossRef] [PubMed]
82. Mosconi, L.; Murray, J.; Tsui, W.H.; Li, Y.; Davies, M.; Williams, S.; Pirraglia, E.; Spector, N.; Osorio, R.S.; Glodzik, L.; et al. Mediterranean Diet and Magnetic Resonance Imaging-Assessed Brain Atrophy in Cognitively Normal Individuals at Risk for Alzheimer's Disease. *J. Prev. Alzheimers Dis.* **2014**, *1*, 23–32.
83. Park, Y.-M.; Steck, S.E.; Fung, T.T.; Zhang, J.; Hazlett, L.J.; Han, K.; Merchant, A.T. Mediterranean diet and mortality risk in metabolically healthy obese and metabolically unhealthy obese phenotypes. *Int. J. Obes.* **2016**, *40*, 1541–1549. [CrossRef]
84. Peñalvo, J.L.; Oliva, B.; Sotos-Prieto, M.; Uzhova, I.; Moreno-Franco, B.; León-Latre, M.; Ordovás, J.M. Greater Adherence to a Mediterranean Dietary Pattern Is Associated With Improved Plasma Lipid Profile: The Aragon Health Workers Study Cohort. *Revista Española de Cardiología (English Edition)* **2015**, *68*, 290–297. [CrossRef] [PubMed]
85. Pocovi-Gerardino, G.; Correa-Rodríguez, M.; Callejas-Rubio, J.-L.; Ríos-Fernández, R.; Martín-Amada, M.; Cruz-Caparros, M.-G.; Rueda-Medina, B.; Ortego-Centeno, N. Beneficial effect of Mediterranean diet on disease activity and cardiovascular risk in systemic lupus erythematosus patients: A cross-sectional study. *Rheumatology* **2021**, *60*, 160–169. [CrossRef] [PubMed]
86. Ruiz-Cabello, P.; Coll-Risco, I.; Acosta-Manzano, P.; Borges-Cosic, M.; Gallo-Vallejo, F.; Aranda, P.; López-Jurado, M.; Aparicio, V. Influence of the degree of adherence to the Mediterranean diet on the cardiometabolic risk in peri and menopausal women. The Flamenco project. *Nutr. Metab. Cardiovasc. Dis.* **2017**, *27*, 217–224. [CrossRef] [PubMed]
87. Salas-Huetos, A.; Babio, N.; Carrell, D.T.; Bulló, M.; Salas-Salvadó, J. Adherence to the Mediterranean diet is positively associated with sperm motility: A cross-sectional analysis. *Sci. Rep.* **2019**, *9*, 3389. [CrossRef]
88. Sotos-Prieto, M.; Luben, R.; Khaw, K.-T.; Wareham, N.J.; Forouhi, N.G. The association between Mediterranean Diet Score and glucokinase regulatory protein gene variation on the markers of cardiometabolic risk: An analysis in the European Prospective Investigation into Cancer (EPIC)-Norfolk study. *Br. J. Nutr.* **2014**, *112*, 122–131. [CrossRef] [PubMed]
89. Tuttolomondo, A.; Casuccio, A.; Buttà, C.; Pecoraro, R.; Di Raimondo, D.; Della Corte, V.; Arnao, V.; Clemente, G.; Maida, C.; Simonetta, I.; et al. Mediterranean Diet in patients with acute ischemic stroke: Relationships between Mediterranean Diet score, diagnostic subtype, and stroke severity index. *Atherosclerosis* **2015**, *243*, 260–267. [CrossRef]
90. Tuttolomondo, A.; Di Raimondo, D.; Casuccio, A.; Velardo, M.; Salamone, G.; Cataldi, M.; Corpora, F.; Restivo, V.; Pecoraro, R.; Della Corte, V.; et al. Mediterranean diet adherence and congestive heart failure: Relationship with clinical severity and ischemic pathogenesis. *Nutrition* **2020**, *70*, 110584. [CrossRef]
91. Tzima, N.; Pitsavos, C.; Panagiotakos, D.B.; Skoumas, J.; Zampelas, A.; Chrysohoou, C.; Stefanadis, C. Mediterranean diet and insulin sensitivity, lipid profile and blood pressure levels, in overweight and obese people; The Attica study. *Lipids Health Dis.* **2007**, *6*, 22. [CrossRef]
92. Veissi, M.; Anari, R.; Amani, R.; Shahbazian, H.; Latifi, S.M. Mediterranean diet and metabolic syndrome prevalence in type 2 diabetes patients in Ahvaz, southwest of Iran. *Diabetes Metab. Syndr. Clin. Res. Rev.* **2016**, *10*, S26–S29. [CrossRef]
93. Viscogliosi, G.; Cipriani, E.; Liguori, M.L.; Marigliano, B.; Saliola, M.; Ettorre, E.; Andreozzi, P. Mediterranean Dietary Pattern Adherence: Associations with Prediabetes, Metabolic Syndrome, and Related Microinflammation. *Metab. Syndr. Relat. Disord.* **2013**, *11*, 210–216. [CrossRef]
94. Zupo, R.; Castellana, F.; Panza, F.; Lampignano, L.; Murro, I.; Di Noia, C.; Triggiani, V.; Giannelli, G.; Sardone, R.; De Pergola, G. Adherence to a Mediterranean Diet and Thyroid Function in Obesity: A Cross-Sectional Apulian Survey. *Nutrients* **2020**, *12*, 3173. [CrossRef]

95. Aridi, Y.S.; Walker, J.L.; Roura, E.; Wright, O.R.L. Adherence to the Mediterranean Diet and Chronic Disease in Australia: National Nutrition and Physical Activity Survey Analysis. *Nutrients* **2020**, *12*, 1251. [CrossRef]
96. Barnaba, L.; Intorre, F.; Azzini, E.; Ciarapica, D.; Venneria, E.; Foddai, M.S.; Maiani, F.; Raguzzini, A.; Polito, A. Evaluation of adherence to Mediterranean diet and association with clinical and biological markers in an Italian population. *Nutrition* **2020**, *77*, 110813. [CrossRef]
97. Karayiannis, D.; Kontogianni, M.D.; Mendorou, C.; Douka, L.; Mastrominas, M.; Yiannakouris, N. Association between adherence to the Mediterranean diet and semen quality parameters in male partners of couples attempting fertility. *Hum. Reprod.* **2016**, *32*, 215–222. [CrossRef]
98. Kesse-Guyot, E.; Ahluwalia, N.; Lassale, C.; Hercberg, S.; Fezeu, L.; Lairon, D. Adherence to Mediterranean diet reduces the risk of metabolic syndrome: A 6-year prospective study. *Nutr. Metab. Cardiovasc. Dis.* **2013**, *23*, 677–683. [CrossRef] [PubMed]
99. Kim, Y.; Je, Y. A modified Mediterranean diet score is inversely associated with metabolic syndrome in Korean adults. *Eur. J. Clin. Nutr.* **2018**, *72*, 1682–1689. [CrossRef] [PubMed]
100. Mahdavi-Roshan, M.; Salari, A.; Ashouri, A.; Alizadeh, I. Association between depression symptoms and Mediterian dietary adherence in adults with cardiovascular disease risk factors in the north of Iran in 2016. *Pol. Ann. Med.* **2018**, *26*, 1–7. [CrossRef]
101. Mattei, J.; Sotos-Prieto, M.; Bigornia, S.J.; Noel, S.E.; Tucker, K.L. The Mediterranean Diet Score Is More Strongly Associated with Favorable Cardiometabolic Risk Factors over 2 Years Than Other Diet Quality Indexes in Puerto Rican Adults. *J. Nutr.* **2017**, *147*, 661–669. [CrossRef] [PubMed]
102. Mayr, H.L.; Itsiopoulos, C.; Tierney, A.C.; Kucianski, T.; Radcliffe, J.; Garg, M.; Willcox, J.; Thomas, C.J. Ad libitum Mediterranean diet reduces subcutaneous but not visceral fat in patients with coronary heart disease: A randomised controlled pilot study. *Clin. Nutr. ESPEN* **2019**, *32*, 61–69. [CrossRef] [PubMed]
103. Mirmiran, P.; Moslehi, N.; Mahmoudof, H.; Sadeghi, M.; Azizi, F. A Longitudinal Study of Adherence to the Mediterranean Dietary Pattern and Metabolic Syndrome in a Non-Mediterranean Population. *Int. J. Endocrinol. Metab.* **2015**, *13*, e26128. [CrossRef]
104. Mohamed, M.; Denis, L.; Rekia, B. Mediterranean Diet and Metabolic Syndrome in Adult Moroccan Women. *J. Res. Obes.* **2015**, *2015*, 15–32. [CrossRef]
105. Roldan, C.C.; Marcos, M.L.T.; Marcos, F.M.; Albero, J.S.; Rios, R.S.; Rodriguez, A.C.; Royo, J.M.P.; López, P.J.T. Adhesion to the Mediterranean diet in diabetic patients with poor control. *Clinica e Investigacion en Arteriosclerosis* **2019**, *31*, 210–217. [CrossRef]
106. Rumawas, M.E.; Meigs, J.B.; Dwyer, J.T.; McKeown, N.M.; Jacques, P.F. Mediterranean-style dietary pattern, reduced risk of metabolic syndrome traits, and incidence in the Framingham Offspring Cohort. *Am. J. Clin. Nutr.* **2009**, *90*, 1608–1614. [CrossRef] [PubMed]
107. Tortosa, A.; Bes-Rastrollo, M.; Sanchez-Villegas, A.; Basterra-Gortari, F.J.; Nuñez-Cordoba, J.M.; Martinez-Gonzalez, M.A. Mediterranean Diet Inversely Associated With the Incidence of Metabolic Syndrome: The SUN prospective cohort. *Diabetes Care* **2007**, *30*, 2957–2959. [CrossRef] [PubMed]
108. Tsartsou, E.; Proutsos, N.; Castanas, E.; Kampa, M. Network Meta-Analysis of Metabolic Effects of Olive-Oil in Humans Shows the Importance of Olive Oil Consumption With Moderate Polyphenol Levels as Part of the Mediterranean Diet. *Front. Nutr.* **2019**, *6*, 6. [CrossRef]
109. Fontana, L.; Eagon, J.C.; Trujillo, M.E.; Scherer, P.E.; Klein, S. Visceral Fat Adipokine Secretion Is Associated With Systemic Inflammation in Obese Humans. *Diabetes* **2007**, *56*, 1010–1013. [CrossRef] [PubMed]
110. Phillips, L.K.; Prins, J.B. The link between abdominal obesity and the metabolic syndrome. *Curr. Hypertens. Rep.* **2008**, *10*, 156–164. [CrossRef]
111. Howard, B.V. Insulin resistance and lipid metabolism. *Am. J. Cardiol.* **1999**, *84* (Suppl. 1), 28–32. [CrossRef]
112. Huo, R.; Du, T.; Xu, Y.; Xu, W.; Chen, X.; Sun, K.; Yu, X. Effects of Mediterranean-style diet on glycemic control, weight loss and cardiovascular risk factors among type 2 diabetes individuals: A meta-analysis. *Eur. J. Clin. Nutr.* **2014**, *69*, 1200–1208. [CrossRef]
113. Mitjavila, M.T.; Fandos, M.; Salas-Salvadó, J.; Covas, M.-I.; Borrego, S.; Estruch, R.; Lamuela-Raventós, R.; Corella, D.; Martínez-Gonzalez, M.Á.; Sánchez, J.M.; et al. The Mediterranean diet improves the systemic lipid and DNA oxidative damage in metabolic syndrome individuals. A randomized, controlled, trial. *Clin. Nutr.* **2013**, *32*, 172–178. [CrossRef]
114. Julibert, A.; Bibiloni, M.D.M.; Gallardo-Alfaro, L.; Abbate, M.; Martínez-González, M.Á.; Salas-Salvadó, J.; Corella, D.; Fitó, M.; Martínez, J.A.; Alonso-Gómez, Á.M.; et al. Metabolic Syndrome Features and Excess Weight Were Inversely Associated with Nut Consumption after 1-Year Follow-Up in the PREDIMED-Plus Study. *J. Nutr.* **2020**, *150*, 3161–3170. [CrossRef]
115. Hołowko-Ziółek, J.; Cięszczyk, P.; Biliński, J.; Basak, G.W.; Stachowska, E. What Model of Nutrition Can Be Recommended to People Ending Their Professional Sports Career? An Analysis of the Mediterranean Diet and the CRON Diet in the Context of Former Athletes. *Nutrients* **2020**, *12*, 3604. [CrossRef] [PubMed]
116. Damasceno, N.R.; Sala-Vila, A.; Cofán, M.; Pérez-Heras, A.M.; Fitó, M.; Ruiz-Gutiérrez, V.; Martínez-González, M.Á.; Corella, D.; Arós, F.; Estruch, R.; et al. Mediterranean diet supplemented with nuts reduces waist circumference and shifts lipoprotein subfractions to a less atherogenic pattern in subjects at high cardiovascular risk. *Atherosclerosis* **2013**, *230*, 347–353. [CrossRef] [PubMed]
117. Hernáez, Á.; Castañer, O.; Fitó, M. Response to Letter Regarding Article, "Mediterranean Diet Improves High-Density Lipoprotein Function in High-Cardiovascular-Risk Individuals: A Randomized Controlled Trial". *Circulation* **2017**, *136*, 342–343. [CrossRef]

118. Notario-Barandiaran, L.; Project, O.B.O.T.I.; Valera-Gran, D.; Gonzalez-Palacios, S.; Garcia-De-La-Hera, M.; Fernández-Barrés, S.; Pereda-Pereda, E.; Fernández-Somoano, A.; Guxens, M.; Iñiguez, C.; et al. High adherence to a mediterranean diet at age 4 reduces overweight, obesity and abdominal obesity incidence in children at the age of 8. *Int. J. Obes.* **2020**, *44*, 1906–1917. [CrossRef]
119. Mata, P.; Alvarez-Sala, L.A.; Rubio, M.J.; Nuño, J.; De Oya, M. Effects of long-term monounsaturated- vs polyunsaturated-enriched diets on lipoproteins in healthy men and women. *Am. J. Clin. Nutr.* **1992**, *55*, 846–850. [CrossRef] [PubMed]
120. Ghobadi, S.; Hassanzadeh-Rostami, Z.; Mohammadian, F.; Nikfetrat, A.; Ghasemifard, N.; Dehkordi, H.R.; Faghih, S. Comparison of blood lipid-lowering effects of olive oil and other plant oils: A systematic review and meta-analysis of 27 randomized placebo-controlled clinical trials. *Crit. Rev. Food Sci. Nutr.* **2018**, *59*, 2110–2124. [CrossRef]
121. Abia, R.; Perona, J.S.; Pacheco, Y.M.; Montero, E.; Muriana, F.J.G.; Ruiz-Gutierrez, V. Postprandial triacylglycerols from dietary virgin olive oil are selectively cleared in humans. *J. Nutr.* **1999**, *129*, 2184–2191. [CrossRef]
122. Berglund, L.; Lefevre, M.; Ginsberg, H.N.; Kris-Etherton, P.M.; Elmer, P.J.; Stewart, P.W.; Ershow, A.; Pearson, T.A.; Dennis, B.H.; Roheim, P.S.; et al. Comparison of monounsaturated fat with carbohydrates as a replacement for saturated fat in subjects with a high metabolic risk profile: Studies in the fasting and postprandial states. *Am. J. Clin. Nutr.* **2007**, *86*, 1611–1620. [CrossRef]
123. Poudyal, H.; Panchal, S.K.; Diwan, V.; Brown, L. Omega-3 fatty acids and metabolic syndrome: Effects and emerging mechanisms of action. *Prog. Lipid Res.* **2011**, *50*, 372–387. [CrossRef]
124. Sleiman, D.; Al-Badri, M.R.; Azar, S.T. Effect of Mediterranean Diet in Diabetes Control and Cardiovascular Risk Modification: A Systematic Review. *Front. Public Health* **2015**, *3*, 69. [CrossRef]
125. Esposito, K.; Maiorino, M.I.; Ceriello, A.; Giugliano, D. Prevention and control of type 2 diabetes by Mediterranean diet: A systematic review. *Diabetes Res. Clin. Pr.* **2010**, *89*, 97–102. [CrossRef]
126. Elhayany, A.; Lustman, A.; Abel, R.; Attal-Singer, J.; Vinker, S. A low carbohydrate Mediterranean diet improves cardiovascular risk factors and diabetes control among overweight patients with type 2 diabetes mellitus: A 1-year prospective randomized intervention study. *Diabetes Obes. Metab.* **2010**, *12*, 204–209. [CrossRef] [PubMed]
127. Georgoulis, M.; Kontogianni, M.D.; Yiannakouris, N. Mediterranean Diet and Diabetes: Prevention and Treatment. *Nutrients* **2014**, *6*, 1406–1423. [CrossRef]
128. Ajala, O.; English, P.; Pinkney, J. Systematic review and meta-analysis of different dietary approaches to the management of type 2 diabetes. *Am. J. Clin. Nutr.* **2013**, *97*, 505–516. [CrossRef] [PubMed]
129. Shimbo, D.; Muntner, P.; Mann, D.; Viera, A.J.; Homma, S.; Polak, J.F.; Barr, R.G.; Herrington, D.; Shea, S. Endothelial dysfunction and the risk of hypertension: The multi-ethnic study of atherosclerosis. *Hypertension* **2010**, *55*, 1210–1216. [CrossRef]
130. Tuttolomondo, A.; Simonetta, I.; Daidone, M.; Mogavero, A.; Ortello, A.; Pinto, A. Metabolic and Vascular Effect of the Mediterranean Diet. *Int. J. Mol. Sci.* **2019**, *20*, 4716. [CrossRef] [PubMed]
131. Bendinelli, B.; Masala, G.; Bruno, R.M.; Caini, S.; Saieva, C.; Boninsegni, A.; Ungar, A.; Ghiadoni, L.; Palli, D. A priori dietary patterns and blood pressure in the EPIC Florence cohort: A cross-sectional study. *Eur. J. Nutr.* **2019**, *58*, 455–466. [CrossRef] [PubMed]
132. Psaltopoulou, T.; Naska, A.; Orfanos, P.; Trichopoulos, D.; Mountokalakis, T.; Trichopoulou, A. Olive oil, the Mediterranean diet, and arterial blood pressure: The Greek European Prospective Investigation into Cancer and Nutrition (EPIC) study. *Am. J. Clin. Nutr.* **2004**, *80*, 1012–1018. [CrossRef] [PubMed]
133. Cowell, O.R.; Mistry, N.; Deighton, K.; Matu, J.; Griffiths, A.; Minihane, A.M.; Mathers, J.C.; Shannon, O.M.; Siervo, M. Effects of a Mediterranean diet on blood pressure: A systematic review and meta-analysis of randomized controlled trials and observational studies. *J. Hypertens.* **2021**, *39*, 729–739. [PubMed]
134. Filippou, C.D.; Thomopoulos, C.G.; Kouremeti, M.M.; Sotiropoulou, L.I.; Nihoyannopoulos, P.I.; Tousoulis, D.M.; Tsioufis, C.P. Mediterranean diet and blood pressure reduction in adults with and without hypertension: A systematic review and meta-analysis of randomized controlled trials. *Clin. Nutr.* **2021**. [CrossRef]
135. Medina-Remón, A.; Tresserra-Rimbau, A.; Pons, A.; Tur, J.; Martorell, M.; Ros, E.; Buil-Cosiales, P.; Sacanella, E.; Covas, M.; Corella, D.; et al. Effects of total dietary polyphenols on plasma nitric oxide and blood pressure in a high cardiovascular risk cohort. The PREDIMED randomized trial. *Nutr. Metab. Cardiovasc. Dis.* **2015**, *25*, 60–67. [CrossRef] [PubMed]
136. Castro-Barquero, S.; Ruiz-León, A.M.; Sierra-Pérez, M.; Estruch, R.; Casas, R. Dietary Strategies for Metabolic Syndrome: A Comprehensive Review. *Nutrients* **2020**, *12*, 2983. [CrossRef] [PubMed]
137. Fontalba-Romero, M.I.; López-Enriquez, S.; Lago-Sampedro, A.; Garcia-Escobar, E.; Pastori, R.L.; Domínguez-Bendala, J.; Alvarez-Cubela, S.; Valdés, S.; Rojo-Martinez, G.; García-Fuentes, E.; et al. Association between the Mediterranean Diet and Metabolic Syndrome with Serum Levels of miRNA in Morbid Obesity. *Nutrients* **2021**, *13*, 436. [CrossRef]
138. Reguero, M.; de Cedrón, M.G.; Wagner, S.; Reglero, G.; Quintela, J.; de Molina, A.R. Precision Nutrition to Activate Thermogenesis as a Complementary Approach to Target Obesity and Associated-Metabolic-Disorders. *Cancers* **2021**, *13*, 866. [CrossRef]
139. Papadaki, A.; Nolen-Doerr, E.; Mantzoros, C.S. The Effect of the Mediterranean Diet on Metabolic Health: A Systematic Review and Meta-Analysis of Controlled Trials in Adults. *Nutrients* **2020**, *12*, 3342. [CrossRef] [PubMed]
140. Hidalgo-Mora, J.J.; Cortés-Sierra, L.; García-Pérez, M.Á.; Tarín, J.J.; Cano, A. Diet to Reduce the Metabolic Syndrome Associated with Menopause. The Logic for Olive Oil. *Nutrients* **2020**, *12*, 3184. [CrossRef]

MDPI
St. Alban-Anlage 66
4052 Basel
Switzerland
Tel. +41 61 683 77 34
Fax +41 61 302 89 18
www.mdpi.com

Nutrients Editorial Office
E-mail: nutrients@mdpi.com
www.mdpi.com/journal/nutrients

www.ingramcontent.com/pod-product-compliance
Lightning Source LLC
LaVergne TN
LVHW070556100526
838202LV00012B/481